Atlas of
Orthopaedic
Pathology

with
Clinical and Radiologic
Correlations

PETER G. BULLOUGH, M.B., Ch.B.
Chief of Orthopedic Pathology
The Hospital for Special Surgery
Professor of Pathology
Cornell University Medical College
New York

VINCENT J. VIGORITA, M.D.
Assistant Attending Pathologist
The Hospital for Special Surgery
Assistant Professor of Pathology
Cornell University Medical College
New York

Foreword by
William F. Enneking, M.D.
Professor of Orthopedics
University of Florida College of Medicine
Gainesville

University Park Press
Baltimore

Gower Medical Publishing
New York • London

A slide atlas of orthopaedic pathology based on the material in this book is also available. Further information regarding the *Slide Atlas of Orthopaedic Pathology* may be obtained from:
Gower Medical Publishing
101 Fifth Avenue
New York, NY 10003
or from:
University Park Press
300 North Charles Street
Baltimore, Maryland 21201

Published in North America by
University Park Press
300 North Charles Street
Baltimore, Maryland 21201

Distributed in Japan by
Maruzen Company Limited
3-10, Nihonbashi 2-chome,
Chuo-ku
Tokyo 103,
Japan

Distributed in all countries
except USA, Canada, and Japan by
Butterworth and Co. (Publishers) Limited
Borough Green,
Sevenoaks,
Kent TN15 8PH
UK

ISBN 0-8391-1915-1 (University Park Press)
ISBN 0-912143-00-2 (Gower)

Library of Congress Cataloging in Publication Data
Bullough, Peter G.
  Atlas of orthopaedic pathology with clinical and radiologic correlations.

  Bibliography: p.
  Includes index.
  1. Bones—Diseases—Atlases. 2. Joints—Diseases—Atlases. I. Vigorita, Vincent. II. Title. [DNLM: 1. Bone diseases—Pathology—Atlases. 2. Bone and bones —Radiography—Atlases. 3. Muscular diseases—Pathology —Atlases. 4. Muscles—Radiography—Atlases. 5. Joint diseases—Pathology—Atlases. 6. Joints—Radiography— Atlases. WE 17 B938a]
RC930.4.B84 1983   616.7'1   83-1707

Printed in Hong Kong by Mandarin Offset International Ltd.

Foreword

This 14-chapter *Atlas of Orthopaedic Pathology* by Bullough and Vigorita is an outstanding contribution to the field of musculoskeletal pathology. It will be of particular interest to students and practitioners of orthopaedic surgery, diagnostic and therapeutic radiology, oncology, and pathology. An even more exciting prospect is the potential effect it will have upon teaching in these fields. The illustrations and text collate the many techniques and basic principles so clearly that even the novice can rapidly assimilate the expertise to appreciate the treasure trove of pertinent information.

The clarity and beauty of the illustrations are unsurpassed. The addition of line diagrams to avoid superimposing letters, arrows, and other symbols adds to already superb reproductions and makes many of the illustrations works of art in addition to their outstanding teaching value.

The availability of a corresponding slide atlas adds a new dimension to this material. It means the illustrations can be individually studied or shown to groups with much greater detail and magnification.

When used in conjunction with the text, the slides provide an individual or group with clearly identified features that permit learning at any pace and to any degree of depth desired. Of even greater potential significance is that the slide atlas provides those responsible for teaching with a source of illustrative material that is far superior to the private teaching collections usually available. It allows multiple instructors to function around a common source, providing the continuity that is so important pedagogically. It also provides a constantly available reference source for departmental libraries that would otherwise be prohibitively expensive in time and resources to individually assemble.

Drs. Bullough and Vigorita are to be highly commended for their monumental contribution. They have obviously spent years painstakingly assembling the illustrative materials drawn from their vast clinical experience. The time and effort they and the publishers have expended to make this material available to all of us is greatly appreciated.

William F. Enneking, M.D.
Professor of Orthopedics
University of Florida College of Medicine
Gainesville

Preface

Musculoskeletal conditions as a whole are the third most frequent acute disease that results in a visit to a doctor, exceeded only by acute respiratory conditions and acute infections. Although not a common cause of death, musculoskeletal diseases are the fifth most frequent cause for hospitalization and the third most frequent cause for surgery. Generally, these diseases impact on the quality of life, with the elderly suffering most, usually from arthritis and/or osteoporosis. As the ratio of older individuals in society continues to increase, the incidence of musculoskeletal disease will, in turn, increase and require increased medical attention.

Unfortunately, medical school curricula and most pathology training programs assign disproportionately little time for the study of the largest organ system—the musculoskeletal system. At autopsy, most attention is devoted to the study of the parenchymal organs, little to the study of the musculoskeletal tissues. Perhaps one reason for this neglect is the fact that gross dissection and histologic sectioning of the skeleton are deemed too difficult and are therefore generally skipped. A great deal of pathology is being overlooked in the process.

From Virchow's time to the present, there has been a devoted group of students for whom musculoskeletal diseases hold a particular interest, and a small number of excellent texts have been written on both the tumorous and nontumorous conditions of bones and joints. Our intent is *not* to present another text, but rather to provide a concise, yet lavishly illustrated account of the pathology of musculoskeletal diseases as encountered in clinical practice and, we hope, to stimulate interest and enthusiasm for this important branch of pathology.

It is our desire that this book be used not only by surgical pathologists but also by orthopaedic surgeons. Radiologists having a special interest in skeletal radiology will also find this book helpful in providing them with pathologic correlations. For these latter groups, we have included an introductory chapter on normal bone, as well as a chapter on the processes involved in injury and repair in general, and of the connective tissues in particular. These chapters are intended to provide sufficient background information to prepare the reader for the pathologic descriptions which follow.

We have attempted to provide a concise clinical, radiologic, and pathologic account of each musculoskeletal condition, accompanied by captioned illustrations which not only complement but indeed augment the text. (For teaching purposes, a slide atlas is being prepared which will include 35-mm slides of all the illustrations in the book.) Labeled line diagrams represent a special feature that accompany many of the roentgenograms and photomicrographs, and serve to isolate the specific structures which are central to the discussion in the text and caption. Both clinical roentgenograms and roentgenograms of the excised specimens are presented, the latter being extremely useful in the study of bone and joint diseases. The Bibliography found in the back of the book is broken down by chapter, and then broken down even further by condition. The number of references per condition are few, but they have been chosen to best amplify the presentations in this book and to provide further access to the literature.

Most of the gross photographs and photomicrographs used in this book have been collected over many years by the senior author: first, as a fellow at the Hospital for Joint Diseases in New York; next, as a lecturer in orthopaedics at the Nuffield Orthopedic Center in Oxford, England; and finally, over the past 14 years, as a pathologist at the Hospital for Special Surgery in New York. Most of the clinical roentgenograms are from the teaching collection of the radiology department at the Hospital for Special Surgery, and are used with the kind permission of Dr. Robert Freiberger. The information presented in this book is based on our experience teaching pathology to orthopaedic residents, and on lectures on the pathology of the skeletal system which the senior author has given to second-year medical students at Cornell University Medical College over the past 14 years, and at the annual Maine Orthopedic Review.

For all our teachers, colleagues, and students who have awakened our interest, enlightened our understanding, and unselfishly shared their experience with us, there are no words to express the debt of gratitude which is most keenly felt.

We are indebted to the staff of the pathology department at the Hospital for Special Surgery—especially Gwen Broome, Jean Kilfoyle, Georgia Clingen, Brigitte Brady, and Tony Labissiere—for their excellent work and support in this and other projects over the years. We would also like to take this opportunity to thank the staff of Gower Medical Publishing for the care that went into the preparation of this book: to Carol Hoidra and Abe Krieger for their editing, to Keith Stout for his satisfying design, and to Tim Hailstone for his keen interest and unflagging support throughout.

Peter G. Bullough
Vincent J. Vigorita   v

Contents

1 Normal Bone

Bone, cartilage, ligaments, and tendons, referred to collectively as the connective tissues, have a mechanical function: they provide for movement, support, and protection. Unlike the parenchymal organs, e.g., the liver or kidneys, which are mainly composed of cellular elements, the connective tissues are mostly formed from an extracellular material (or matrix) that is made up of substances well suited to the mechanical functions of the tissue. A knowledge of the matrix components and the ability to recognize changes in them are essential to the understanding of diseases of the connective tissue.

THE MATRIX

Collagen fibers, the principal extracellular components of the connective tissue, are made up of bundles of fibrils, which in turn are composed of stacked molecules formed from polypeptide chains arranged in a helical pattern (Fig. 1.1). Collagen is well suited to resist pulling; however, it does not resist bending or compression, and since bone and cartilage are subjected to these latter types of forces, they contain, in addition to collagen, stiffening substances.

In bone this stiffening substance appears in the form of crystals of calcium phosphate (hydroxyapatite) (Fig. 1.2).

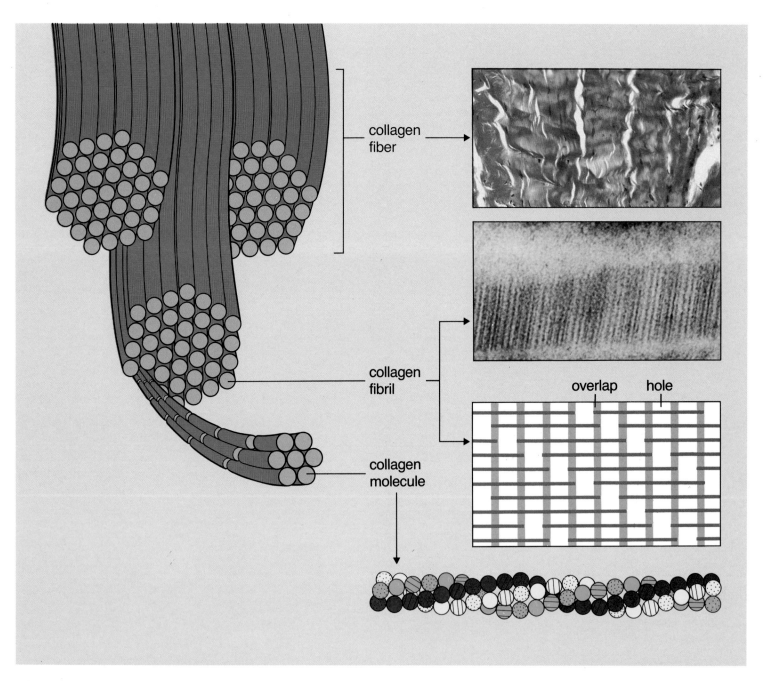

collagen fiber

collagen fibril

overlap   hole

collagen molecule

Fig. 1.1 In histologic sections stained with hematoxylin and eosin, the collagen is seen as wavy homogeneous strands of pink material that represent bundles of collagen fibers. The collagen molecule is a triple helix formed of polypeptide chains, which in turn are formed of repeating tripeptide sequences of glycine-x-y-glycine-x-y, etc., in which x and y are frequently proline and hydroxyproline.

By transmission electron microscopy the individual collagen fibrils are visualized, and are seen to have two orders of banding. As can be seen from the drawing, the larger bands result from the gaps between the individual molecules of collagen, which then overlap the adjacent molecules.

The bone mineral is an analogue of hydroxyapatite, $Ca_{10}(PO_4)_6(OH)_2$. The crystals are too small to be seen by light microscopy, but they can be visualized by electron microscopy in nonmineralized tissue. They are approximately $2 \times 9 \times 25$ nm in size.

In cartilage the filler between the collagen fibers is a large, negatively charged molecule of proteoglycan, with a molecular weight of several million and a spatial configuration reminiscent of a test tube brush (Figs. 1.3 and 1.4). The proteoglycan macromolecule is formed from long chains of repeating disaccharides, which are covalently linked to a protein backbone. The entire structure is attached to a hyaluronic acid core.

The matrix components of the connective tissues are manufactured by cells that, of themselves, occupy only a small volume of the tissues. Nevertheless, these cells, i.e., fibroblasts (cells that produce fibrous collagenized tissue), osteoblasts (cells that produce bone), and chondroblasts (cells that produce cartilage), are essential to the production and maintenance of a healthy matrix. Cellular disease may lead to the production of abnormal matrix constituents. The breakdown of matrix constituents, either physiologically or pathologically, may occur through the action of enzymes derived from either the connective tissue cells themselves or from blood-borne inflammatory cells.

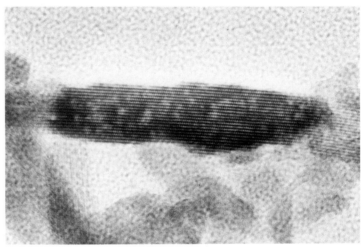

Fig. 1.2 Electron micrographs of bone mineral crystals: at a magnification factor of 101,500 × *(left)*, the crystal structure can be clearly seen, and at higher magnification 2,110,000 × *(right)*, the lattice formation of the crystals can be appreciated. (The various stains for demonstrating calcium salts in undecalcified sections are described at the end of this chapter.)

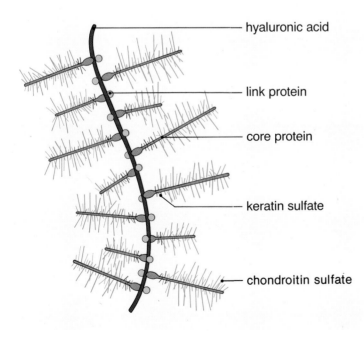

- hyaluronic acid
- link protein
- core protein
- keratin sulfate
- chondroitin sulfate

Fig. 1.3 Schematic drawing of the proteoglycan macromolecule. The proteoglycan in histologic sections may be stained by various techniques, including safranin 0, alcian blue, and toluidine blue.

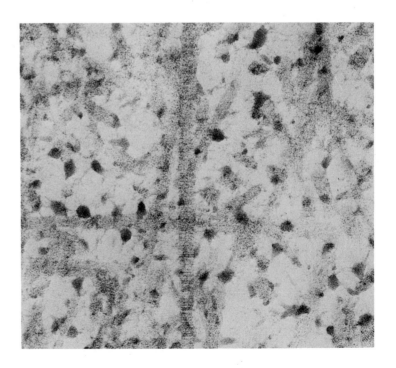

Fig. 1.4 Electron microscopic examination of cartilage demonstrates amorphous electron-dense deposits of proteoglycan between collagen fibers (102,900 ×).

CELLULAR CONTROL OF THE MATRIX

The bone matrix is synthesized by a layer of cells on the surface of the bone (Fig. 1.5). These cells, the osteoblasts (Fig. 1.6), are mesenchymal in origin and contain abundant endoplasmic reticulum as well as the enzyme alkaline phosphatase. As the osteoblasts produce bone matrix, they become surrounded by the matrix that they have formed, and thus they are buried within the surface of the bone (Fig. 1.7). In this way, the osteoblasts become osteocytes.

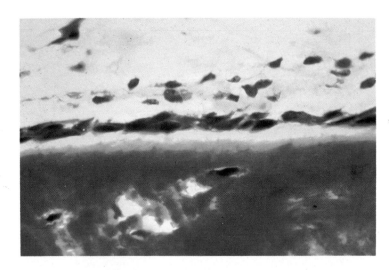

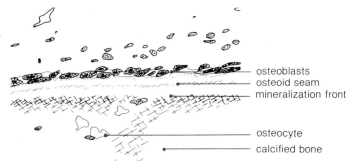

Fig. 1.5 Photomicrograph of bone tissue shows a layer of active osteoblasts on the surface, and, within the substance of the bone, osteocytes. The following five photographs show detailed views of these cells (and their processes) and the bone matrix.

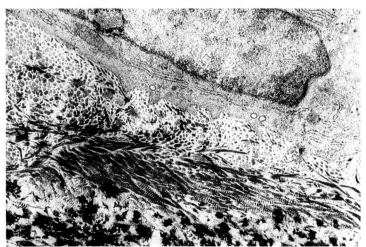

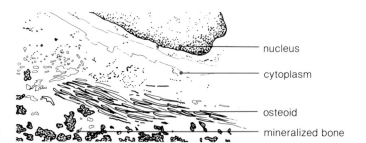

Fig. 1.6 Electron photomicrograph shows a portion of an osteoblast in the upper half. The cytoplasm is rich in rough endoplasmic reticulum. Underlying the cell is a layer of nonmineralized collagenous matrix (osteoid), which in light microscope sections is seen as a smooth pink layer on the bone surface. Directly under the region of the osteoid seam is a thin layer of mineralized bone.

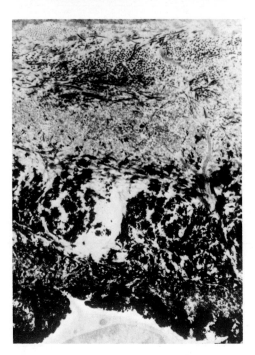

Fig. 1.7 Electron photomicrograph includes in the field a portion of an osteoblast (*top*); a nonmineralized osteoid seam; and mineralized bone with part of an osteocyte in it. Portions of osteocytic processes are seen in both the mineralized bone matrix and the osteoid seam (10,000 ×).

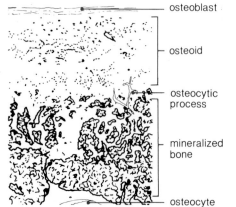

By the use of special techniques, it can be demonstrated that the osteocytes unite with each other and with the osteoblasts on the surface of the bone by a series of connecting cell processes that run in the canals permeating the bone tissue (Figs. 1.8 to 1.10). These canals are called the osteocytic canaliculi, and they are of great importance in serving the body's need for calcium homeostasis. *Note that the osteocytic canaliculi do not cross the cement lines.* (See Fig. 1.26 for description of cement lines.)

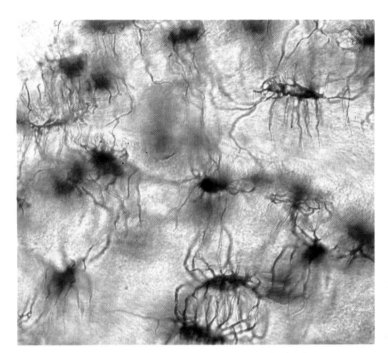

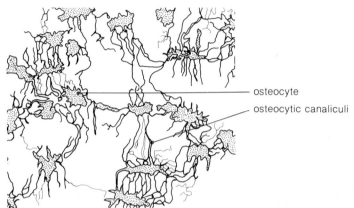

Fig. 1.8 Photomicrograph of osteocytes and osteocytic canaliculi seen by transmitted light in ground bone section (10×).

osteocyte

osteocytic canaliculi

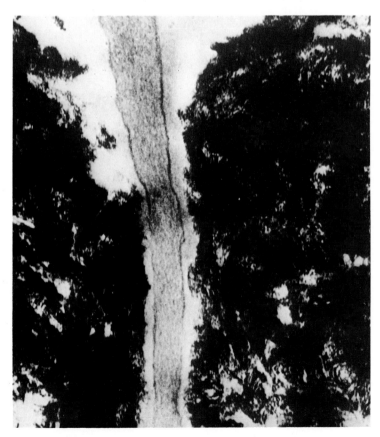

Fig. 1.9 Electron photomicrograph of a portion of an osteocytic process in an osteocytic canaliculus in mineralized bone (50,000×).

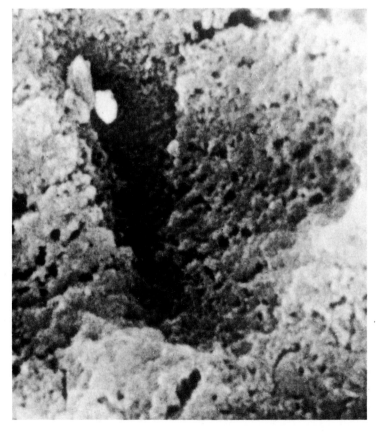

Fig. 1.10 Scanning electron microscope photograph of the bone surface shows the opening of the canaliculi only onto the surface (7,000×).

Associated with cells that are actively forming bone matrix, one may see, underlying the cellular layer, a thin layer of nonmineralized bone matrix (osteoid) (Fig. 1.11). The recognition of osteoid in histologic sections usually depends upon the preparation of undecalcified sections, and the ability to identify this nonmineralized bone is a key factor in the diagnosis of certain metabolic disturbances in the bone (e.g., osteoporosis and osteomalacia).

It can be demonstrated on histologic examination that actively forming bone surfaces, as well as inactive formed surfaces, are smooth. However, some bone surfaces have an irregular or "gnawed out" appearance, and these

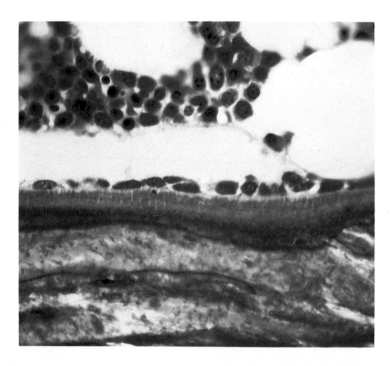

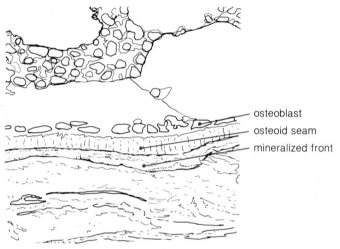

Fig. 1.11 Photomicrograph of a section of undecalcified bone shows a prominent layer of active osteoblasts lying on an osteoid seam, with underlying mineralized bone. The calcification front is seen as a deeply staining basophilic line.

osteoblast
osteoid seam
mineralized front

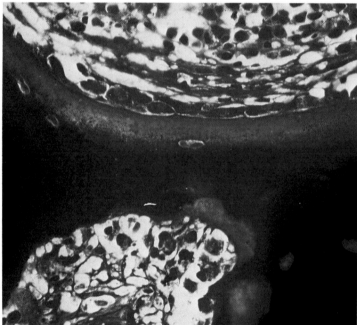

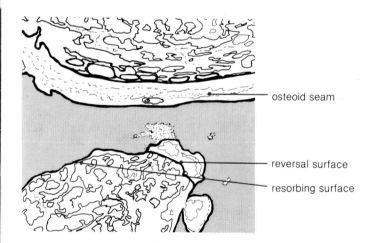

Fig. 1.12 Photomicrograph shows contrast of bone-forming surface with osteoid seam (*upper*) with a resorbing surface (*lower*). At the lower left an irregular previously resorbed surface is seen to have been covered by a layer of osteoid, and this appearance is referred to as a reversal surface.

osteoid seam

reversal surface
resorbing surface

surfaces either have been resorbed or are actively resorbing (Fig. 1.12). The cells concerned with resorption are the osteoclasts, and they frequently lie in cavities in the bone surface known as Howship's lacunae (Fig. 1.13).

Under an electron microscope the osteoclast can be seen to have a ruffled border adjacent to the bone, and to contain many lysosomal bodies, mitochondria, and vesicular inclusions (Fig. 1.14). The osteoclast is generally a multinucleate cell, but mononuclear forms of resorbing cells can also be seen. Although complete agreement as to the origin of the osteoclast has not yet been reached, the cell probably derives from blood-borne monocytes.

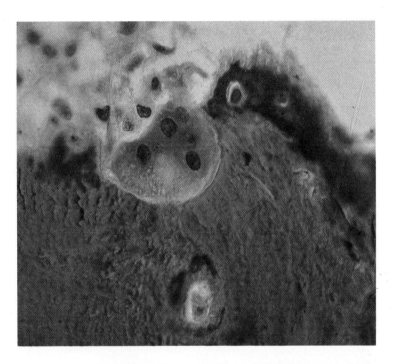

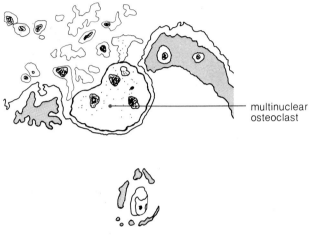

Fig. 1.13 Photomicrograph shows an osteoclast in a Howship's lacuna. Osteoclasts are identified by their abundant cytoplasm and multiple nuclei.

multinuclear osteoclast

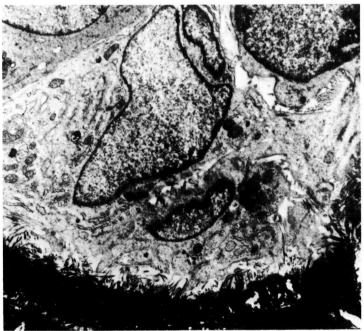

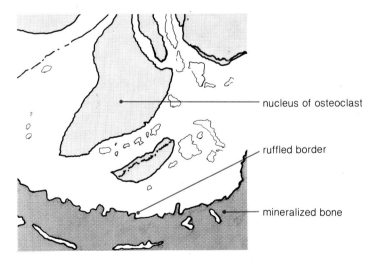

Fig. 1.14 Electron photomicrograph of an osteoclast. Note the interdigitating ruffled border of the osteoclast and the underlying mineralized bone (6,500×).

nucleus of osteoclast

ruffled border

mineralized bone

THE BONES

Gross Structure and Function. Each bone has a limiting surface shell known as the cortex. Enclosed by the cortical shell are plates and rods of bone tissue known as the spongy, cancellous, or trabecular bone (Figs. 1.15 to 1.17).

The thickness of the cortex varies considerably both within a single bone and in different bones. For example, in the normal vertebral bodies the cortex is very thin, whereas in the long bones such as the femur and the tibia the cortex may reach more than one quarter of an inch in thickness. Even in the long bones, however, there is great variation in thickness between the ends of the bone (in which the cortex is thin) and the midshaft of the bone (in which the cortex is thick).

A moment's reflection will make the reason for these differences obvious. The thick cortical bone is well constructed to resist bending, and it is in the middle of the

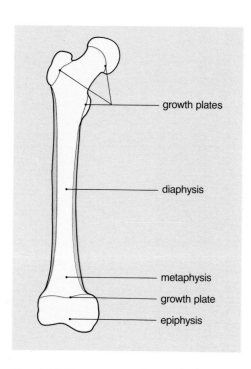

Fig. 1.15 Bone compartments in femur.

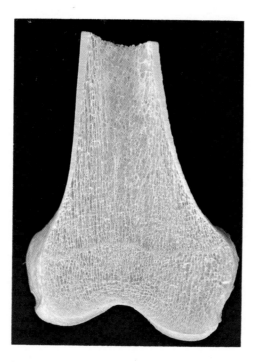

Fig. 1.16 A cleaned and macerated specimen of the lower femur demonstrates the distribution of cancellous bone and the thickening of the cortex approaching the diaphysis (*left*). Roentgenogram of the

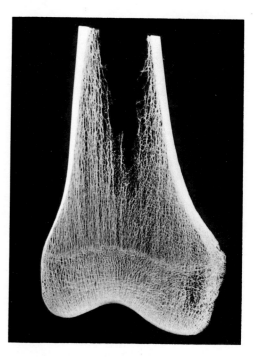

same specimen (*right*). Note the horizontal plate of bone which marks the site of the previous cartilage growth plate (the "epiphyseal scar").

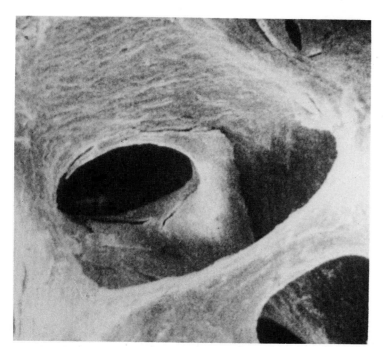

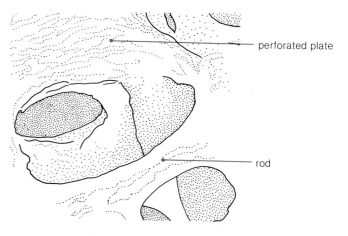

Fig. 1.17 Scanning electron microscope picture of the plates and rods of bone in the epiphysis.

long bones that this force occurs. In contrast, the cancellous or trabecular bone is concentrated where compressive forces predominate, i.e., in the vertebral bodies and in the expanded ends of long bones. It can therefore be appreciated that, in both the skeleton and the connective tissues in general, the architecture of the matrix reflects its function. This concept of organized distribution is summarized in Wolff's law: bone elements place or displace themselves in the direction of functional pressure (Fig. 1.18).

The bones are often compartmentalized by the morphologist into three indistinct zones—the epiphysis, or region above the growth plate (or, in adults, the zone above the closed growth plate); the metaphysis, the region immediately below the growth zone; and the diaphysis, the region between the growth zones, i.e., the shaft of the long bones. The terms epiphysis, metaphysis, and diaphysis are useful in the description of diseases, since many diseases have predilections for one or another of these compartments.

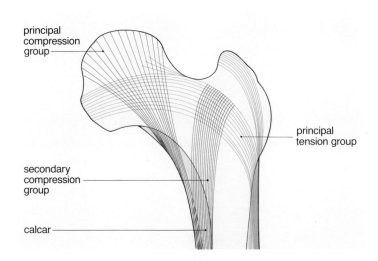

Fig. **1.18** (*upper*), Wolff's law is well demonstrated in the head and neck of the femur, in which it can be seen that the bone trabeculae radiate from the articular surface down onto the medial cortex of the femoral neck (the calcar), which is much thicker than the cortex on the lateral side of the femoral neck.

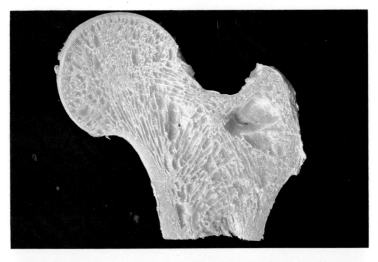

Fig. **1.18** (*center*), In this slice through the upper end of the femur, the marrow fat has been washed out of the specimen in order to better demonstrate the distribution of the cancellous bone.

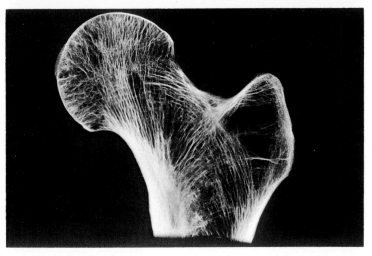

Fig. **1.18** (*lower*), However, the best way to demonstrate the arrangement of the bone trabeculae is by roentgenograms of the specimen.

PERIOSTEUM: Except at the musculotendinous insertions and at their articular ends, the bones are covered by a thin but tough fibrous membrane, the periosteum. At the articular margins and tendinous insertions the periosteum blends imperceptibly with the surface fibers of those tissues.

On microscopic examination, the periosteum is seen to have two layers; an outer fibrous layer and an inner layer, the cambium layer, which forms bone. In children the cambium layer provides for the increasing diameter of the bone with growth (Fig. 1.19). In adults the bone-forming potential of the periosteum is reactivated after trauma and infection, and in association with some tumors. In children the periosteum is only loosely attached to the underlying bone, whereas in adults it is firmly attached. This observation correlates well with the clinical extent of periosteal reaction, which in similar conditions is much greater in children than in adults (Fig. 1.20).

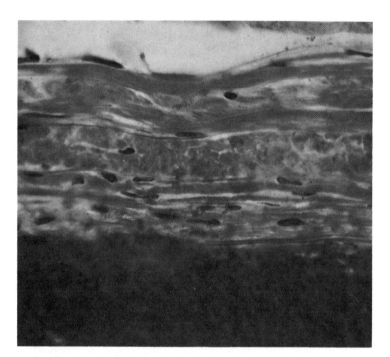

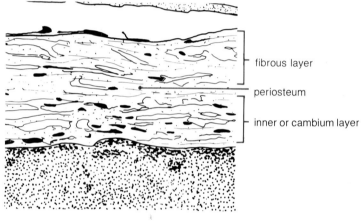

Fig. 1.19 Photomicrograph of the periosteum and underlying cortical bone. Note the double layer, of which the inner or cambium layer is more active in producing bone.

fibrous layer

periosteum

inner or cambium layer

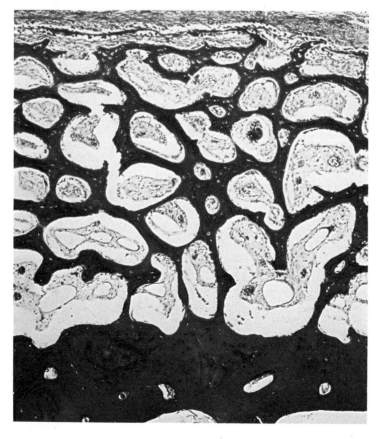

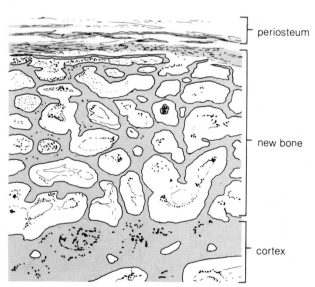

Fig. 1.20 Photomicrograph of periosteal new bone layer produced by the cambium of the periosteum following trauma in a child.

periosteum

new bone

cortex

BLOOD SUPPLY: Numerous capillaries enter the bone through the periosteum (Fig. 1.21). This periosteal blood supply augments the principal nutrient arteries, which enter the medullary cavity by penetrating the cortex (usually at about the middle of the diaphysis), and the epiphyseal and metaphyseal vessels at the ends of the bone (Fig. 1.22).

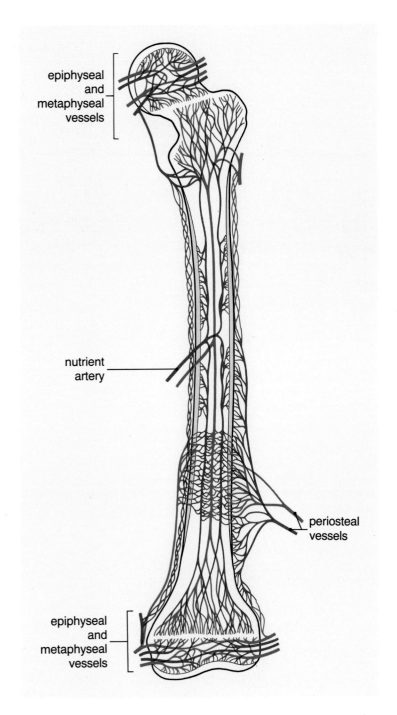

Fig. 1.21 Diagram of the blood supply to the bone.

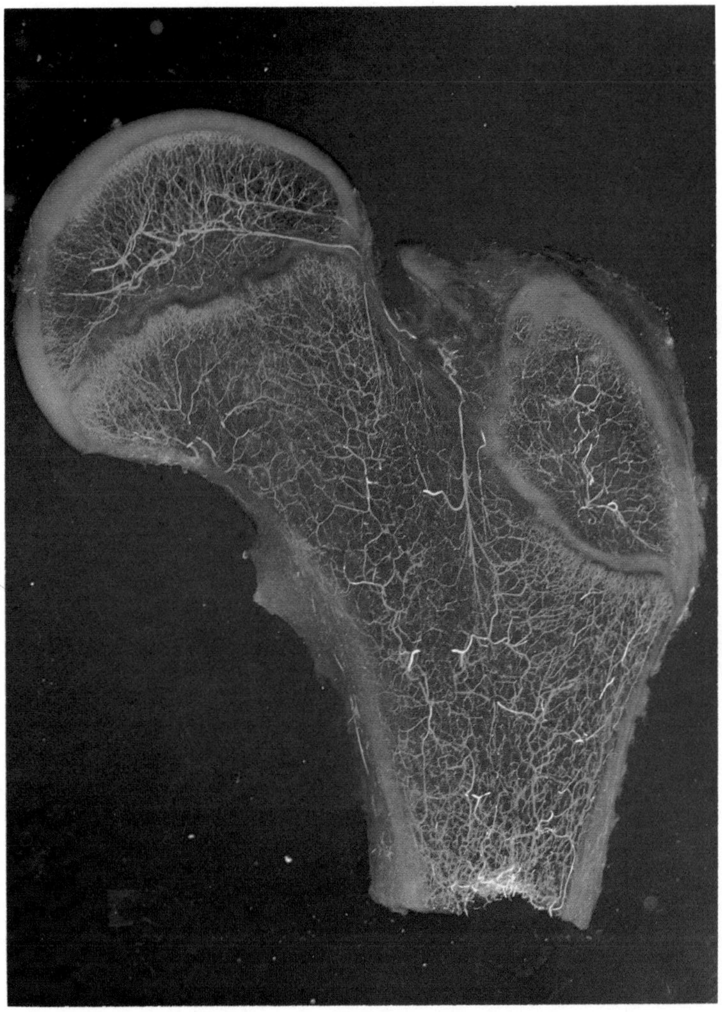

Fig. 1.22 Coronal section of femur showing blood supply. Note separate vascular supply to diaphysis, femoral epiphysis, and trochanteric apophysis. (Courtesy of H.V. Crock.)

Histology. MATURE BONE: In mature bone tissue the collagen fibers of the matrix are arranged in layers or lamellae (hence "lamellar bone"), and in each of these layers the collagen bundles lie parallel to each other (Figs. 1.23 and 1.24). However, the orientation of the collagen bundles changes significantly from one layer to another, in a way similar to the structure of plywood. Therefore, bone tissue gains much strength from its internal construction.

In cortical bone the lamellae are arranged concentrically around a vascular core (haversian canal) to form an osteon (Fig. 1.25). On histologic examination it can be seen

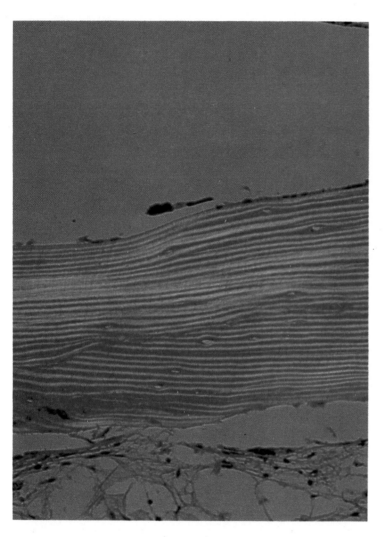

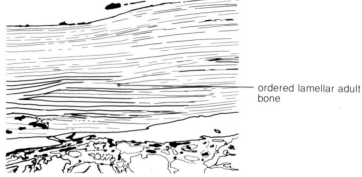

Fig. 1.23 A segment of trabecular bone microscopically examined with polarized light.

ordered lamellar adult bone

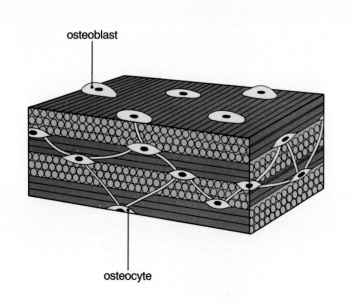

osteoblast

osteocyte

Fig. 1.24 Diagrammatic representation of the layered (lamellar) appearance of bone shows how the alternating dark and light layers are explained by the change in direction of the collagen fibers in each layer.

that surrounding each osteon, and also irregularly distributed throughout the trabecular bone, there are distinct lines that appear deep blue after hematoxylin and eosin staining. These lines are the cement lines (Fig. 1.26). When histologic sections are examined by polarized light, it can be seen that there is a discontinuity of the collagen on either side of the cement line. From this observation it can be inferred that the bone is constructed of separate pieces like a three-dimensional jigsaw puzzle. (It has been demonstrated experimentally that fractures occur along the cement lines.)

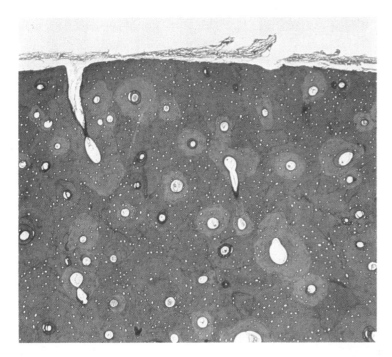

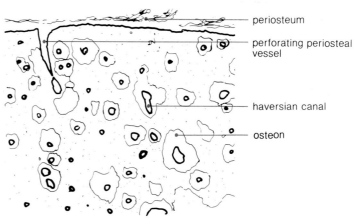

Fig. 1.25 Photomicrograph of cortical bone shows lamellae surrounding haversian canals to form osteons.

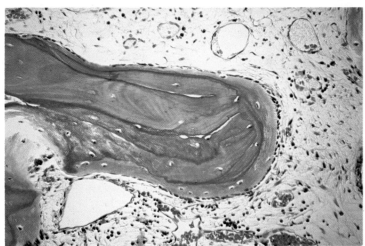

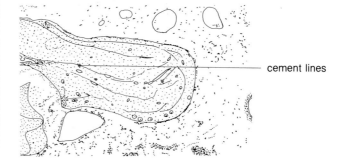

Fig. 1.26 Photomicrograph of trabecular bone (*upper*) taken by transmitted light. The cement lines are blue (hematoxylin and eosin stain). When the same histologic field is photographed through polarized light (*lower*), the cement lines appear as dark lines running through the bone tissue. On either side of the cement lines the collagen bundles run in different directions.

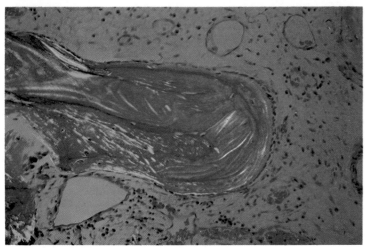

IMMATURE BONE: In addition to lamellar bone there is another form of bone tissue in which the collagen matrix is irregularly arranged in a woven pattern resembling the warp and woof threads in fabric (Figs. 1.27 and 1.28). The cells within this matrix are larger, more rounded, and closer together than those seen in normal bone. This type of bone, which has been variously called woven bone, primitive bone, fiber bone, and immature bone, is seen during development, in fracture callus, in bone-forming tumors, and in conditions in which the rate of formation of bone is highly accelerated (e.g., Paget's disease and other hypermetabolic states). *The recognition of this kind of bone by the pathologist is important, because it usually indicates the presence of a disease process.*

MARROW: The bone marrow is the organ of hematopoiesis, and it contains many cells not related to bone function. Further definition of bone marrow cytology is beyond the scope of this work; nevertheless, there are certain principles that merit attention since they are of importance in the understanding of the pathology of bones and joints.

Although hematopoietic tissue is found in all the bones at birth, with maturation the tissue is confined for all practical purposes to the axial skeleton; that is, the skull, ribs, vertebral column, sternum, and pelvic girdle. The appearance of cellular marrow at other sites during adult life is abnormal and warrants investigation. (Interestingly, although in disease states hyperplastic marrow may be seen in long bones, it is often arrested at the site of the closed epiphyseal plate.)

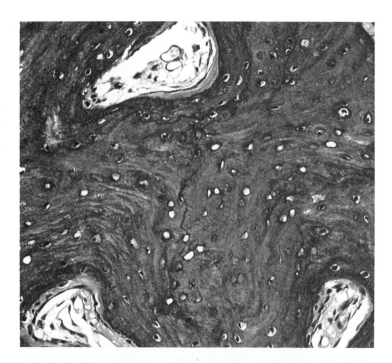

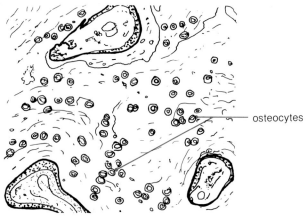

Fig. 1.27 Photomicrograph of immature bone from a patient with osteogenesis imperfecta. Note the crowded oval to round osteocytes (hematoxylin and eosin stain).

osteocytes

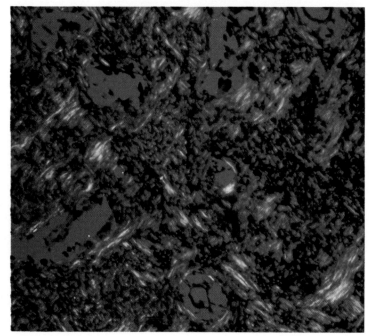

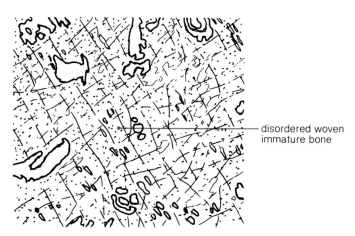

Fig. 1.28 Photomicrograph of immature bone taken with polarized light demonstrates the irregular woven appearance of the collagenous matrix.

disordered woven immature bone

THE JOINTS

Gross Structure. The ends of contiguous bones, together with their soft tissue components, constitute a functioning unit: the joint. Of the three types of joints the most common form is the diarthrodial joint, which has a cavity and forms a movable connecting unit between two bones (Fig. 1.29). Hyaline cartilage (articular cartilage) covers the articulating surfaces of the diarthrodial joints, with the exception of the sternoclavicular and temporomandibular joints, which are covered by fibrocartilage. The second type of joint is the amphiarthrodial joint, which is characterized by limited mobility, e.g., the intervertebral disc (Figs. 1.30 and 1.31). Finally, there are the synarthroses, such as the skull sutures, which are nonmovable.

Cartilage. The articular ends of the bones are covered by hyaline cartilage, which is a nerveless, bloodless, firm and yet pliable tissue. In young people hyaline cartilage is translucent and bluish-white, and in older individuals it is opaque and slightly yellowish (Fig. 1.32). Hyaline cartilage deforms under pressure, but on removal of the deforming pressure, it recovers its original shape. (In growing children, it provides the precursor for the bony skeleton, and also the means by which the bones increase in length.)

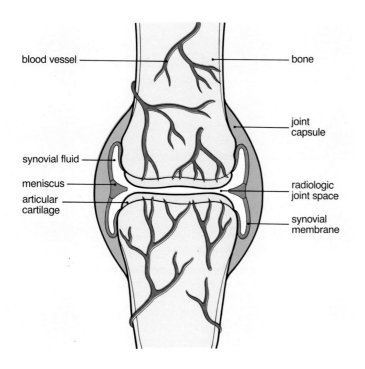

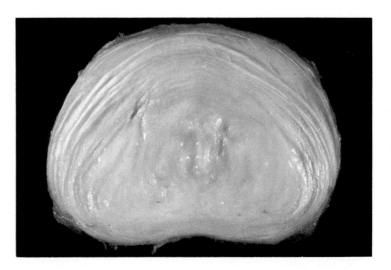

Fig. 1.30 Intervertebral disc seen from above. Note the circumferential fibers in the annulus fibrosus. The nucleus pulposus is seen at the center. The nucleus pulposus, which is rich in proteoglycan and water, acts to resist compression. The circumferential fibers of the annulus prevent lateral spread of the nucleus.

Fig. 1.29 Diagram of the knee joint. The radiologic joint space consists of the radiolucent articular cartilage plus the joint cavity.

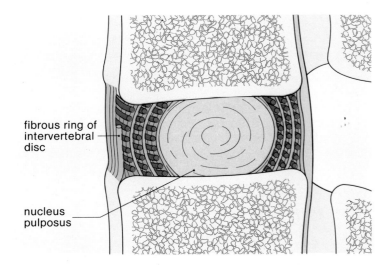

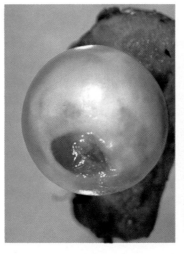
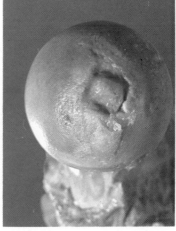

Fig. 1.31 Longitudinal section of intervertebral disc. The vertical fibers in the annulus fibrosus run between the adjacent vertebral bodies and prevent hyperextension or hyperflexion of the spine.

Fig. 1.32 Femoral head from an 18-year-old shows a translucent bluish-white cartilage (*left*), and from a 65-year-old shows an opaque slightly yellowish cartilage (*right*).

Articular cartilage is characterized on histologic examination by its abundant glassy extracellular matrix with isolated, sparse cells situated in well defined spaces (lacunae). It is often described as having four layers or zones: the superficial, intermediate, deep, and calcified layers.

In the superficial layer the cells are flat, the collagen fibers tend to be horizontally disposed, and the matrix tends to contain less proteoglycan. In the intermediate zone the cells are spherical and evenly spaced. In the deep zone the cells have a tendency to form radial groups that follow the pattern of collagen disposition. And in the calcified zone, that is, the zone adjacent to the bone, the cells are apparently nonviable and the matrix is heavily calcified (Fig. 1.33).

A combination of polarizing microscopy, transmission electron microscopy, and scanning electron microscopy has shown that the principal orientation of collagen in articular cartilage is vertical through most of its thickness and horizontal at the surface (Fig. 1.34). The distribution of proteoglycans in the cartilage matrix varies markedly from joint to joint, geographically within a single articular

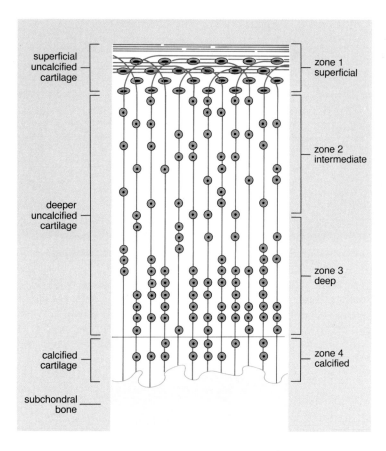

Fig. 1.33 The zones of adult articular cartilage (uncalcified matrix = white, cells = black, collagen = red).

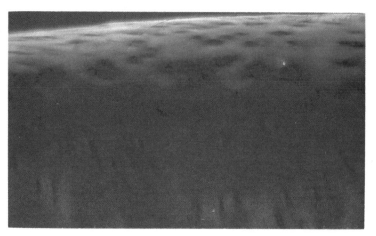

Fig. 1.34 Photomicrograph of the articular cartilage using polarized light and a first order red compensating filter. The fibers at the surface of the cartilage are seen as blue, the fibers in the lower part of the cartilage, red, and between the two layers there is less polarization. These observations can be interpreted as demonstrating that at the surface the fibers are horizontally disposed, in the deep part of the cartilage they are vertical, and in between there is a crossover of fibers.

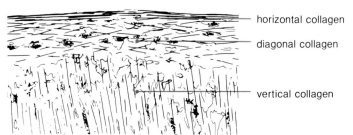

Fig. 1.35 A portion of cartilage stained by toluidine blue shows intense metachromasia around the chondrocytes in the deep part of the noncalcified cartilage. This appearance represents staining of the proteoglycan, and it should be noticed that there is much less staining in the interterritorial matrix than around the cell. Even less staining is seen in the calcified cartilage.

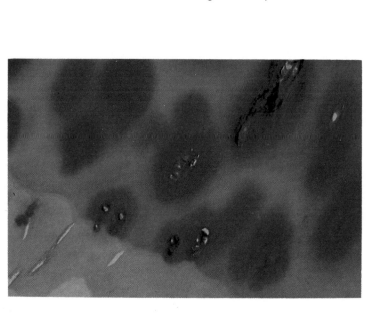

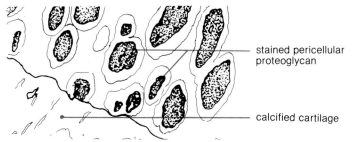

cartilage, and also as a function of age. (Generally proteoglycan distribution is more diffuse in children than in adults.) The surface layers of the cartilage contain much less proteoglycan than the deeper layers. In the deeper layers there is a higher concentration of staining with safranin O and toluidine blue around the cells (the pericellular matrix) than between the cells (the intercellular matrix) (Fig. 1.35).

In histologic sections stained with hematoxylin and eosin, the junction between the calcified cartilage and the noncalcified cartilage is marked by a basophilic line known as the tidemark. This basophilic line is not seen in the developing skeleton, but it is clearly visible in the adult (Figs. 1.36 and 1.37).

Mechanical failure of the cartilage rarely, if ever, gives rise to the separation of bone and cartilage. However, should it occur, this failure is seen as a horizontal cleft at the junction of the calcified and noncalcified cartilage (at the tidemark) (Fig. 1.38). Presumably failure occurs at the tidemark because of the considerable change in the rigidity of the cartilage at this juncture.

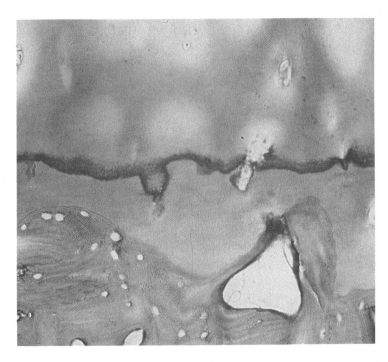

Fig. 1.36 Photomicrograph of the junction of articular cartilage with bone shows the basophilic line (tidemark) that separates the noncalcified from the calcified cartilage. This line represents the mineralization front of the calcified cartilage. In normal adult cartilage, it is clearly defined and relatively even, but in arthritic conditions the line may become widened and diffuse, with duplication of the line a common finding.

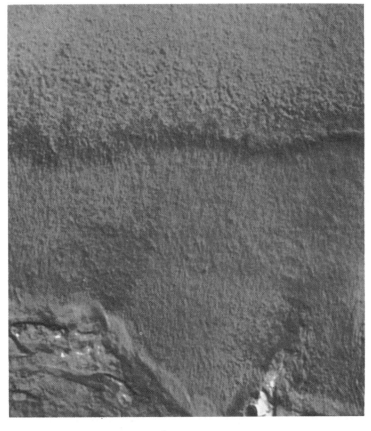

Fig. 1.37 Photomicrograph demonstrates the tidemark at a somewhat higher power than in Fig. 1.36, using differential interference contrast (DIC) microscopy. By the use of this technique a granular appearance of the tidemark can be appreciated.

Fig. 1.38 Photomicrograph demonstrates a traumatic separation of the cartilage that has occurred in the region of the tidemark. This defect has become filled by reparative fibrous tissue.

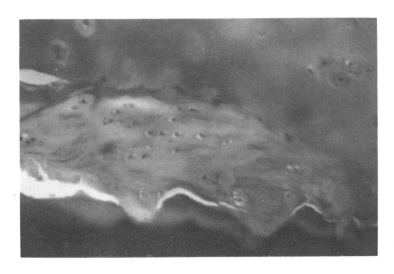

At its base, adult articular cartilage is bordered by the subchondral bone plate. The collagen fibers of the cartilage are not anchored into the bone, but the cartilage tissue is keyed into the irregular surface of the underlying bone, again like a jigsaw puzzle. Because the cartilage adjacent to the bone is calcified and has a rigidity similar to that of bone, the keying is rigid (Fig. 1.39). The insertions of ligaments and tendons into the bone are effected by a similar keying, and at their insertions ligaments and tendons are also calcified (Fig. 1.40).

In addition to hyaline cartilage, of which articular cartilage is composed, two other forms of cartilage are recognized in histologic examinations. *Fibrocartilage* is a tissue in which the matrix contains a high proportion of collagen, the fibers of which are usually visible by transmitted light microscopy. Fibrocartilage is found in

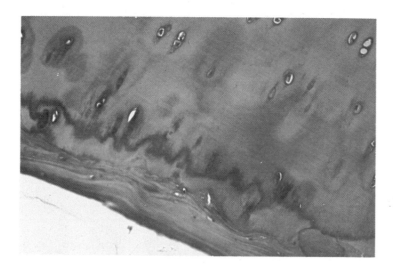
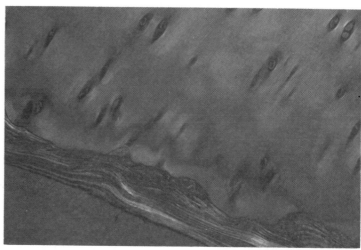

Fig. 1.39 Photomicrographs of the bone-cartilage interface. In the section on the left the tidemark, which indicates the upper edge of the calcified cartilage, can be seen as a wavy blue line, but the bone-cartilage interface is poorly visualized. When the same histologic field is examined by polarized light using a first order red compensator filter (*right*) the bone, which is seen as red, and the cartilage (blue) are easily differentiated and the tidemark may still be seen.

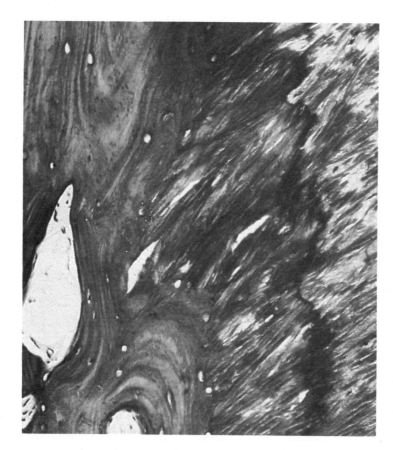
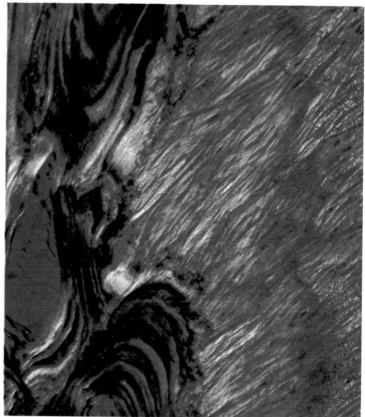

Fig. 1.40 Photomicrographs of the insertion of a ligament into bone. In the section on the left the wavy blue line, which represents the edge of the calcified portion of the ligament, is clearly seen, but the interface of ligament and bone is not well visualized. When the same histologic field is examined by polarized light (*right*), the interface of calcified ligament and bone is clearly demonstrated.

the menisci of the knee, the annulus fibrosus, and at the insertions of ligaments and tendons into the bone (Fig. 1.41). The second type of nonhyaline cartilage is *elastic cartilage,* in which the matrix contains a high proportion of elastic tissue. Elastic fibers are found in the ligamentum flavum, external ear, and epiglottis (Fig. 1.42).

Both the fibrocartilage and elastic cartilage incorporate the term "cartilage" because the cells are rounded and lie in lacunae, which gives them a superficial resemblance to the cells of hyaline cartilage. However, the mechanical functions of these tissues are very different from those of hyaline cartilage. Both fibrocartilage and elastic cartilage function principally as resistors of tension, whereas hyaline cartilage is mainly subject to and resists compressive forces.

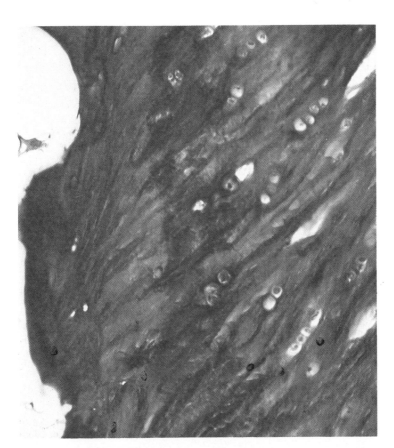

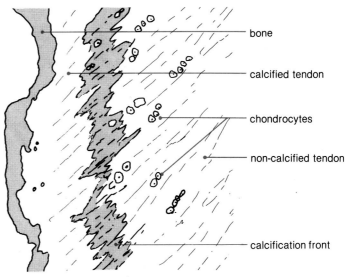

Fig. 1.41 Photomicrograph of tendon insertion. Note that the cells of the tendon are rounded and lie in lacunae. This appearance is described as fibrocartilage.

bone

calcified tendon

chondrocytes

non-calcified tendon

calcification front

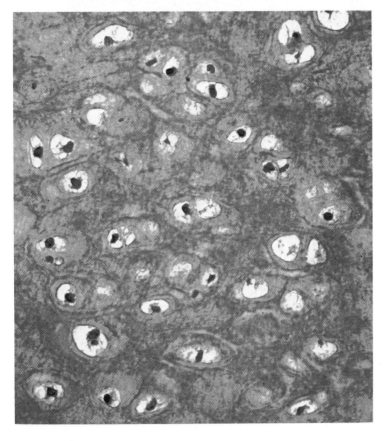

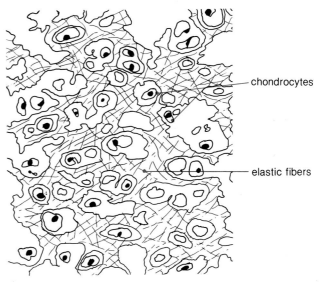

Fig. 1.42 Photomicrograph of ear cartilage. Although the cells resemble those seen in hyaline cartilage, the matrix contains many elastic fibers that appear bright red in this section stained with phloxine and tartrazine.

chondrocytes

elastic fibers

Synovial Membrane. The synovial membrane lines the inner surface of the joint capsule and all other intra-articular structures, with the exception of articular cartilage and the meniscus. Synovial membrane consists of two parts. The first component of synovial membrane is the synovial lining (or intimal layer) bounding the joint space. This layer is predominantly cellular. The second component is a subintimal, supportive, or backing layer that is formed of fibrous and adipose tissues in varying proportions.

The surface of the synovial lining is smooth, moist, and glistening, with a few small villi and fringelike folds.

The cellular elements of the joint lining consist of intimal cells (or synoviocytes) and other connective tissue cells, including fat cells, fibroblasts, histiocytes, and mast cells. (Mast cells are omnipresent in connective tissue.) Sections of synovial membrane show along the edge facing the synovial cavity a single row or sometimes multiple rows of closely packed cells with large elliptical nuclei (Fig. 1.43).

Electron microscopic studies have revealed two principal types of synovial cells, which are designated as types A and B. (Many cells have features of both types and have been called intermediate.) The predominant cell (type A) has many of the features of a macrophage, and there is good evidence that it is structurally adapted for phagocytic functions (Fig. 1.44). The less common type B cells are richly endowed with rough endoplasmic reticulum, they contain Golgi systems, and often show pinocytotic vesicles (Fig. 1.45). In normal synovial intima far more type A cells are found than type B.

The synovial membrane has three principal functions: the secretion of synovial fluid hyaluronate (B cells); the phagocytosis of waste material derived from the various components of the joint (A cells); and the regulation of the movement of solutes, electrolytes, and proteins by the capillaries into the synovial fluid.

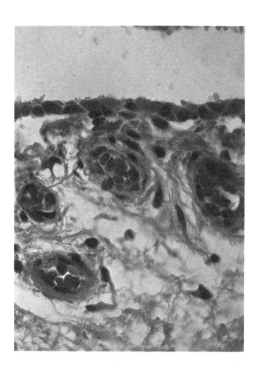

Fig. 1.43 Photomicrograph of synovium shows a delicate synovial lining resting on a fibroadipose subintimal layer that is rich in capillaries, lymphatics, and nerve endings.

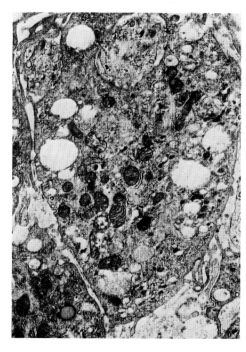

Fig. 1.44 Electron photomicrograph of an A cell shows abundant mitochondria and dense inclusion bodies.

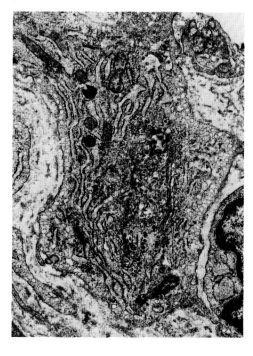

Fig. 1.45 Electron photomicrograph of a B cell shows abundant rough endoplasmic reticulum and many pinocytotic vesicles.

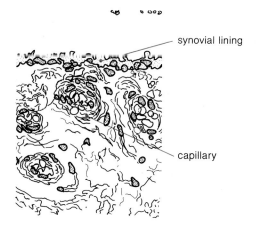

synovial lining

capillary

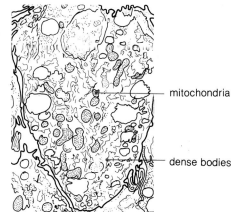

mitochondria

dense bodies

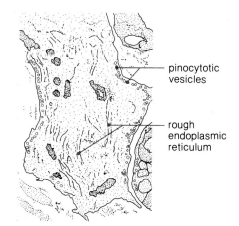

pinocytotic vesicles

rough endoplasmic reticulum

BONE GROWTH AND DEVELOPMENT

Unlike most tissues, bone can grow only by apposition on the surface of an already existing substrate such as bone and/or calcified cartilage. In contrast, cartilage grows by interstitial cellular proliferation and matrix formation. It is perhaps because of the capacity of cartilage for interstitial growth that most of the embryonic skeleton is first formed in the cartilage, and furthermore, that cartilage proliferation plays such an important role in skeletal growth and development.

Even before any bone tissue formation has occurred, it can be seen in an embryonic cartilage skeleton that the cartilage cells towards the middle of the bone model are larger and more separated by interstitial matrix than those towards the end of the bone model, which are fairly small and closely packed together (Fig. 1.46). As the cells in the center of the bone shaft continue to enlarge, the cartilage matrix lying between the cells becomes calcified, and the cells die (Fig. 1.47). The mechanisms that are responsible for the calcification of the matrix are not completely understood, but it is generally believed that the initiators of calcification are small membrane-bound vesicles known as matrix vesicles, which are found in the interstitial matrix between the cells.

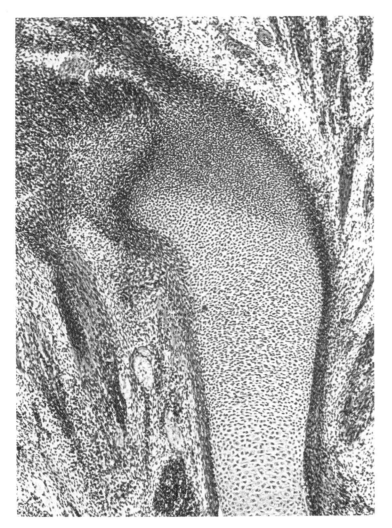

Fig. 1.46 Photomicrograph of the upper end of the femur and hip joint in a 5-week fetus. The bone is already modeled in cartilage and covered by a condensation of mesenchymal cells, which will eventually become the periosteum. Notice that the cells in the diaphysis of the cartilage model of the bone are larger and paler than those at the end of the bone.

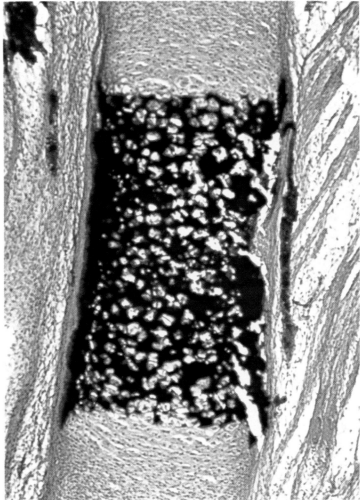

Fig. 1.47 Photomicrograph of the shaft of the long bone in a 7-week fetus; cut, undecalcified, and stained with von Kossa stain. Notice the calcification of the cartilage matrix (black) that occurred in the diaphysis of the bone.

Following the calcification of the cartilage matrix, the periosteum surrounding this portion of the bone begins to produce a primitive bone matrix that is quickly formed into a cuff of bone (Fig. 1.48). After the formation of this cuff of bone, small capillaries can be seen penetrating through the periosteum and the periosteal bone cuff into the calcified cartilage matrix, destroying the now empty cartilage lacunae and establishing a vascular network through the calcified cartilage (Fig. 1.49). Cells perhaps derived from the vessel walls are seen lining up on the surface of the remaining calcified cartilage and depositing a bony matrix.

This process, that is, cartilage calcification followed by vascular invasion and deposition of bony matrix on the remaining calcified cartilage, is known as endochondral ossification, and it is the normal route by which cartilage is transformed into bone. The bone that is first laid down, that is, with a core of calcified cartilage and

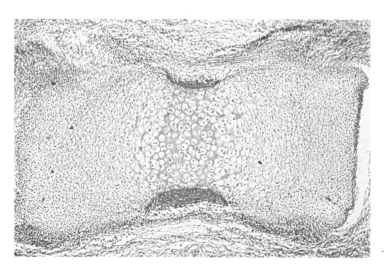

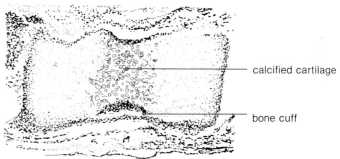

Fig. 1.48 Photomicrograph of a section through a metacarpal bone from a 7-week fetus. In the diaphysis the cartilage matrix stains with a deeper blue, indicating that it is calcified. Around the calcified cartilage matrix can be seen a narrow cuff of immature bone.

— calcified cartilage

— bone cuff

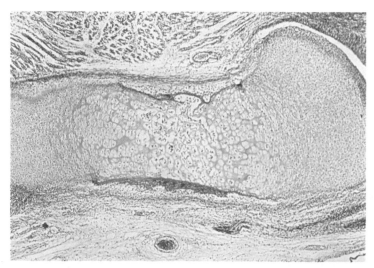

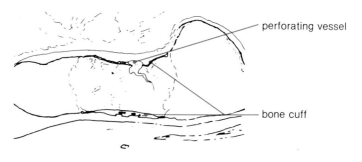

Fig. 1.49 (*upper*) Photomicrograph of a long bone removed from a 10-week fetus.

— perforating vessel

— bone cuff

Fig. 1.49 (*lower*) Close-up shows the calcified cartilage below, and the diaphyseal bone cuff above, covered by the condensed mesenchymal tissue that forms the periosteum. Penetrating through the bone cuff into the calcified cartilage is a blood vessel. This blood vessel will eventually erode through the calcified cartilage entirely, bringing in osteoblasts to form the earliest primary spongiosa.

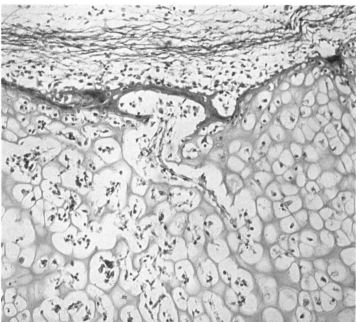

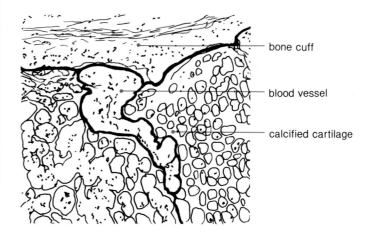

— bone cuff

— blood vessel

— calcified cartilage

primitive bone on the surface, is commonly known as the primary spongiosa (Fig. 1.50; see also Fig. 1.57). As the primary spongiosa is remodeled and the calcified cartilage removed, the bony trabeculae come to be formed entirely of bony tissue, and in this stage they are generally called the secondary spongiosa.

In the embryo the process of endochondral ossification continues until a considerable portion of the shaft of the bone is converted into an osseous tissue and only the ends of the bone are formed of cartilage (Fig. 1.51). The cartilage at the bone ends can be seen to be continuously proliferating and lengthening by interstitial growth. The cartilage cells, as they approach the midshaft of the bone, undergo enlargement and degeneration; the cartilage matrix calcifies, and eventually vascular invasion and the formation of a primary spongiosa occurs. Thus it is that the bone grows in length (Fig. 1.52).

Fig. 1.50 A portion of the primary spongiosa taken from the diaphysis of a long bone in a 10-week fetus. Notice the delicate cores of calcified cartilage covered by plump cells (osteoblasts), which are forming thin seams of immature bone matrix.

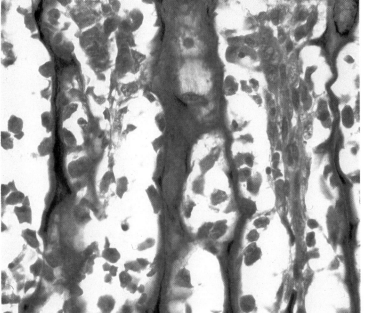

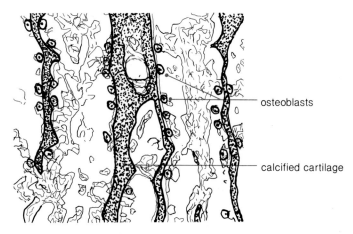

Fig. 1.51 Gross photograph of a femur taken from a 6-month stillborn baby. At this stage the epiphyseal ends of the bone are still entirely cartilaginous.

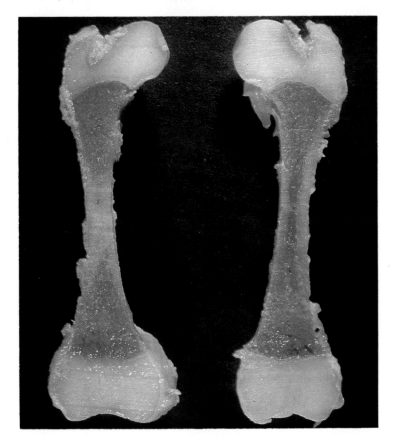

Fig. 1.52 Photomicrograph of the upper end of the femur shows the junction between the newly formed bone and the epiphyseal cartilage. The bone grows in length by the process of endochondral ossification, in which the calcified cartilage is invaded by blood vessels and replaced by bone.

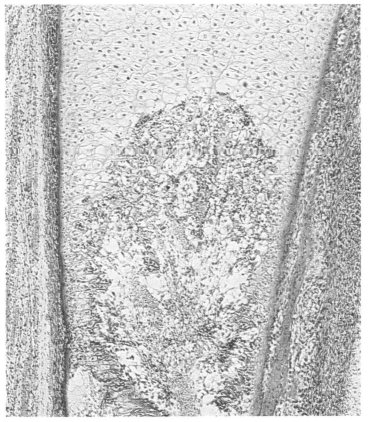

1.23

At some point during development a secondary center of ossification is formed within the cartilaginous end of the bone (Figs. 1.53 and 1.54). Initially, calcification occurs at the middle of the secondary center. This area is then invaded by blood vessels and the process of subchondral ossification ensues. The vessels leading to the degenerated and calcified cartilage in the center of the epiphysis are carried in canals that develop from the surface covering of the embryonal bone (Fig. 1.55). As the secondary center of ossification grows, the only remaining cartilage is the cartilage covering the articular end of the bone, and a thin layer or plate of cartilage

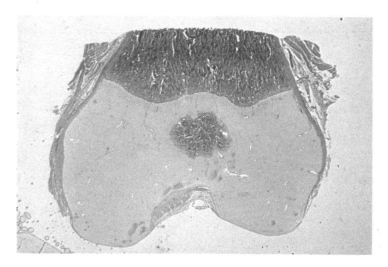

Fig. 1.53 The secondary center of ossification is demonstrated in the lower end of the femur. This area increases in size by the process of maturation and calcification of the cartilage around the secondary center, with subsequent endochondral ossification.

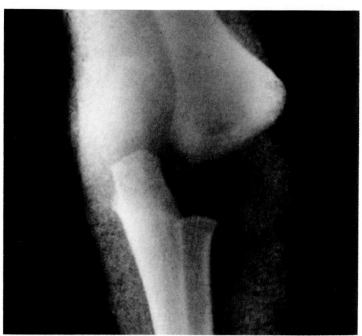

Fig. 1.54 This post-traumatic roentgenogram of a 2-year-old child illustrates the importance of knowing when and where the secondary centers of ossification appear. At first sight, it might appear that there has been a dislocation of the elbow. However, since the ossification center of the capitulum is still in place, it can be inferred that the joint is intact and that the displacement of the humerus results from a fracture through the region of the growth plate.

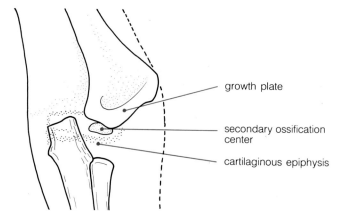

growth plate

secondary ossification center

cartilaginous epiphysis

Fig. 1.55 The vessels that feed the ossification center are carried in canals through the epiphyseal cartilage, and one of these canals is demonstrated here in high power.

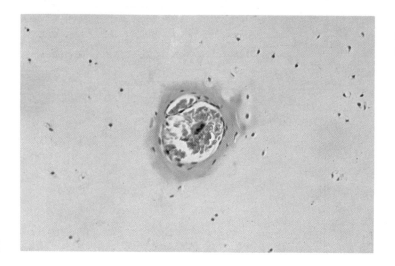

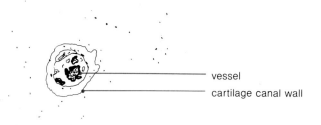

vessel

cartilage canal wall

lying between the secondary center of ossification and the main part of the bone shaft. This plate is known as the growth plate or physis (Figs. 1.56 to 1.58).

The epiphysis is therefore that portion of the bone that is above the growth plate or physis. The metaphysis is that portion just below the growth plate, the area occupied by the primary spongiosa. And in general, the metaphysis corresponds to the flared zone in the shaft below the growth plate. The diaphysis is the portion that lies between the two growth plates.

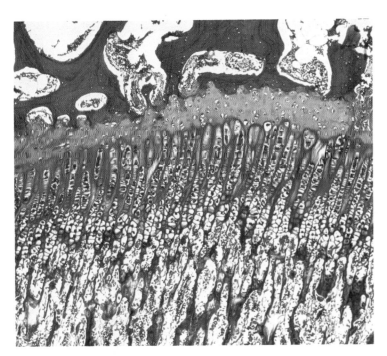

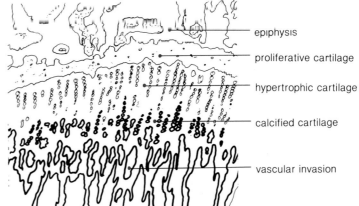

Fig. 1.56 Photomicrograph demonstrates the appearance of the growth plate during active bone growth. At the top of the field there is a portion of the epiphysis, and the cartilage cells in this region are proliferating cells. Further down the cells begin to palisade into vertical columns, and, as they approach the metaphysis, the cells hypertrophy and the matrix calcifies. The calcified matrix is then invaded by blood vessels.

epiphysis
proliferative cartilage
hypertrophic cartilage
calcified cartilage
vascular invasion

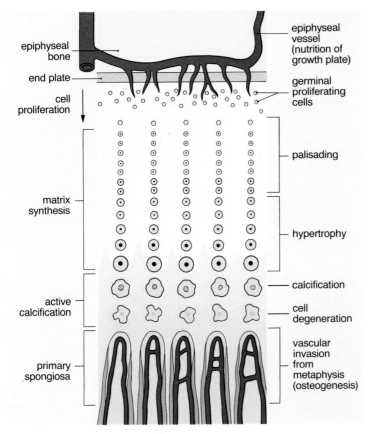

epiphyseal bone
end plate
cell proliferation
matrix synthesis
active calcification
primary spongiosa

epiphyseal vessel (nutrition of growth plate)
germinal proliferating cells
palisading
hypertrophy
calcification
cell degeneration
vascular invasion from metaphysis (osteogenesis)

Fig. 1.57 Diagram of the growth plate.

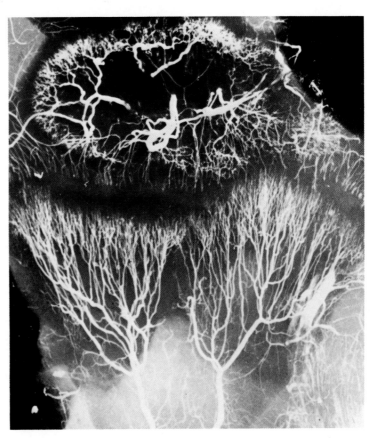

Fig. 1.58 Specimen of the upper end of the tibia in an immature pig. The vessels have been injected with barium sulfate and the bone decalcified. The ramifying vessels in the metaphysis that provide for endochondral ossification are clearly seen.

The cartilage of the growth plates continues to proliferate and to undergo endochondral ossification until apparent growth ceases at adolescence. At adolescence the growth plate is perforated by blood vessels and becomes obliterated (Fig. 1.59). However, a trace of the growth plate scar continues in the form of an epiphyseal bony plate, which is recognizable on radiologic examination and in anatomic specimens throughout life (Fig. 1.60). Acute illness may result in a temporary cessation of growth, and the stigma of this cessation may

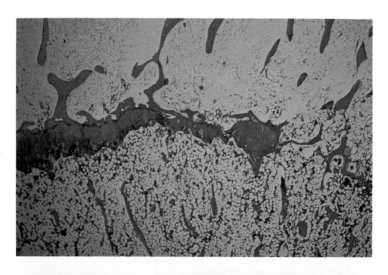

Fig. 1.59 Photomicrograph of the epiphyseal growth plate from the upper end of the tibia in a 17-year-old boy. Although the growth plate is still open on the left side of the field, it can be seen that at the right side a bony continuity has been established between the metaphysis and the epiphysis, and at this point growth can be said to have ceased. In general, the plate first closes in its central portion, and the peripheral portion of the plate is the last part to close.

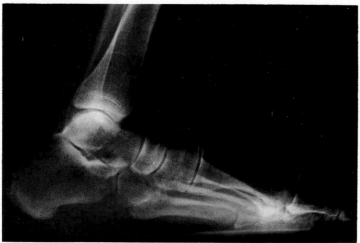

Fig. 1.60 Roentgenogram of the ankle in an adult shows the epiphyseal scar in the lower end of the tibia.

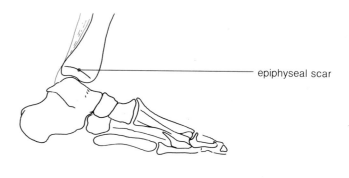

epiphyseal scar

Fig. 1.61 Roentgenogram of the tibia in a child with an open epiphyseal plate. In the shaft of the tibia can be seen clearly a number of radiopaque lines that represent episodes of growth arrest.

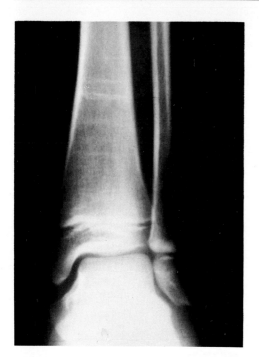

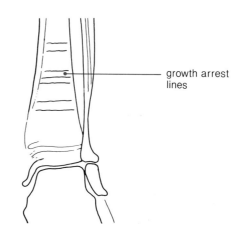

growth arrest lines

remain for many years as a linear density paralleling the epiphyseal scar in the shaft of the bone, known as a Harris line or growth arrest line (Fig. 1.61).

The bones of the skull, some of the facial bones, and most of the clavicle form like the initial bone cuff, i.e., without a pre-existing cartilage model, from undifferentiated connective tissue cells (mesenchyme). These bones are termed membranous bones, and they grow only by the apposition of new bone on the surface. *They have no cartilaginous growth plates* (Figs. 1.62 to 1.64).

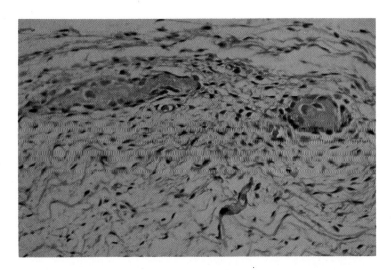

Fig. 1.62 Photomicrograph of a section taken through the skull area of an 11-week fetus. The bone presents first as cellular condensations that secrete an extracellular matrix of immature bone.

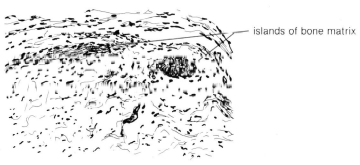

islands of bone matrix

Fig. 1.63 Drawing of a macerated specimen of the parietal bone demonstrates how individual foci of secreted bone matrix fuse together to form first a network of bone, and later a plate.

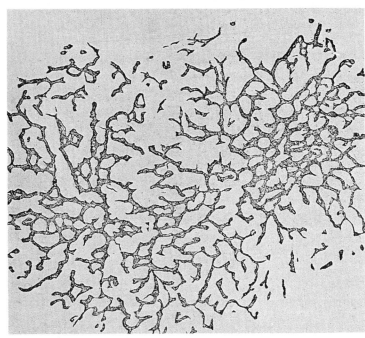

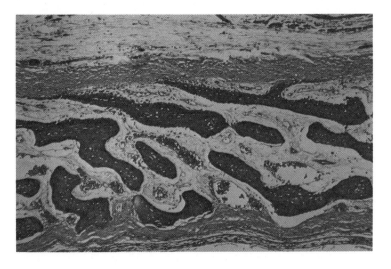

Fig. 1.64 Photomicrograph of a calvarial bone from a 19-week fetus shows a section through the bone plate. The dural surface is on the lower border of the field, and the epidermal surface is on the upper border. Notice the resorptive activity along the dural surface and the blastic activity along the epidermal surface, which allows for the expansion of the cranium.

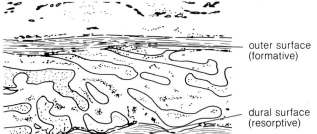

outer surface (formative)

dural surface (resorptive)

METHODS OF EXAMINATION OF SKELETAL TISSUE

Gross Examination. Bone specimens received by the surgical pathologist often consist only of fragments, the anatomic site of which cannot be recognized. On the other hand, when a larger piece of bone is submitted, anatomic landmarks should be carefully sought. Large specimens should be cut with a band saw into parallel slices 3 to 5 mm thick, so that the interior appearance of the bone may be examined.

On occasion the color of the bone may be particularly helpful. For example, necrotic bone is an opaque yellow, in contrast to the rather translucent and pink appearance of living bone. The pathologist should examine the specimen for evidence of generalized or localized increase in porosity or sclerosis. When multiple pieces of bone are received, the pieces chosen for embedding should preferably be those that appear to show the greatest departure from normal.

Radiologic Examination. A particularly useful adjunct to gross examination is the preparation of radiographs of the surgical specimens, using low voltage x-rays (Faxitron, Field Emission Corporation, McMinnville, Oregon 97128, USA) and industrial film (Kodalith Ortho film, Type 3). Such radiographs not only help in choosing the areas to section, but they are also frequently helpful in the interpretation of histologic material, e.g., finding a nidus in osteoid osteoma or defining an infarct.

Because bone and cartilage are somewhat translucent it is frequently difficult to produce acceptable black and white photographs. This problem can be overcome by using a monochromatic shortwave light source, such as an ultraviolet lamp.

Microscopic Examination. The histologist uses various staining techniques to demonstrate the components of the matrix.

Collagen may be demonstrated by a trichrome stain, or the van Gieson stain, and also by the use of polarized light. This latter technique is particularly useful because, not only does it clearly show the collagen fibers, but it also allows one to determine the orientation of the collagen and to study the microarchitecture of the tissue. This information can be particularly helpful in the interpretation of diseased tissue, e.g., Paget's disease or scars.

The proteoglycans can be demonstrated by the use of the safranin O stain, alcian blue stain, and less specifically by toluidine blue and PAS (periodic acid-Schiff).

Mineral components can be demonstrated only in undemineralized tissue. It is possible, by embedding the tissue in plastic and using specially hardened knives, to cut histologic sections that still contain the minerals within the bone matrix. Undecalcified sections are particularly important in the assessment of metabolic disturbances. The mineral may be stained by two techniques: alizarin red, which will stain the calcium components of the hydroxyapatite red, and the von Kossa method, which will stain the phosphate component as well as other salts, e.g., carbonate and oxalate, black.

The distribution of mineral in the tissue may also be studied by the technique of microradiography. Using low kilovoltage x-rays from an x-ray tube with a very fine focal spot, roentgenograms are made from thin slices of bone that have been cut with a diamond saw at approximately 100 μm.

It cannot be too strongly emphasized that an essential component in the interpretation of bone and joint histology is a careful correlation with the clinical radiographs and history.

HISTOLOGIC TECHNIQUES: Often a major problem for the individual wishing to study bone and bone disease lies in the preparation of adequate histologic sections. There are some simple techniques that should be followed in order to achieve good tissue sections.

First, adequate fixation of the tissue requires that larger pieces of bone be cut into slices between 3 and 5 mm thick. This can be achieved using a band saw. After using the band saw it is important to carefully wash the cut surface of the bone under running water, brushing the surface gently with a soft brush. This procedure will ensure that any fragments of bone and bone dust generated by the saw are washed out of the interstices of the marrow. If this cleaning is not done, artifacts may be apparent on the histologic sections.

The tissue should be fixed in adequate amounts of buffered formalin. Buffered formalin will prevent: (1) the formation of formalin pigment (which may interfere with the proper interpretation of other pigments that may be present, e.g., iron or gold), and (2) the formation of formic acid, which might result in undesirable decalcification.

If decalcification is desired, then 5 per cent nitric acid following adequate fixation of the tissue will produce good results. However, an adequate volume of acid should be used—approximately ten times that of the tissue—and since the acid is neutralized as the calcium is removed from the bone, the acid should be changed, preferably twice a day. To ensure access of the acid, gentle agitation on a shaker is a helpful procedure. By the use of this technique, most bones will be decalcified in one or two days.

After decalcification has been achieved, it is essential that the tissue be adequately washed in running water for at least 12 hours, in order to assure good differentiation of the hematoxylin and eosin stains. In many laboratories the bone tissue is either overdecalcified or the acid is inadequately removed; in both cases poor staining results.

Better sections of bone are achieved after vacuum embedding of the tissue. A guide to the preparation of undecalcified sections and the stains applicable to such sections will be presented in Chapter 2 under "Quantitative Histologic Assessment of Bone."

2 Diseases Resulting from Disturbances in the Formation and Breakdown of Bone I

Morphologic alterations in the skeleton result from genetic or acquired defects in the formation or breakdown of components of the bone matrix (collagen, proteoglycan, or mineral) by the cells.

DEFINITION OF TERMS

Before consideration of specific pathologic states, it is necessary to define the terms by which they are generally described. Osteopenia is a radiologic term that indicates relative radiolucency of the skeleton. Osteosclerosis refers to a relative increase in density of the skeleton (Fig. 2.1). Osteoporosis describes a reduction in bone tissue mass but normal mineralization of the organic matrix. The condition referred to as osteomalacia is brought about by a disturbance in the rate of mineralization of bone. On morphologic examination, patients with this condition are found to have increased osteoid or non-mineralized bone throughout the skeleton (Fig. 2.2).

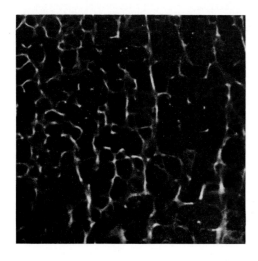 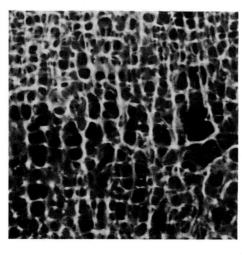 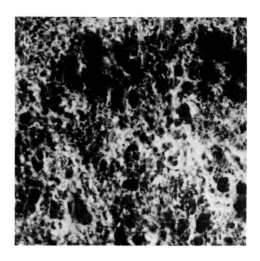

Fig. 2.1 Radiographs of osteopenic (*left*), normal (*center*), and osteosclerotic (*right*) vertebrae demonstrate the relative radiolucency (*left*) and density (*right*) of bone in two pathologic conditions. The normal vertebra has readily identifiable vertical and horizontal bone trabeculae.

Osteopenia (*left*) in the vertebral column is seen as a loss of bone tissue. Note that the horizontal trabeculae are thinner or have disappeared completely. Before severe loss of bone has occurred, there may be a compensatory thickening of the vertical trabeculae.

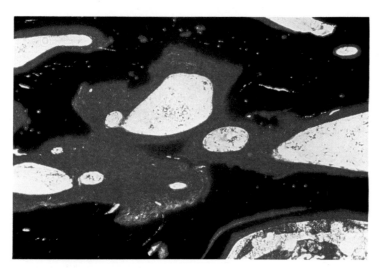

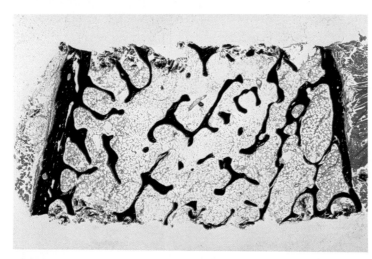

Fig. 2.2 Adult ilial bone (von Kossa stain). Note that nonmineralized bone or osteoid, pink in the von Kossa stain, covers most of the trabecular bone surface and constitutes a substantial portion of the bone tissue in states of osteomalacia (*upper*). In normal adult bone (*lower*) less than 20 per cent of the trabecular bone surfaces are covered by osteoid. (Low power view, undecalcified section.)

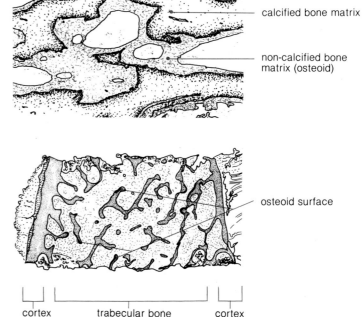

calcified bone matrix

non-calcified bone matrix (osteoid)

osteoid surface

cortex   trabecular bone   cortex

QUANTITATIVE HISTOLOGIC ASSESSMENT OF BONE

Since the accurate diagnosis of metabolic bone disease requires systematic and reliable bone sampling and processing, an outline of current methodology is presented.

The standard biopsy is of bone removed from the ilium, which is generally accepted as an accessible bone that is representative of the overall condition of the skeleton. Most investigators use a sample that is obtained from a site 2 cm below the iliac crest and 2 cm behind the anterior superior iliac spine. Such standardization of the site is necessary because of the variance of bone throughout the ilium (Fig. 2.3). A four-component bone biopsy trephine is used in the procedure (Fig. 2.4). This instrument produces a cortex-to-cortex cylindrical specimen which, depending on the particular instrument used, may be from 3 to 8 mm in diameter (Fig. 2.5).

The biopsy tissue is fixed immediately after its removal from the iliac crest in 10 per cent neutral buffered formalin. Tissue that has been double-labeled with tetracycline is fixed in 70 per cent ethanol to better preserve the label. All tissue is subsequently dehydrated and then infiltrated with embedding medium. This process is accomplished by consecutive infiltration of the specimen with absolute acetone and methyl methacrylate monomer, clean methyl methacrylate monomer, and finally with polymerized methyl methacrylate embedding medium.

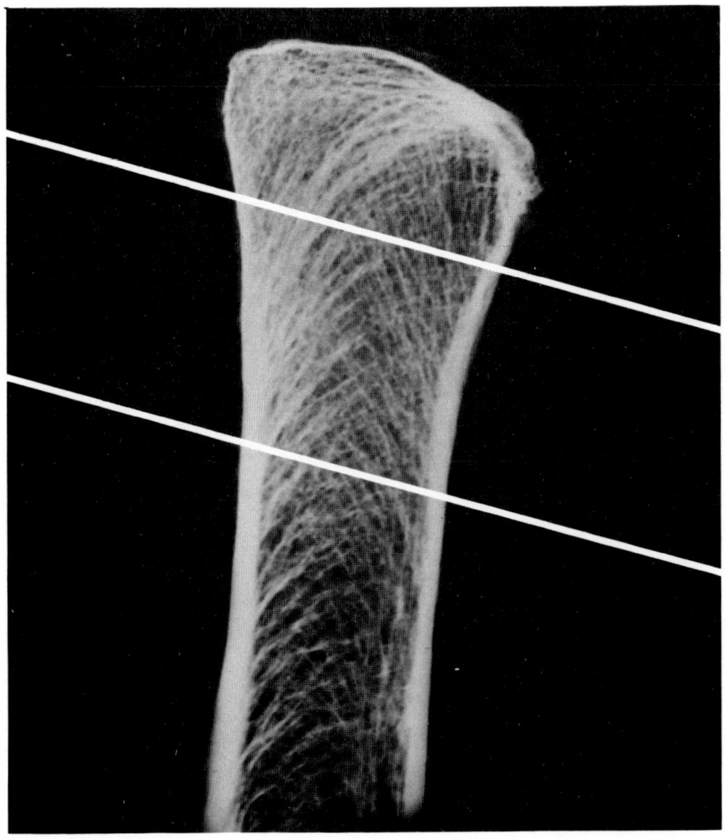

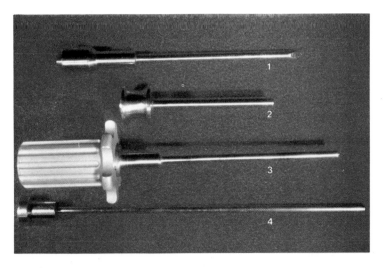

Fig. 2.4 A four-component bone biopsy instrument. A guide (1) is used to place an outer cannula or sleeve (2), which provides fixation to the periosteum. Once the cannula is in place on the periosteum, the guide is removed and the tubular trephine (3), which has a cutting edge, is used to obtain the biopsy. The biopsy sample is removed from the trephine by means of an obturator (4).

Fig. 2.3 Roentgenogram of a coronal section of the ilial bone demonstrates the site variation in thickness of cortical bone and the cancellous bone density. The preferred site for biopsy (between lines) is approximately 2 cm below the iliac crest. Here the cortex is well defined on both sides.

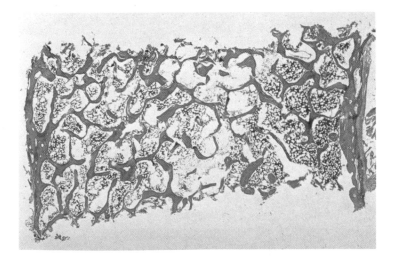

Fig. 2.5 Transilial biopsy (hematoxylin and eosin stain). A full-thickness, cortex-to-cortex sample with no crushing or other artifacts is a satisfactory specimen for histomorphometry.

Tissue blocks are cut with a carbide-tipped blade on a Jung microtome, model K, both knife and block having been wetted with 70 per cent ethanol. Five-micrometer sections are placed on Haupt's gelatinized slides. In addition to routine stains, von Kossa's stain, which specifically differentiates calcium salts (and therefore mineralized bone), is also employed.

The actual determination of the amount of bone present in the sample (the degree of osteopenia) requires systematic, reliable, and reproducible quantitation. In the past this quantitation had been accomplished by the use of an integrated eyepiece that enabled the juxtaposition of a grid over the tissue to be examined. The intersections encompassing the constituent to be examined (bone, osteoid, etc.) were calculated and presented either as raw data or as percentages of the total number of intersections.

Modern techniques employ the use of more exact equipment. One such apparatus is the Zeiss MOP-AM03 computer (Fig. 2.6). Slides are viewed under a standard

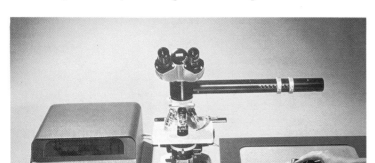

Fig. 2.6 The Zeiss MOP-AM03 computer. To the right a technician is holding a graphic cursor. An image of the activated cursor is superimposed on the histologic section by means of the black tubular arm (optical drawing tube) attached to the microscope. The digitizing tablet is activated by a signal produced by the graphic pen, and the signals from the digitizing tablet are analyzed by the previously programmed MOP3 analyzer on the left.

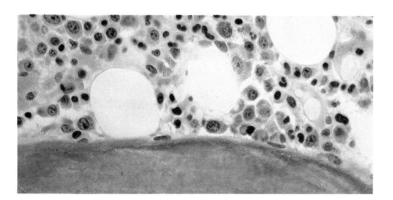

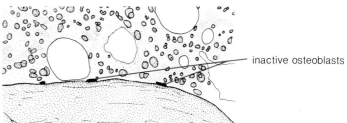

Fig. 2.7 Inactive bone surface (hematoxylin and eosin stain). Smooth surface with flat lining cells (inactive osteoblasts).

inactive osteoblasts

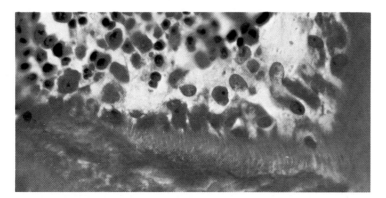

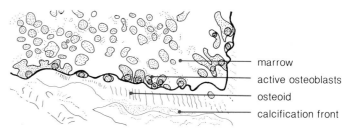

Fig. 2.8 Active bone surface (hematoxylin and eosin stain). Prominent osteoid and active osteoblasts.

marrow
active osteoblasts
osteoid
calcification front

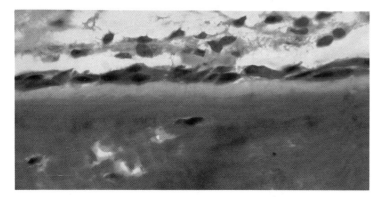

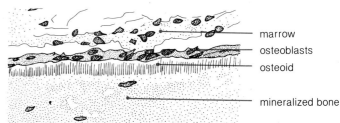

Fig. 2.9 Active bone surface (hematoxylin and eosin stain). Osteoid and relatively less active osteoblasts.

marrow
osteoblasts
osteoid
mineralized bone

2.4

microscope fitted with an appropriate objective, which is attached to an optical drawing tube for binocular observation. This arrangement allows the viewer to see both the specimen and a cursor, which can be used to trace the bone surfaces. When the cursor is activated, a graphic tablet sends coordinates to the MOP-AM03, which is programmed to calculate values for the desired parameters.

An assessment of the state of activity of the bone may be accomplished by evaluating quantitatively both the type and number of bone cells present and the morphology of the bone surface. A surface actively undergoing resorption is scalloped or jagged and contains osteoclasts. Inactive resorption surfaces are also jagged but contain no cells. Smooth surfaces that are covered by osteoblasts are considered the surfaces of bone undergoing active bone formation (Figs. 2.7 to 2.12). Fig. 2.13 demonstrates that a microscopic field may be a complex amalgam of resorption and formation.

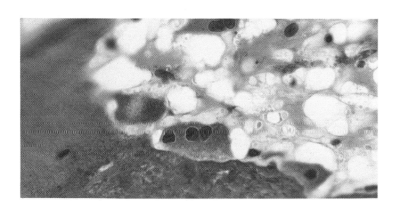

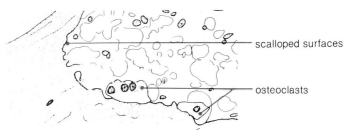

Fig. 2.10 Active resorptive bone surface (hematoxylin and eosin stain). Scalloped surface with many osteoclasts.

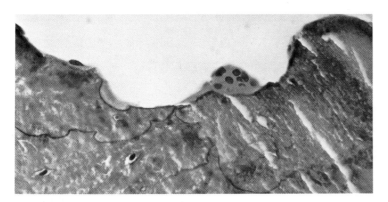

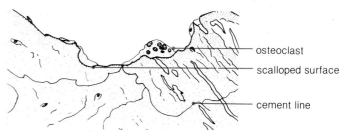

Fig. 2.11 Quiescent resorptive bone surface (hematoxylin and eosin stain). Scalloped surface with few osteoclasts.

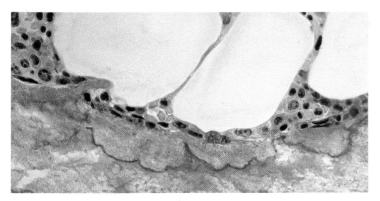

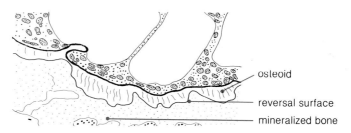

Fig. 2.12 Reversal bone surface (hematoxylin and eosin stain). A previously resorbed (scalloped) surface has been covered with a new layer of osteoblasts that are depositing osteoid.

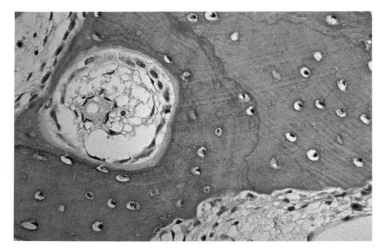

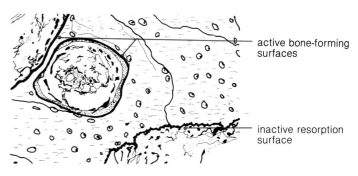

Fig. 2.13 Microscopic field shows variety of bone surfaces.

Once the total amount of bone surfaces present on the tissue is determined, percentages of each of several parameters can be calculated. For example, the percentage of resorbing surface is the percentage of total bone surface showing scalloped zones.

Specific quantities of bone mass can be derived by calculating the area of the tissue occupied by bone and non-mineralized bone (osteoid). Similar calculations can be made of the percentage of cancellous bone and the percentage of cortical bone (Fig. 2.14).

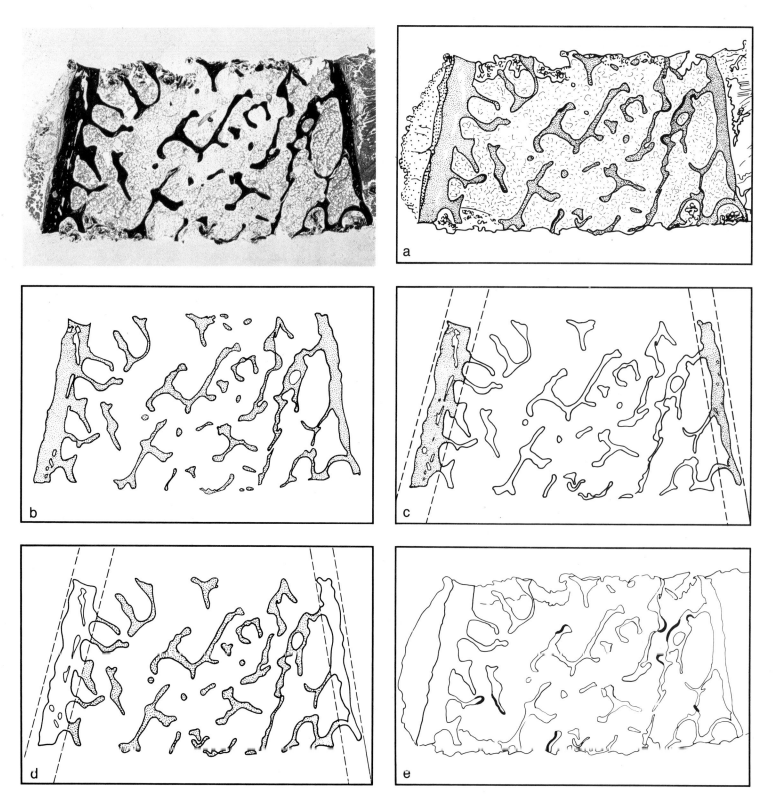

Fig. 2.14 Adult transilial bone biopsy (von Kossa stain). Accompanying diagrams show (a) Total bone and marrow (100% of area), (b) Total bone (26.8% of area), (c) Cortical bone (11.4% of area),

(d) Trabecular bone (15.4% of area), (e) Osteoid (14.5% of surface, 1% of area).

DYNAMIC ANALYSIS OF BONE ACTIVITY

In addition to data derived from the histomorphometric analysis of a single biopsy, it is possible to make more dynamic statements about bone morphology by utilizing the ability of autofluorescent tetracycline antibiotics to chelate to calcium at sites of active bone formation. The areas of tetracycline labeling can subsequently be studied by fluorescence microscopy (Fig. 2.15). The analysis of rates of bone formation is optimally accomplished by the procedure that employs two sequentially administered doses of tetracycline. Bone-forming surfaces will reveal, albeit focally, two discrete fluorescent lines. The distance between the two labels can be calculated to yield the rate of bone formation. Surfaces taking up tetracycline may be considered "active" surfaces. A number of parameters can be calculated in further delineating bone dynamics (Table 2.1).

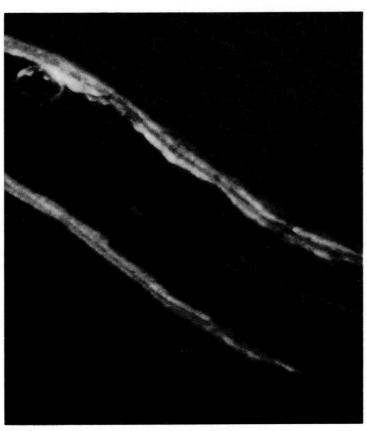

Fig. 2.15 Adult transilial bone, double tetracycline-labeled, fluorescent microscopy. By measuring the distance between two fluorescent tetracycline labels administered at known times it is possible to calculate the proportion of bone surface taking up the label, a true indicator of an active surface, as well as rates of bone formation. In this photomicrograph both surfaces of a trabeculum have been labeled.

Parameter		Definition
Fractional labeled surface	%	The extent of tetracycline-labeled surfaces as a percentage of the total trabecular bone surface
Apposition rate	μm/day	The distance between tetracycline labels divided by the number of days separating the two labeled cases
Bone formation rate	μm/day	Apposition rate × Fractional labeled surface

Table 2.1 Parameters that can be calculated from double tetracycline-labeled bone

marrow space

second label

first label

second label

HYPERPARATHYROIDISM
Osteitis fibrosa cystica, von Recklinghausen's disease of bone

The overproduction of parathyroid hormone may be either a primary or a secondary condition. In primary hyperparathyroidism, an adenoma, carcinoma, or parathyroid hyperplasia of obscure etiology leads to marked hypercalcemia, and usually to hypophosphatemia (Figs. 2.16 to 2.19). Patients are usually between the third and fifth decades of life, and they may present with a history of recurrent kidney stones, peptic ulcers, or nonspecific complaints such as nausea, vomiting, weakness, or headaches; however, the symptoms are subtle and may go unnoticed for years. On rare occasions the patient presents with a hypercalcemic crisis. Although kidney disease is the most common clinical presentation of primary hyperparathyroidism, bone disease is present in approximately one quarter of the patients. The surgical removal of the neoplastic gland is the treatment of choice.

In chronic renal failure, phosphate retention leads to hypocalcemia, which initiates compensatory or "secon-

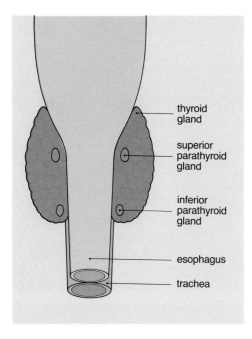

Fig. 2.16 Posterior aspect of laryngeal junction with pharynx, and commencement of the esophagus and trachea. Note the position of the parathyroid glands, normally measuring no more than 4 to 5 mm.

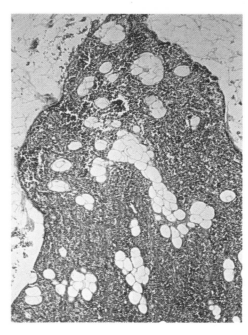

Fig. 2.17 Photomicrograph of parathyroid gland shows glandular tissue admixed with fat.

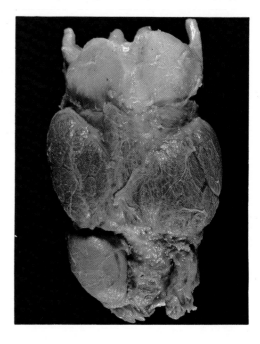

Fig. 2.18 Parathyroid adenoma: large tan nodule measuring approximately 2 cm on the left side of the lower pole.

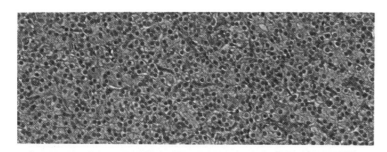

Fig. 2.19 Photomicrograph of parathyroid adenoma shown in Fig. 2.18. The cells are of one type, chief cells, partially arranged in small acini and cords. Characteristically no fat is visible in the adenomatous tissue (hematoxylin and eosin stain).

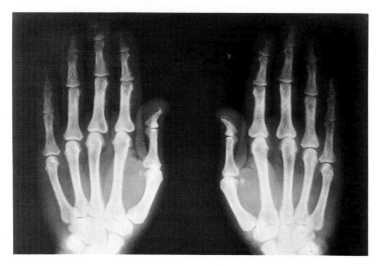

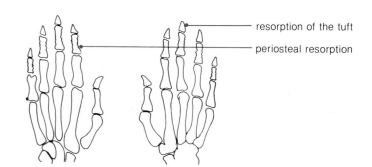

Fig. 2.20 Clinical roentgenogram of the hands shows resorption of the tufts of the terminal phalanges and characteristic subperiosteal resorption of the middle and proximal phalanges. This resorption is more marked on the radial side of the phalanges.

dary" hyperparathyroidism. Medical treatment to reduce excessive levels of serum phosphate should be attempted first, since a subtotal parathyroidectomy may lead to significant postoperative hypoparathyroidism.

Whether hyperparathyroidism occurs as a primary or secondary condition, the radiologic and pathologic features are similar. On radiologic examination one may note diffuse osteopenia and/or circumscribed lucent areas. However, the most characteristic changes are seen in roentgenograms of the hand, and these changes in-

clude the erosion of the tufts of the phalanges and subperiosteal cortical resorption, especially on the radial side of the middle phalanges (Fig. 2.20). Other sites of erosive resorption are the symphysis pubis (Fig. 2.21), the distal clavicles (Fig. 2.22), and the end plates of the vertebral bodies (Fig. 2.23), as well as the loss of the lamina dura (that is, the layer of the dense bone at the root of the teeth). The skull may show a granular demineralization, the so-called "salt and pepper" appearance (Fig. 2.24).

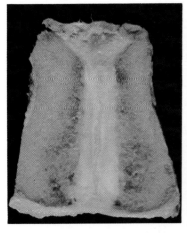 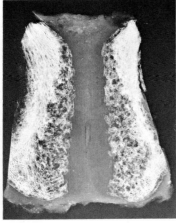

Fig. 2.21 (*left*), Gross appearance of the symphysis pubis shows hyperemia and resorption of the bone on each side of the symphysis. Roentgenogram of the specimen (*right*).

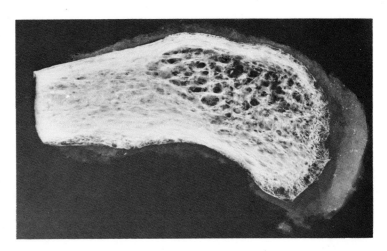

Fig. 2.22 A characteristic anatomic site in which to note erosion in hyperparathyroidism is the distal clavicle. In this specimen roentgenogram resorption is clearly seen, with loss of the smooth cortex and replacement by a lacy irregular outline.

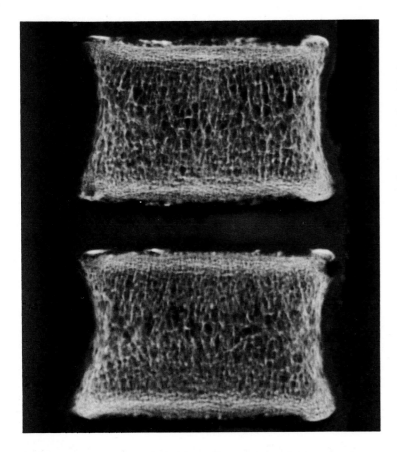

Fig. 2.23 Specimen roentgenogram of a slice taken through the vertebral bodies in a young person with hyperparathyroidism shows the irregularity and resorption of the cortical bone, particularly in the end plates of the vertebral bodies.

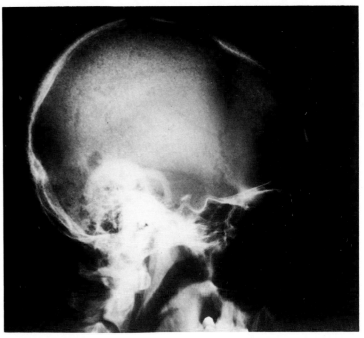

Fig. 2.24 Hyperparathyroidism: clinical roentgenogram of a skull showing salt and pepper appearance.

On histologic examination, one sees an increased number of osteoclasts on the bone surfaces (even on periosteal surfaces), and characteristically there is a "tunneling" or "dissecting" resorption of trabeculae (Fig. 2.25). Other findings include the resorption of pericellular bone by osteocytes (osteocytic osteolysis), increased woven bone, and marrow fibrosis, especially abutting trabecular surfaces (Fig. 2.26). This last finding should be distinguished from the more generalized fibrosis seen in association with myelofibrosis.

Occasionally patients with hyperparathyroidism will present on radiologic examination with a lytic lesion that suggests a tumor (Fig. 2.27). The lesion is seen especially in the diaphysis of long bones, the jaw, or the skull. This entity is the so-called "brown tumor" (brown because of old and recent hemorrhage), and on microscopic examination it shows numerous giant cells in a fibrous cellular stroma (Fig. 2.28). With the achievement of control of the hyperparathyroidism, whether surgically or medically, there is a dramatic regression of the radiologic and histologic changes.

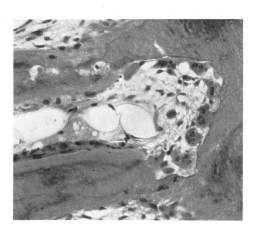

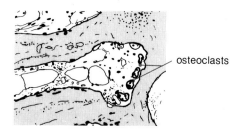

osteoclasts

Fig. 2.25 Photomicrograph shows tunneling resorption of trabecular bone. Note that the apex of the tunnel is lined by numerous osteoclasts, and that behind the osteoclasts is some fibrosis. (Medium power hematoxylin and eosin stain, undecalcified section.)

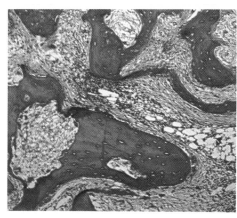

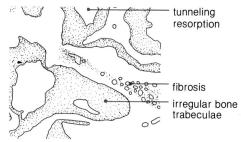

tunneling resorption

fibrosis

irregular bone trabeculae

Fig. 2.26 Photomicrograph shows marrow fibrosis, tunneling resorption, and irregular new bone formation in a patient with secondary hyperparathyroidism. (Low power hematoxylin and eosin stain, decalcified section.)

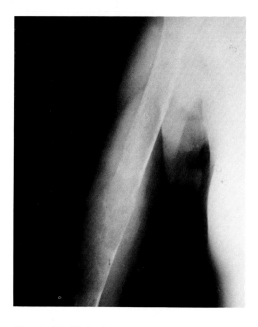

Fig. 2.27 Clinical roentgenogram shows large destructive lesion in lower end of the humerus. This patient presented initially with pain in the arm, and the radiologic examination suggested the presence of primary or secondary neoplasm. Further investigation revealed hypercalcemia and other radiologic changes consistent with hyperparathyroidism.

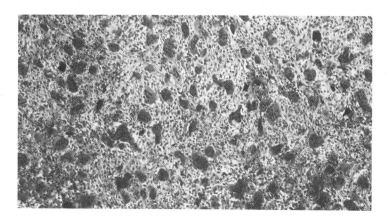

Fig. 2.28 Photomicrograph of tissue curetted from the lesion shown in Fig. 2.27. Many giant cells are scattered throughout a cellular fibrous stroma. Note that giant cells are more dense around interstitial extravasation of red blood cells, a characteristic finding of brown tumor of hyperparathyroidism. In such cases the histologic appearance alone suggests the diagnosis of giant cell tumor.

Table 2.2 Causes of Osteomalacia
Vitamin D disturbances
Inadequate endogenous production
Deficient exposure to sunlight
Dietary deficiency of vitamin D
Inadequate intestinal absorption of vitamin D
Malabsorption syndrome
Postgastrectomy
Celiac disease
Inflammatory bowel disease
Aberrant metabolism of vitamin D
Liver
Cirrhosis
Dilantin therapy
Renal disease
Kidney disease
Chronic renal failure
Renal tubular disorders
Acidosis
Hypophosphatemia
Familial errors in metabolism
Familial hypophosphatemia
Hypophosphatasia

OSTEOMALACIA

Osteomalacia results from metabolic disturbances that lead to an increase in nonmineralized bone. Osteomalacia may have a number of etiologies (Table 2.2). The availability of vitamin D, upon which calcium absorption is dependent, may be disturbed by poor nutritional intake, lack of sunlight, intestinal malabsorption, and renal or hepatic disease. (Both the kidney and the liver are sites of vitamin D metabolism.) In addition, renal disease leading to deficient reabsorption of phosphate and calcium into the blood may cause osteomalacia. (In children this disease is known as renal rickets.)

The most common symptom of osteomalacia in adults is bone pain, which may be vague initially but gradually becomes severe, and sometimes localized. There may also be muscle weakness, often profound. On radiologic examination one usually finds generalized osteopenia, and classically there are multiple bilateral and symmetrical cortical lucent areas (Fig. 2.29). These lucent areas, which are typically perpendicular to the long axis of the bone, are often referred to as Looser's zones, and on microscopic examination these Looser's zones are shown to be cortical fractures filled in with poorly mineralized callus and fibrous tissue. In general the axial skeleton (the vertebrae, pelvis, ribs and sternum) is more affected than the peripheral skeleton.

Upon histologic examination one notes a marked increase in the amount of nonmineralized matrix (osteoid) on the surfaces of the bone trabeculae and lining the haversian canals of the cortical bone (Fig. 2.30). In order to determine the extent of osteomalacia, one must use quantitative histomorphometry. Patients with osteomalacia typically have most, if not all, of their trabecular and cortical bone surfaces covered by osteoid, and on quantification at least 10 per cent of their bone mass consists of nonmineralized bone matrix (Fig. 2.31). Specific therapy depends upon the etiology of the condition.

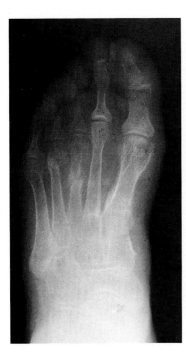
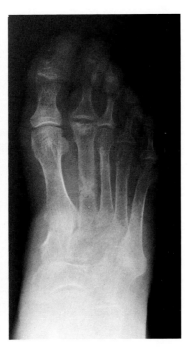

Fig. 2.29 Roentgenogram of the feet of a patient with osteomalacia shows bilateral fractures of the metatarsals.

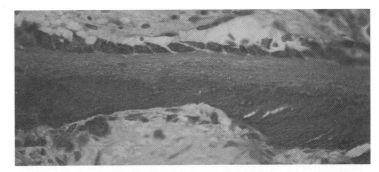
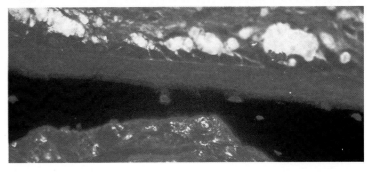

Fig. 2.30 Photomicrographs of a bone trabecula lined by osteoblasts on the upper surface and resorbing on the lower surface. A thick layer of nonmineralized bone matrix (osteoid) is present. The upper section has been stained with hematoxylin and eosin, the lower section with von Kossa's stain.

Fig. 2.31 Low power photomicrograph of a specimen from a patient with osteomalacia demonstrates that all the bone surfaces are covered by a thick layer of osteoid, which constitutes more than 10% of the total bone volume.

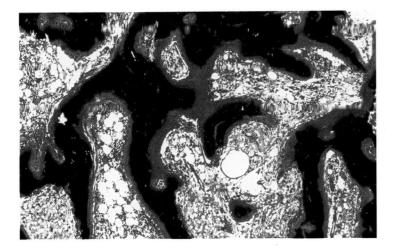

RICKETS

Rickets is the childhood manifestation of a defect in mineralization. The disease is characterized by widespread skeletal deformities, particularly typical epiphyseal changes. Classic rickets was that resulting from a deficiency of vitamin D, but it is no longer commonly seen in Western society. The most common cause of rickets in the United States is renal tubular dysfunction.

Rickets may be observed in a patient as early as 6 months of age, at which time thinning and softening of the calvarium and bulging fontanelles may be evident. These cranial changes usually diminish by two years of age, but they are followed by other dramatic skeletal changes, including beading of the costochondral junctions of the ribs (the so-called rachitic rosary) (Figs. 2.32 and 2.33), a depression along the line of the rib diaphragm attachment (Harrison's groove), and a chicken-breasted appearance. Both the wrists and ankles may be enlarged, owing to the widening of the epiphysis consequent upon failure of the primary spongiosa to mineralize (Fig. 2.34).

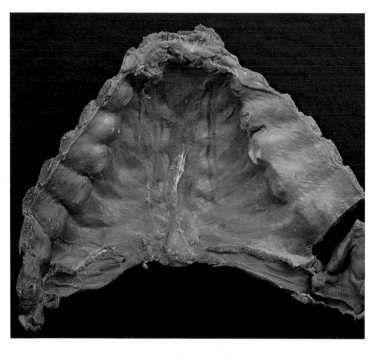

Fig. 2.32 Rickets: dissected specimen of the rib cage shows marked prominence of the costochondral junctions, which gives rise to the so-called rachitic rosary.

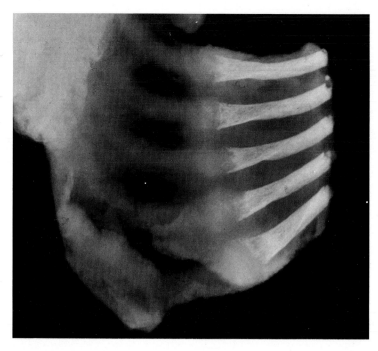

Fig. 2.33 Roentgenogram of a portion of this specimen demonstrates the irregularity and poor mineralization of the metaphysis of the rib.

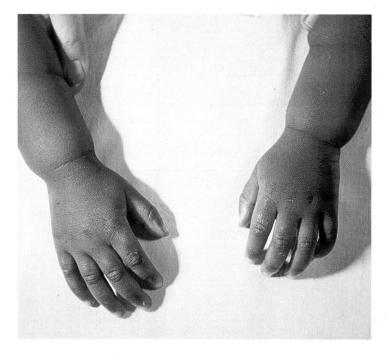

Fig. 2.34 Rickets: hand and forearm of a young child show prominence above the wrist, consequent upon the flaring and poor mineralization of the lower end of the radius and ulna.

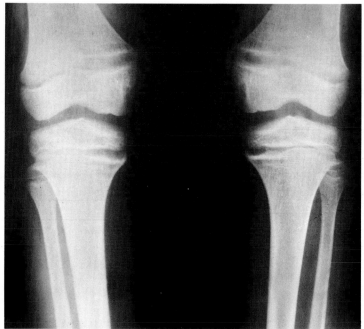

Fig. 2.35 Roentgenogram of the legs of a young patient with vitamin D resistant rickets. Note the widening of the growth plates of the lower tibia. This patient has probably received some treatment.

Eventually curvature, especially anterior curvature, of the long bones develops. Spinal abnormalities including dorsal kyphosis, scoliosis, and lumbar lordosis may serve to diminish height.

On radiologic examination, one sees a markedly widened and irregular epiphyseal growth plate zone, often with a cup-shaped concavity and flaring of the metaphyseal end of the bone (Fig. 2.35). These changes are correlated in histologic studies by the presence of irregular, disorderly columns of proliferating cartilage in the growth plate and tongues of proliferating irregular cartilage extending into the adjacent bone (Figs. 2.36 and 2.37). These changes are associated with an absence of the calcified zone of the cartilage and a poorly formed primary spongiosa (Fig. 2.38).

The most striking histologic change is in the presence of large amounts of nonmineralized bone throughout the skeleton. The presence of pseudofractures similar to those seen in osteomalacia may also be noted.

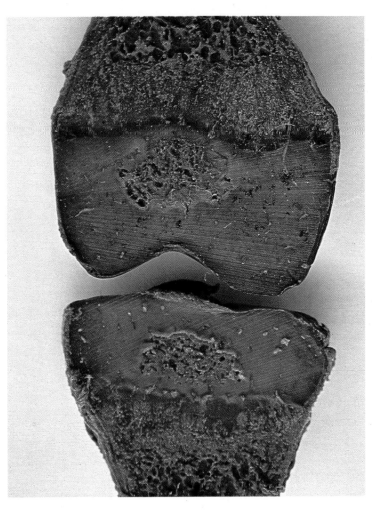

Fig. 2.36 Rickets: section through the lower end of the femur and the upper end of the tibia in a young child shows widening of the epiphyseal growth plate region, together with irregularity of the metaphysis and tongues of cartilage, which are seen penetrating into the metaphyseal bone.

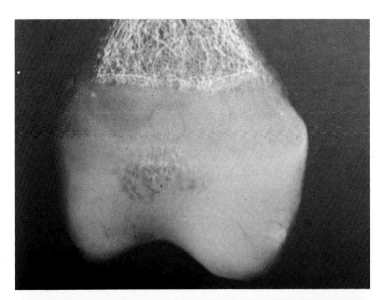

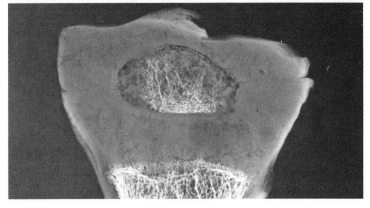

Fig. 2.37 Roentgenograms of the specimen shown in Fig. 2.36 demonstrate the widening of the epiphyseal region and the irregularity of the metaphyseal bone.

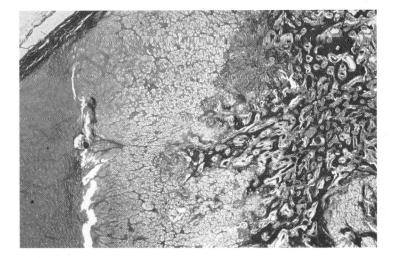

Fig. 2.38 Photomicrograph of the costochondral junction in a patient with rickets shows widening of the growth cartilage region with irregularity at the cartilage-bone interface and poorly mineralized, disorganized primary spongiosa.

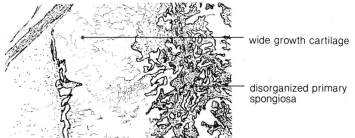

wide growth cartilage

disorganized primary spongiosa

HYPOPHOSPHATEMIA

Phosphate serves the body significantly as a buffer, and it also plays a major role in calcium homeostasis. Since 85 per cent of total body phosphorus is located in the skeleton, a decrease in the number of phosphate ions in the serum (hypophosphatemia) may be expected to affect the skeleton.

Hypophosphatemia may result from any number of causes, both congenital and acquired. These causes include increased urinary phosphate loss (as seen in hyperparathyroidism), renal tubular defects, or the administration of diuretic therapies. The condition may also be traced to decreased intestinal absorption, as seen in vitamin D deficiency malabsorption syndromes, or it may be iatrogenically induced by the use of phosphate-binding antacids. The disorder also occurs after a shift of phosphorus from the serum into the cells, as seen after insulin administration, in states of respiratory alkalosis, and in salicylate poisoning.

Acquired hypophosphatemia is sometimes seen in association with some bone tumors. The most outstanding feature of the disease is impaired renal tubular phosphate reabsorption, the mechanism of which is unclear. Laboratory studies in patients with acquired hypophosphatemia reveal normal glomerular filtration rates, normal to low levels of serum calcium, a markedly lowered level of serum phosphorus, and elevated levels of alkaline phosphatase.

FAMILIAL HYPOPHOSPHATEMIA
Vitamin D resistant rickets, refractory rickets

Familial hypophosphatemia is a genetically determined x-linked disorder that is usually manifested by the second year of life. It is characterized by deficient renal phosphate transport, and probably also by intestinal phosphate transport disturbances. Typically, the patient's urinary excretion of phosphorus is increased.

Roentgenographic and pathologic findings are similar to those seen in patients with rickets caused by vitamin D deficiency.

Most states of hypophosphatemia can be corrected medically, and do not lead to severe skeletal aberrations. However, chronic states of hypophosphatemia may lead to severe sequelae, especially in growing children.

FANCONI'S SYNDROME
Renal glycosuric rickets

Fanconi's syndrome is a recessively transmitted genetic disorder characterized by marked aminoaciduria. The disorder may be accompanied by an associated metabolic defect in cystine metabolism, the so-called Lignac-Fanconi disease. Patients with these conditions exhibit normal glomerular function, a decrease in the level of serum carbon dioxide, normal to low levels of serum calcium, low levels of serum phosphorus, and elevated levels of alkaline phosphatase.

On roentgen examination, one may note the presence

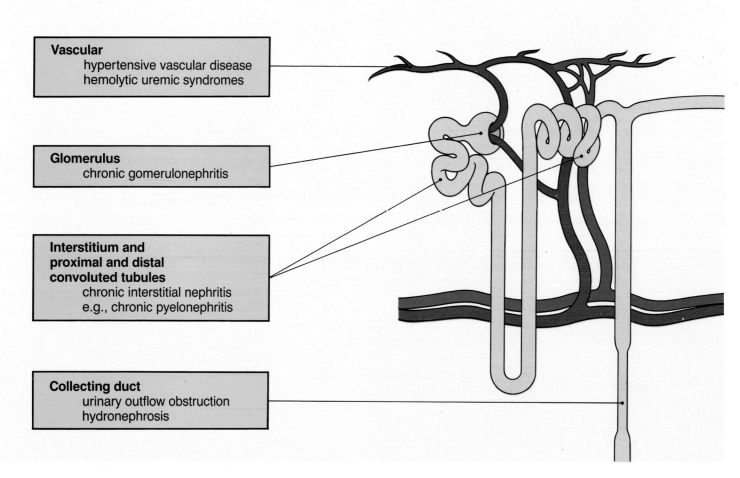

Fig. 2.39 Causes of chronic renal failure.

of diffuse osteopenia, stress fractures, and rickets-like changes in the epiphysis.

Irregular and widened epiphyseal cartilage zones are clearly seen in pathologic studies in children, but the dramatic increase in nonmineralized bone seen in patients with rickets is not apparent.

The condition is considered to result principally from a failure in collagen synthesis, stemming from the amino-acid deficiency.

It should be noted that in those patients with Fanconi's syndrome associated with cystinosis, cystine deposits are present in the bone and in the visceral organs.

RENAL OSTEODYSTROPHY

Because of the important role of glomerular filtration and renal tubular reabsorption in both processing serum calcium and phosphorus and maintaining acid-base equilibrium, and the important mechanism of in-

termediary vitamin D metabolism in the kidney, chronic renal disease (glomerular, tubular, or interstitial) may give rise to marked skeletal abnormalities (Fig. 2.39). These aberrations result from hyperparathyroid effects and osteomalacia.

In practice, the skeletal manifestations of chronic renal disease (renal osteodystrophy) are complex in etiology and morphologic presentation.

OSTEOSCLEROSIS

In many patients with chronic renal failure, one may note increased density of the skeleton on radiographic examination. This increased density is manifested on histologic studies as increased woven or immature bone superimposed on the general picture of hyperparathyroidism (Figs. 2.40 to 2.42). Both the radiologic and histologic changes may be confused with those of Paget's disease.

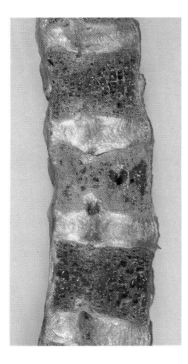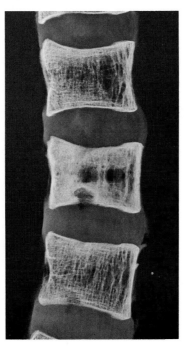

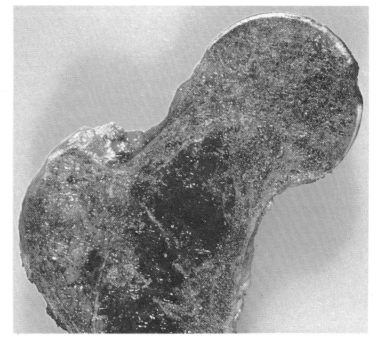

Fig. 2.40 (*left*), A segment of the lower thoracic and upper lumbar spine from a patient with renal osteodystrophy shows loss of the normal trabecular appearance of the bone with increased sclerosis and some collapse. Roentgenogram of the specimen (*right*).

Fig. 2.41 Upper end of the femur from the patient shown in Fig. 2.40. Again the disorganization of the bony architecture is apparent, and the cortex is seen to be hyperemic and irregular. These gross changes, both those seen in the vertebral bodies and in the femur, may suggest Paget's disease.

Fig. 2.42 Photomicrograph of a portion of the bone shown in Fig. 2.41 demonstrates increased osteoclastic resorption, marked increase in osteoblastic deposition of the bone, and increased osteoid seams on the surface of the bone (hematoxylin and eosin stain, undecalcified section).

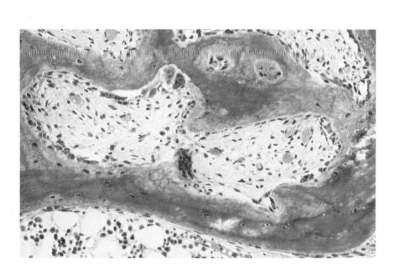

Soft Tissue Calcification

(See Chapter 14 for a discussion of soft tissue ossification.)
Calcification in Injured Tissue. Dead tissue that does not undergo rapid absorption frequently becomes calcified. This type of calcification, which is *not related to any disturbance in general calcium homeostasis*, is called dystrophic calcification. Calcification is common in areas of coagulation necrosis, as occurs in infarction. It is also common in caseous necrosis, which is seen in patients with tuberculosis. Of particular interest to orthopaedic surgeons is the calcification that is common in tendons, ligaments, and bursae (Figs. 2.43 and 2.44).

A common clinical setting for dystrophic calcification is a painful shoulder corresponding anatomically to the insertion of the supraspinatus muscle into the humerus. On gross examination one observes amorphous chalky white deposits or circumscribed gritty calcifications. These crystalline deposits have been shown by x-ray diffraction studies to be hydroxyapatite crystals. Histologic studies reveal that the calcium may be isolated in fibrous or fatty tissue, or it may be present with chronic inflammatory cells, including, at times, multinucleated giant cells.

Metastatic Calcification. Metastatic calcification is caused by an increased calcium phosphate product in the blood, and therefore the condition results from both hypercalcemia and hyperphosphatemia. The mineral deposition is particularly likely to occur in the kidneys

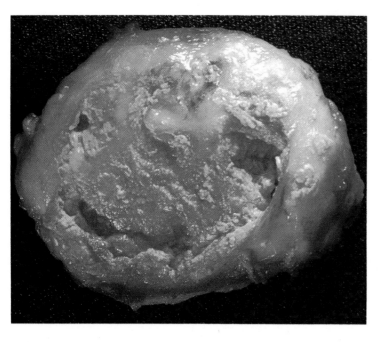

Fig. 2.43 The cut surface of a grossly thickened achromial bursa with extensive calcium deposits.

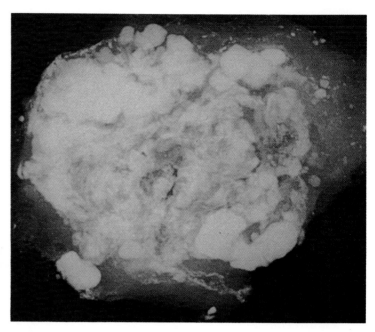

Fig. 2.44 Roentgenogram of the specimen shown in Fig. 2.43 clearly reveals the extent of calicification.

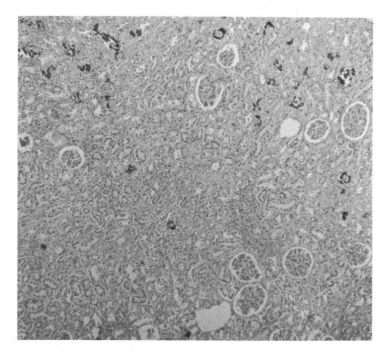

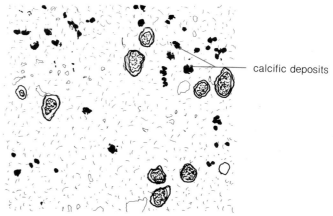

Fig. 2.45 Photomicrograph of the kidney in a patient with prolonged hypercalcemia resulting from a parathyroid adenoma. Extensive calcium deposits are seen in relation to the glomeruli and the proximal tubules.

calcific deposits

(Fig. 2.45), alveolar walls of the lungs, the media and intima of the blood vessels, the cornea, conjunctiva, and gastric mucosa. The calcification is both intracellular and extracellular, and it is seen in association with hyperparathyroidism, sarcoidosis, metastatic carcinoma, and myeloma. Metastatic calcification is a particular problem in patients with hypermetabolic states who have had prolonged bed rest.

TUMORAL CALCINOSIS

Tumoral calcinosis is a rare condition that primarily affects black people in otherwise good health. The disease usually presents in the second decade of life, and it is characterized by the deposition of painless calcific masses around the hips, elbows, shoulders, and gluteal areas (Figs. 2.46 to 2.49). A familial incidence has been reported.

The lesions may be massive, are often bilateral, and they affect multiple sites. The patient's serum phosphate level may be elevated. Surgical excision is the most successful form of treatment, although recurrences are not uncommon.

A microscopic examination of the tissue from these patients reveals calcific deposits with focal mild mononuclear and, occasionally, multinucleated giant cell reaction. With the use of x-ray diffraction studies, one can identify the presence of hydroxyapatite.

Attempts to treat this disorder with low calcium and phosphate diets and phosphate-combining antacids have had some success.

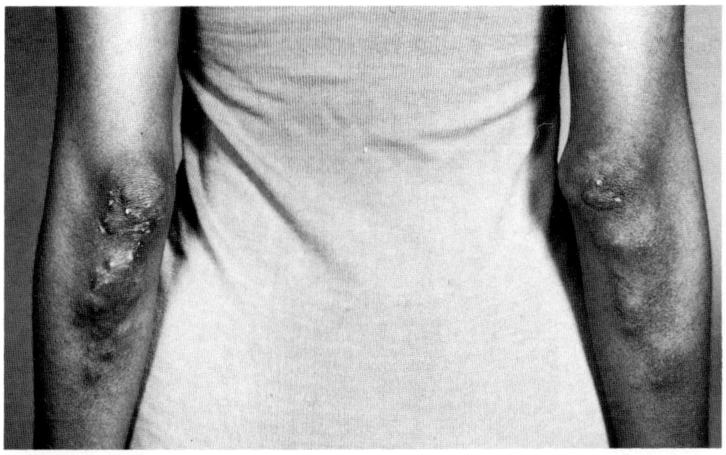

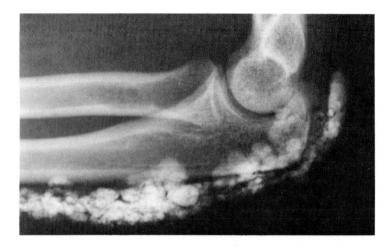

Fig. 2.47 Roentgenogram of this patient's arm shows the extent of the calcified masses.

Fig. 2.46 Photograph of a young black woman with extensive subcutaneous calcium deposits (tumoral calcinosis) around the elbows and along the extensor surfaces of the forearm.

Fig. 2.48 Cut surface of the excised specimen from the patient shown in Figs. 2.46 and 2.47.

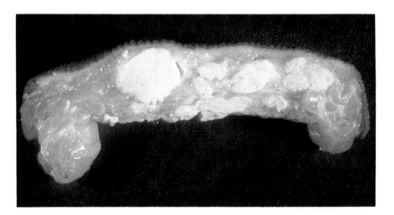

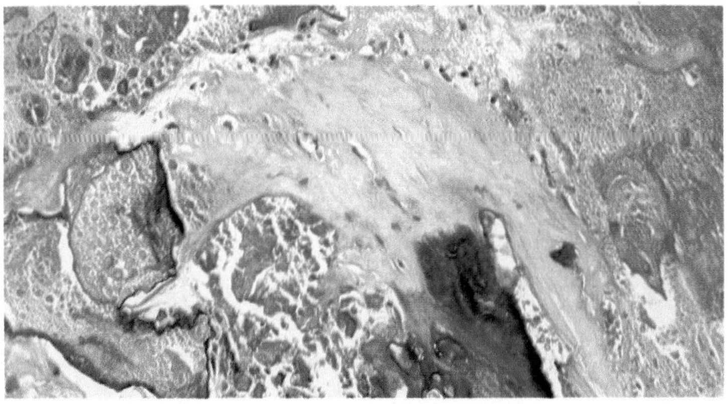

Fig. 2.49 Microscopic appearance of the calcified tissue shown in Fig. 2.48. Note that, although most of the tissue is necrotic and calcified, there is some viable fibrous connective tissue in the center of the field.

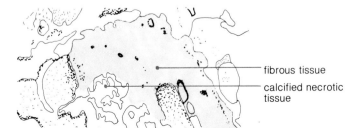

fibrous tissue

calcified necrotic tissue

2.17

OSTEOPOROSIS

Decreased density of the skeleton is a nonspecific condition that may result from any of a number of causes, including mineral and collagen disturbances, hematologic and endocrine abnormalities, neoplastic disorders, or immobilization (Table 2.3).

It is also well known that the amount of bone present in the skeleton decreases with age, more significantly in women, and in whites rather than blacks. The presence of roentgenographically evident osteopenia that has resulted in fracture (usually vertebral crush fractures, Colles fractures, or femoral neck fractures) is generally consid-

ered senile osteoporosis. Clinically significant osteoporosis may also develop early in some post-menopausal women.

In those patients with osteoporosis there are characteristic roentgenographic features, such as the thinning of cortical bone and the generalized rarefaction of the skeleton. In the vertebral column one sees thinning and eventual disappearance of the transverse trabeculae, with subsequent thickening of the vertical trabeculae, and later the thinning of these trabeculae as well (Fig. 2.50). Compression fractures occur, giving rise to the

Table 2.3 Causes of Osteopenia
Malnutrition
Mineral disturbances 　Osteomalacia
Collagen disturbances 　Scurvy 　Osteogenesis imperfecta 　Homocystinemia
Endocrine 　Acromegaly 　Hyperthyroidism 　Hyperparathyroidism 　Hypogonadism 　Cushing's syndrome 　Steroid therapy
Local tissue effect 　Heparin 　Mastocytosis 　Prostaglandin 　Vascular
Mechanical 　Disuse 　Immobilization
Proliferative disorders 　Hematologic 　Neoplastic
Idiopathic

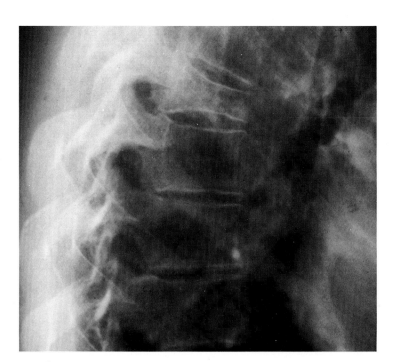

Fig. 2.50 Lateral roentgenogram of the thoracic spine from a 30-year-old man with idiopathic osteoporosis. The marked osteopenia is accompanied by some exaggeration of the vertical striations in the bone, and by a crush fracture of one vertebral body.

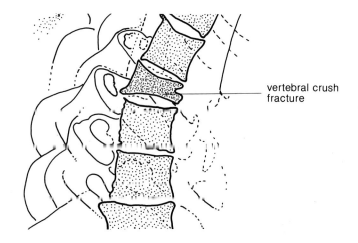

vertebral crush fracture

2.18

widening of the intervertebral disc, the so-called "cod-fish" appearance. In general the low thoracic and upper lumbar vertebrae are most affected.

Since vertebral bone loss has been calculated to approximate 30 per cent before roentgenographic detection, radiologists have long sought special techniques by which to evaluate bone mass, density, and calcium content. Methods that employ monoenergetic radiation, such as single and dual photon absorptiometry, have met with considerable success, particularly in generating useful data in serial exams on individual patients. Other techniques involving radionuclide uptake, neutron activation, and computed axial tomography are still in the experimental stage. It is important to realize that, at the present time, only a bone biopsy can adequately evaluate the degrees of nonmineralized bone and the cellular activities of osteoclasts and osteoblasts—factors that are critical in the appreciation of the morphologic heterogeneity of osteoporosis.

In morphologic terms, osteoporosis is defined as decreased bone mass, the bone itself having a normal biochemical makeup (Figs. 2.51 and 2.52). Morphometric

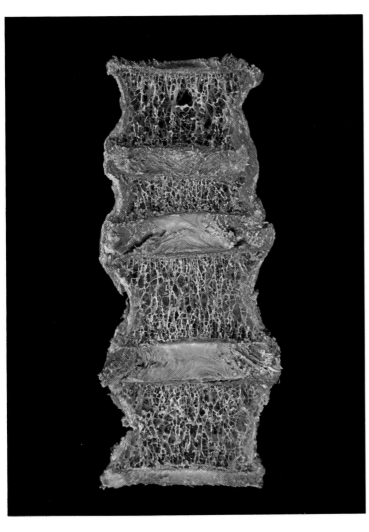

Fig. 2.51 Frontal section of a portion of the lumbar, lower thoracic, and upper lumbar vertebrae, taken at autopsy in a patient with osteoporosis. The bone marrow has been carefully washed out of the interstices of the bone to better demonstrate the trabecular pattern. Note the marked loss of bone tissue and the compression fracture.

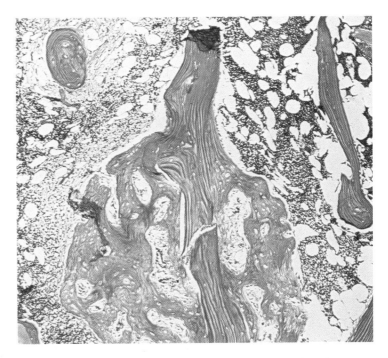

Fig. 2.52 Photomicrograph taken from a vertebral body in a patient with osteoporosis shows a microfracture of one of the trabeculae. Surrounding the fractured trabecula is a small microcallus. In patients with osteoporosis such microfractures are abundant in the vertebral bodies.

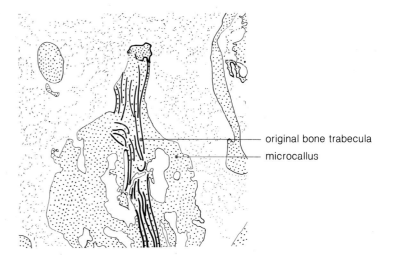

original bone trabecula
microcallus

analyses of the cellular parameters, the amount of bone present, and the degree to which osteoid is present on the surfaces of the trabecular and cortical bone have led to the characterization of some of the types of osteoporosis (Figs. 2.53 to 2.56).

Although cellular activity, i.e., relative and absolute osteoblast and osteoclast counts, is usually low in idiopathic osteoporosis, indicating a relatively "inactive" state, it may sometimes be high. In more than 15 per cent of the patients this increased activity is associated with normocalcemic, normophosphatemic hyperparathyroidism. An additional subgroup of patients is noted to have increased osteoid surfaces. In disuse osteoporosis the most dramatic finding initially is an increase in the number of resorptive surfaces. In steroid-induced osteoporosis, osteoclastic activity is high, with relatively normal bone formation.

The treatment of osteoporosis should, insofar as it is possible, be directed toward the underlying etiology. In patients with idiopathic osteoporosis, a number of therapeutic agents have been used with varying degrees of success. Exercise is crucial in maintaining skeletal integrity. Calcium supplementation corrects the relative calcium deficiency in the post-menopausal state. In conjunction with sodium fluoride, an effective bone stimulant, new bone formation has been documented.

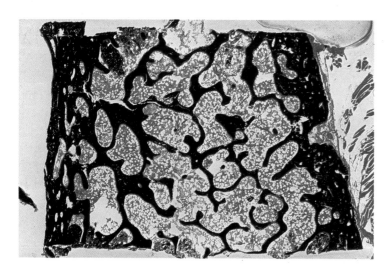

Fig. 2.53 Transilial biopsy of normal bone demonstrates a cortical bone volume of 20.3% and a trabecular bone volume of 37.2%.

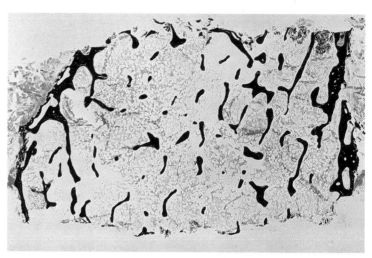

Fig. 2.54 Transilial biopsy of a patient with moderate to severe osteoporosis. Morphometric analysis shows a cortical bone volume of 7% and a trabecular bone volume of 13%.

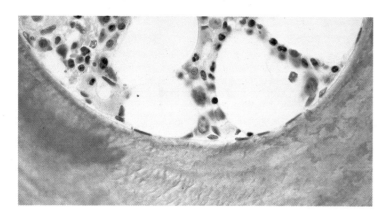

Fig. 2.55 Photomicrograph of a representative area of bone trabecula in a patient with idiopathic osteoporosis. The cells lining the trabecula are flat with little osteoid surface activity, a morphologic subtype best described as inactive.

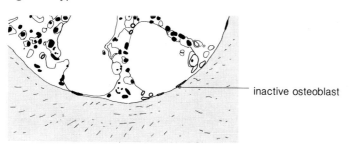

inactive osteoblast

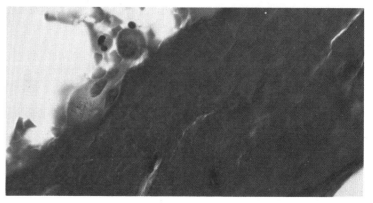

Fig. 2.56 Photomicrograph of a specimen from a patient with active osteoporosis shows increased resorptive surfaces.

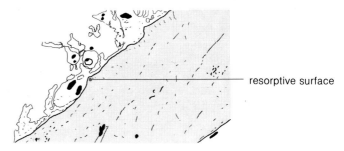

resorptive surface

Vitamin D metabolites assist calcium absorption and, in fact, their deficient production may explain many cases of osteoporosis. Although estrogen replacement therapy is theoretically sound, its link with atypical endometrial changes has limited its widespread use. Other agents in experimental protocols have been used to suppress bone resorption (e.g., calcitonin and diphosphonates) or to stimulate bone formation (e.g., anabolic steroids). Long-term corticosteroid therapy, excessive alcohol intake, and endocrinopathies such as hyperthyroidism account for a significant number of cases of osteoporosis and should be corrected medically.

Localized (Transient) Osteoporosis. In 1900 Sudeck described a transient yet painful osteoporosis of the lower extremity that occurred without obvious cause, though possibly related to trauma (Figs. 2.57 and 2.58). Similar localized radiolucent areas have since been described elsewhere, and various names have been used to describe them, including Sudeck's atrophy, transient osteoporosis, and reflex sympathetic dystrophy. The lesions tend to be juxta-articular in location. Interestingly, areas of osteoporosis may spontaneously remit with subsequent remineralization, and yet appear later elsewhere on the skeleton; i.e., they appear to be "migratory" in nature.

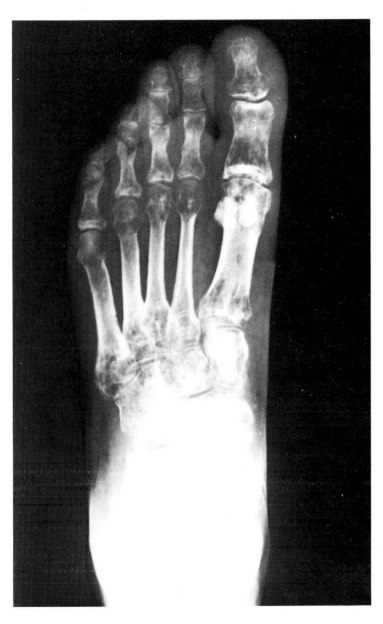

Fig. 2.57 Localized osteoporosis: roentgenogram of a foot in a patient with painful osteoporosis localized to the foot and ankle. Note the marked juxta-articular osteoporosis.

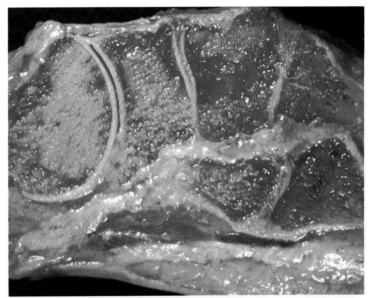

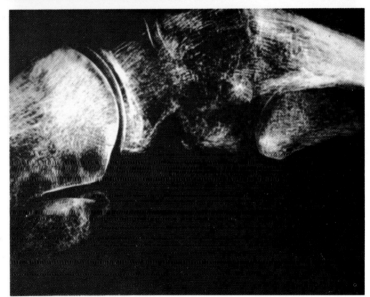

Fig. 2.58 (*upper*), Localized osteoporosis: gross specimen of a section through the foot shows marked hyperemia in patches, but particularly juxta-articularly. Roentgenogram of a slice of the specimen (*lower*).

Patients with this condition characteristically have acute localized pain that is often debilitating. Laboratory findings are unremarkable. The involved areas show an increased uptake of isotope on technetium bone scanning, and this increased uptake may predate the radiologic evidence of osteoporosis by some months. The histopathologic findings have been only infrequently reported; however, the examination of histologic sections has shown thinned bone trabeculae with evidence of osteoclastic bone resorption (Fig. 2.59).

Since the lesions usually remit spontaneously within one year, the importance of this disorder rests in recognizing its benign nature. It should not be confused with diseases such as osteomyelitis or metastatic cancer, which it may mimic roentgenographically on initial presentation.

MASSIVE OSTEOLYSIS
Phantom bone, disappearing bone, Gorham's disease
Progressive localized osteoporosis with eventual disappearance of mineralized bone occurs in patients with this rare disease. Microscopic examination of biopsy tissue has shown an overgrowth of thin-walled dilated blood vessels (Fig. 2.60). The clinical course of the disease may be protracted over a period of years, but it usually stabilizes. The disease may be confined to a single bone, or it may affect two or more bones centered around a joint. (A further discussion of this disease appears in Chapter 10.)

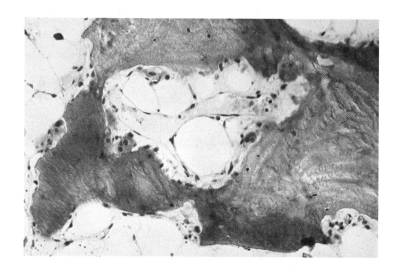

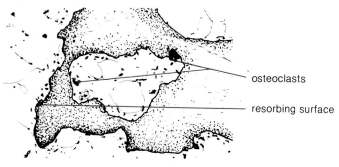

Fig. 2.59 Localized osteoporosis: histologic section shows marked focal osteoclastic resorption.

osteoclasts

resorbing surface

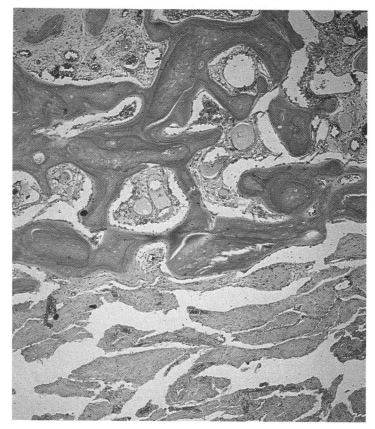

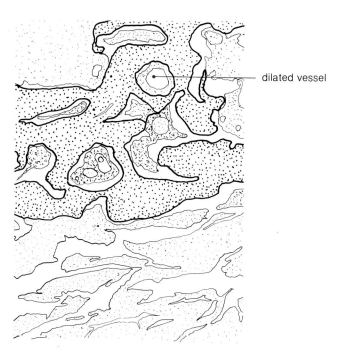

Fig. 2.60 Bone biopsy taken from a patient with disappearing bone disease, adjacent to the site of involvement. Note the presence of large dilated vessels in the marrow spaces.

dilated vessel

3 Diseases Resulting from Disturbances in the Formation and Breakdown of Bone II

OSTEOGENESIS IMPERFECTA

Clinical Evaluation. Many investigators would agree that the disease called osteogenesis imperfecta includes a number of distinct syndromes, some of which are inherited as an autosomal dominant trait, others as a recessive trait, and still others occurring as spontaneous mutations. The various syndromes have in common the features that the majority of patients are short in stature and have an increased propensity to fracture (Fig. 3.1).

The standard treatment of fractures by immobilization results in disuse osteoporosis, which in turn increases the tendency to fracture, thereby setting up a vicious cycle (Fig. 3.2). So, once having fractured a bone, these unfortunate patients have a tendency to repeated fractures in the same area.

Most patients will also have blue sclerae, poorly formed dentin, and ligamentous laxity, all of which indicate that

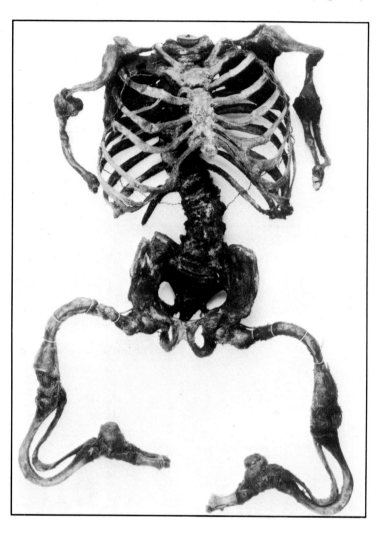

Fig. 3.1 Skeleton of an older child with osteogenesis imperfecta congenita. There are deformities in all four limbs, together with scoliosis, and chest and pelvic deformities.

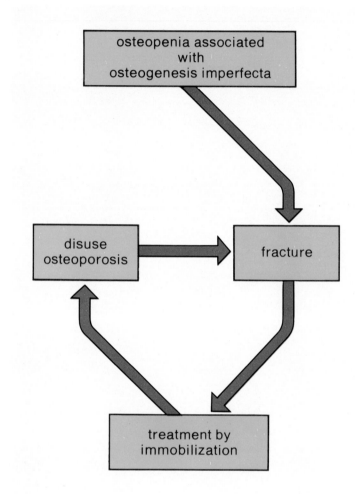

Fig. 3.2 Fracture cycle in patients with osteogenesis imperfecta. Patients with osteogenesis imperfecta have a tendency to fracture. The standard treatment of fractures by immobilization results in disuse osteoporosis, which in turn increases the tendency to fracture.

Fig. 3.3 Osteogenesis imperfecta: clinical photograph showing blue sclerae. The color results from the thinness of the sclerae.

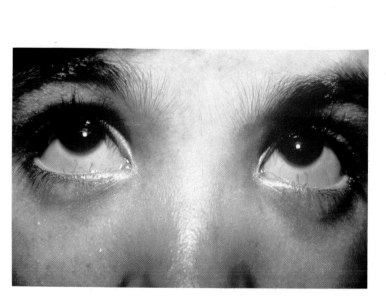

the disease is not confined to the skeleton, but is rather a generalized disorder of the connective tissues (Figs. 3.3 and 3.4). Collagen, in particular, may be considered a significant factor in osteogenesis imperfecta, as it appears to be deficient quantitatively and may also differ qualitatively from that seen in normal patients.

Two clinical forms of the disease are generally recognized. The more severe (congenita) type is manifest at birth and associated with generalized osteoporosis, multiple fractures with deformities, micromelia, and caput membranacea (Fig. 3.5).

Patients afflicted by the less severe (tarda) type, which may or may not be manifest at birth, are separated into two groups depending on functional disability (Fig. 3.6). The tarda I patients have deformities usually confined to the lower limbs that limit ambulation. The tarda II patients, though short, are without significant limb deformity, and therefore are functionally much less disabled.

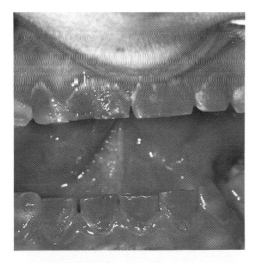 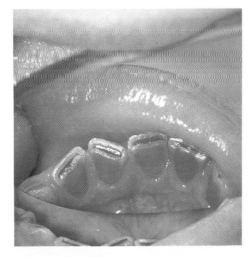

Fig. 3.4 Two examples of the appearance of teeth in patients with osteogenesis imperfecta. Brown short teeth result from failure in the formation of dentin. The enamel appears to be normal.

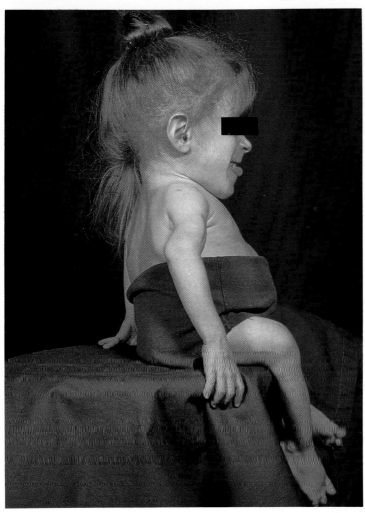 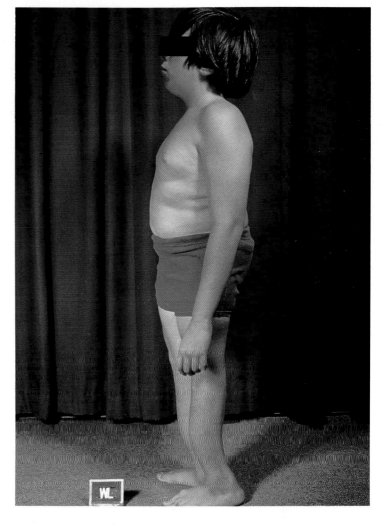

Fig. 3.5 Patient with osteogenesis imperfecta congenita shows defects of all four limbs and an increased anteroposterior diameter of the chest. Note also the spinal deformity.

Fig. 3.6 Patient with osteogenesis imperfecta tarda I shows anterior bowing of the tibia and short lower limbs. In comparison, the upper limbs appear relatively normal.

Roentgenographic Features. The characteristic roentgen findings in osteogenesis imperfecta are osteopenia and fractures and/or bone deformities (bowing) (Fig. 3.7). Long bones, apart from being smaller in size than one would expect, are often slender as well. The spine shows variable degrees of deformity, usually scoliosis, owing to compression fractures and wedging of the vertebral bodies (Fig. 3.8). In the severely affected congenita type of patients, multiple centers of ossification are observed in the skull (so-called wormian bones) (Fig. 3.9).

In the epiphyseal ends of the bones, collections of scalloped radiolucent areas with sclerotic margins are

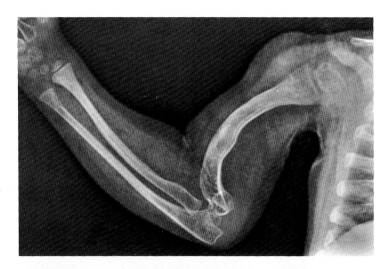

Fig. 3.7 Roentgenogram of the upper limb in a patient with osteogenesis imperfecta congenita shows severe osteoporosis, slender bones, and multiple healed fractures.

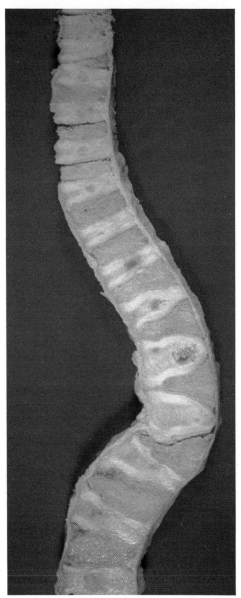 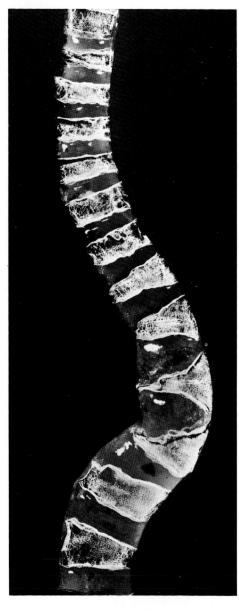

Fig. 3.8 (*left*), Dissected specimen of spine shows scoliosis subsequent to multiple compression fractures. (*right*), Specimen roentgenogram of spine. Scoliosis subsequent to multiple compression fractures resulting from osteoporosis.

present in about two-thirds of the children classified as having the congenita form, and in less than half of those classified as tarda I (Figs. 3.10 and 3.11). These lesions are not seen in association with the tarda II form of the disease. The lesions are most common in the lower limbs, and, in order of descending frequency, they are seen in the distal femur, proximal tibia, distal tibia, and proximal femur. In the upper extremity, lesions occur most frequently in the proximal and distal humerus.

Gross Pathologic Features. Upon gross examination, the bones show a loss of bone tissue with thin eggshell-like cortices and very little medullary spongy bone. Many specimens will demonstrate either recent or healed fractures, with angulation and/or bowing (Fig. 3.12).

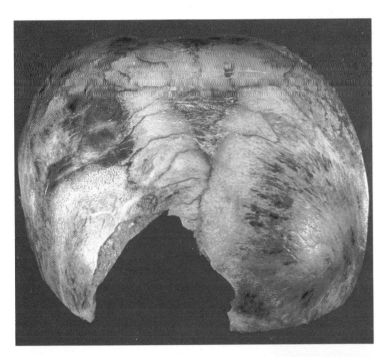

Fig. 3.9 Skull from a 9-year-old child shows posterior fontanelle and multiple wormian bones.

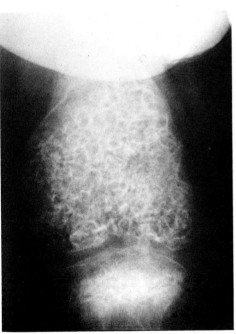

Fig. 3.10 Roentgenogram of knee joint in an 8-year-old child with osteogenesis imperfecta congenita. The epiphysis and metaphysis of the femur are filled with nodular lesions with radiolucent centers and a radiodense margin, resembling popcorn. No growth plate can be seen in the femur. In the tibia the growth plate can be visualized; however, the central portion is somewhat disrupted. The image of the buttock obscures the femoral diaphysis.

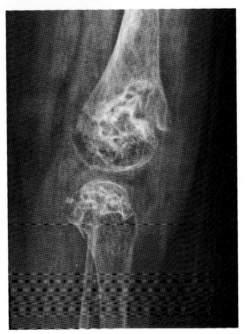

Fig. 3.11 Roentgenogram of the knee in a patient with osteogenesis imperfecta congenita. There is irregularity and disruption of both the femoral and tibial growth plates, though less severe than that shown in Fig. 3.10.

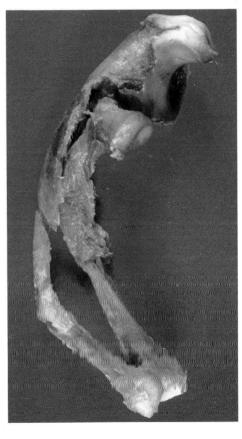

Fig. 3.12 Dissected specimen of forearm bones shows multiple fractures, including fracture dislocation of the radial head.

3.5

The Epiphysis. In general, the epiphyseal ends of the long bones, including the articular surfaces, retain a recognizable shape, although in proportion to the rest of the bone they appear larger and some show irregularity of the articular surface (Fig. 3.13). The secondary centers of ossification are often decidedly distorted, and they contain small cartilaginous nodules of 1 to 4 mm in diameter (Fig. 3.14). The growth plate is of variable appearance, ranging from normal, to having one or more indentations into the metaphysis, to total disruption of its regular outline (Figs. 3.15 to 3.17). These changes correspond to the scalloped lesions seen on radiographic examination.

The microscopic examination of the growth plate may show a disorganization of the proliferative and hypertrophic zones, a permeation of the cartilage by

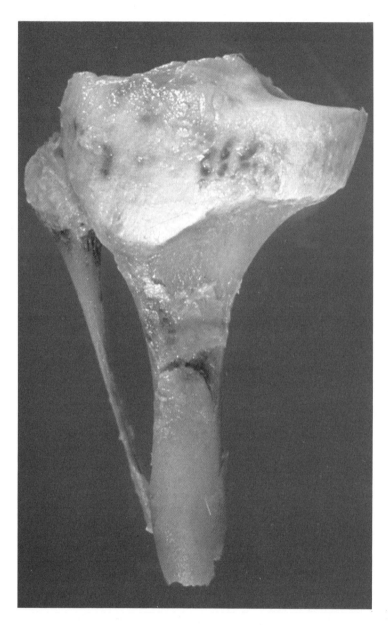

Fig. 3.13 Upper end of tibia shows relative enlargement of the cartilaginous end of the bone and marked narrowing of the shaft of the fibula.

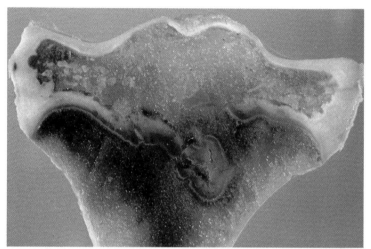

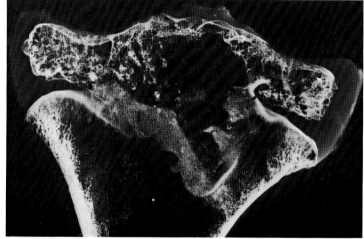

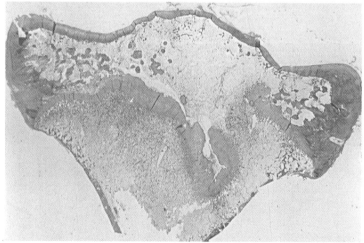

Fig. 3.14 *(upper),* Dissected specimen of the upper end of the tibia shows multiple cartilaginous nodules in the epiphysis and disruption of the growth plate. Roentgenogram of the specimen *(center).* Histologic section *(lower).*

metaphyseal blood vessels, and a decreased thickness of the calcified zone of the growth plate cartilage. The primary spongiosa on the metaphyseal side is extremely scanty, and is usually of the woven variety.

The large cartilage masses that are seen both on radiographic and gross examinations in the region of the metaphysis result from the fragmentation of the growth plate, and show, on microscopic examination, polarized maturation with columnization of the chondrocytes, and some evidence of endochondral ossification. It seems likely that these epiphyseal changes occur secondary to trauma, and that they are not developmental in origin. The resulting fragmentation of the growth plate might be expected to interfere with growth.

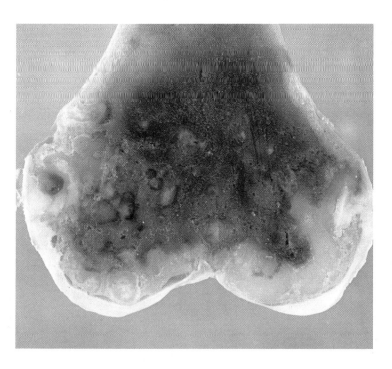

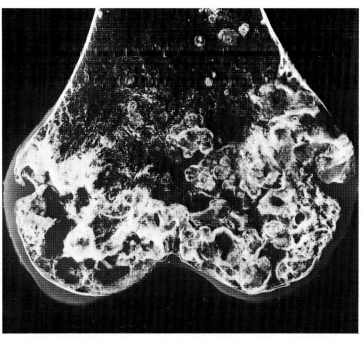

Fig. 3.15 Dissected specimen of the lower end of the femur shows complete disruption of the growth plate with multiple nodules of cartilage in the epiphysis and metaphysis.

Fig. 3.16 Roentgenogram of the specimen shown in Fig. 3.15. Note complete disruption of the growth plate and multiple nodules of cartilage in the epiphysis and metaphysis.

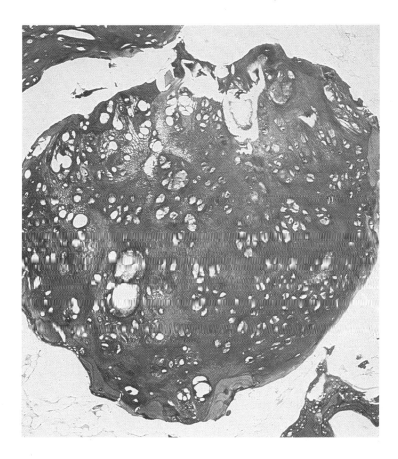

Fig. 3.17 Histologic section of one of the cartilage nodules illustrated in Figs. 3.15 and 3.16 shows hypercellularity and disorganization. A thin rim of bone is present around each of the nodules, giving rise to the rim of radiodensity seen in the roentgenogram.

Biopsy specimens of the iliac crest in patients with osteogenesis imperfecta congenita are characterized by large areas of osseous tissue that is devoid of an organized trabecular pattern. Plump osteoblasts are crowded along prominent osteoid seams, and large oval osteocytes are surrounded by small amounts of matrix, which often lacks a lamellar pattern. Even in areas in which a lamellar pattern is seen, the lamellae are thin. The osteoclasts appear to be morphologically normal, although both they and the resorption surfaces are more numerous (Figs. 3.18 and 3.19).

Bone from patients with osteogenesis imperfecta tarda is characterized by a predominantly fine lamellar pattern with only small areas of woven bone. Osteoblasts are increased in number, but they appear smaller, more spherical, and less numerous than their counterparts in the congenita group. Osteoid seams are also prominent. The osteocytes, although more mature in appearance than those in patients with osteogenesis imperfecta congenita, are more numerous, larger, and less homogeneously arranged throughout the trabeculae than the osteocytes in normal patients. Osteoclasts appear morphologically normal, but increased in number, when compared with those in individuals not affected by osteogenesis imperfecta.

The histologic appearances of the bone suggest that at least one reason for the reduced bone mass is a decreased amount of production of collagen by the osteoblasts, evident morphologically as crowded osteocytes. The disruption of the growth plate, as has been described, will also interfere with growth and contribute to these patients' short stature.

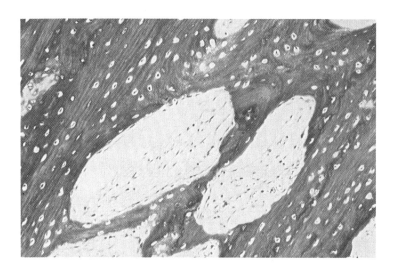

Fig. 3.18 Osteogenesis imperfecta congenita: bone biopsy showing marked hypercellularity of the bone with a fine lamellar pattern.

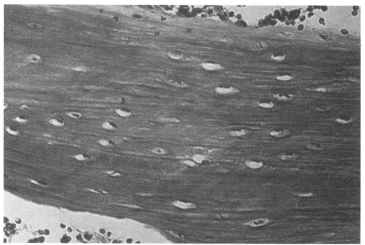

Fig. 3.19 Osteogenesis imperfecta congenita: bone biopsy shows features illustrated in Fig. 3.18 at higher power.

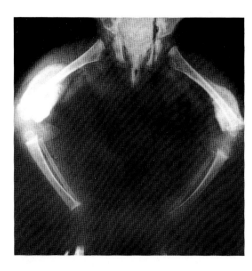

Fig. 3.20 Roentgenogram of a young child shows extensive periosteal elevation in both femurs, with epiphyseal separation of the lower femoral epiphyses.

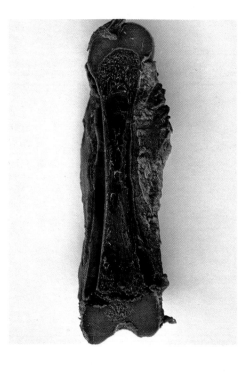

Fig. 3.21 Photograph of a specimen showing periosteal elevation and subperiosteal hemorrhage. Separation of the lower femoral epiphysis has occurred.

SCURVY

An important step in the intracellular synthesis of collagen is the hydroxylation of the amino acids proline and lysine. This process is dependent on the presence of vitamin C. In the absence of vitamin C, the conversion of proline and lysine to hydroxyproline and hydroxylysine does not take place, with a resulting failure of collagen synthesis.

Scurvy, which results from a deficient intake of vitamin C, is characterized clinically by hemorrhage into a variety of tissues, including the skin, mucous membranes, and bones. The patients may have an anemia, and problems with the gums associated with loosening of the teeth. They may also manifest poor wound healing.

The bone lesions in young children are characterized by subperiosteal hemorrhage that may be massive (Figs. 3.20 to 3.23). In addition, because the primary spongiosa fails to form adequately, there frequently occurs a fracture through the metaphysis, with a resulting separation of the epiphysis. In those times in which infantile scurvy was commonly seen, the disorder was frequently associated with rickets.

Because the periosteum is more securely attached to the bone in adults, subperiosteal hematomas were not a characteristic part of the clinical syndrome in that group. However, because of the defect in collagen synthesis, the patients frequently exhibited marked osteoporosis.

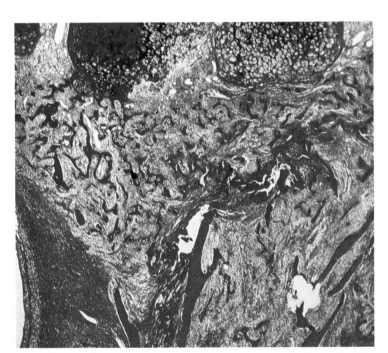

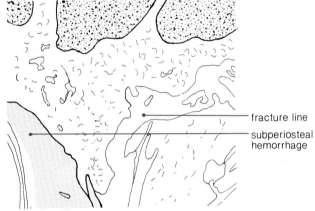

Fig. 3.22 Photomicrograph of the region of the growth plate and metaphysis in a patient with scurvy. Subperiosteal hemorrhage and a fracture through the metaphysis are apparent.

fracture line
subperiosteal hemorrhage

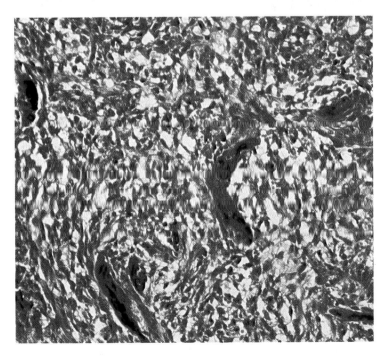

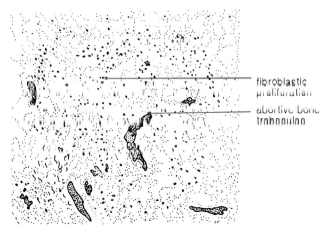

Fig. 3.23 Photomicrograph at a higher power of the same specimen shown in Fig. 3.22. There is extensive fibroblastic proliferation, with minimal bone and collagen production. The extravasation of red blood cells can be seen throughout the tissue.

fibroblastic proliferation
abortive bone trabeculae

MUCOPOLYSACCHARIDOSIS

The extracellular and extrafibrillar amorphous component of the tissue matrix is often referred to as the ground substance. It is particularly prominent in the connective tissues, and it plays an important role in the mechanical properties and form of cartilage and bone. The ground substance is not a single substance. It is rather a mixture of many components, and in different tissues it has quite different composition. In general, however, it is formed of polysaccharides combined with proteins.

There are a number of heritable diseases that are characterized by a failure in the metabolism of these mucopolysaccharides and the subsequent storage of mucopolysaccharides, and/or urinary excretion of excessive amounts of mucopolysaccharides. In the majority of these diseases, marked skeletal abnormalities occur, probably because protein polysaccharides are so important in the formation of the cartilage.

At least ten and probably more syndromes exist. Many of these syndromes are characterized by the storage of dermatan sulfate and heparin sulfate in various tissues, strikingly in the reticuloendothelial system, the heart, and the central nervous system (Fig. 3.24). Morquio's syndrome, known as mucopolysaccharidosis IV, is characterized by excessive amounts of keratin sulfate and chondroitin sulfate in the urine. This disease appears to be phenotypically, genetically, and chemically distinct, probably involving a defect in the metabolism of the proteoglycans of the cartilage (Fig. 3.25).

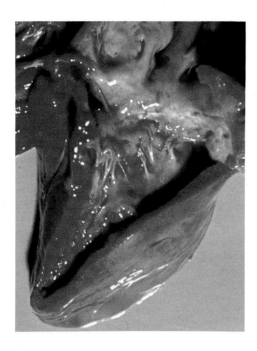

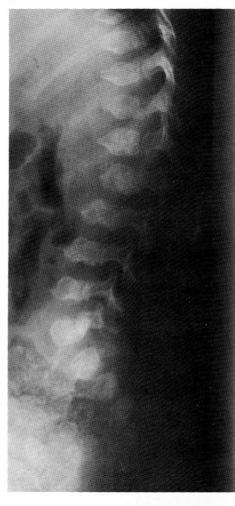

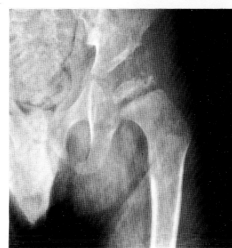

Fig. 3.24 The heart from a child with Hurler's syndrome. Note the thickening of the chordae tendineae cordis and the opacity of the endothelial lining of the heart, both resulting from the accumulation of macrophages filled with polysaccharides.

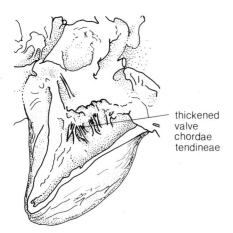

thickened valve chordae tendineae

Fig. 3.25 Roentgenograms of the spine and hip in a child with Morquio's syndrome. These children, who have short stature, show marked abnormalities at the epiphyseal ends of the long bones with deformed secondary centers of ossification, which in later life will lead to arthritic changes. In the spine there are characteristic deformities of the vertebral bodies with tongue-like extensions on the anterior surface and occasionally hemivertebrae, which give rise to spinal deformities.

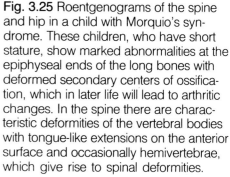

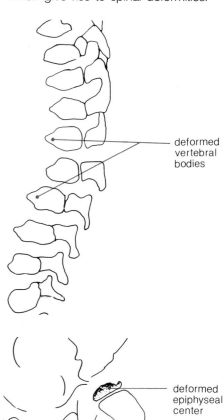

deformed vertebral bodies

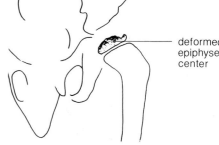

deformed epiphyseal center

HYPOPHOSPHATASIA

Hypophosphatasia is a rare, genetically transmitted error of metabolism in which there is a disturbance in the synthesis of the enzyme alkaline phosphatase. Two forms of the disease have been described; the first inherited as an autosomal recessive trait that manifests in children, who are severely affected, and the second as an autosomal dominant characteristic that becomes evident in adults, in whom the disease is less severe.

In infants the disorder is manifested as a failure to thrive, growth retardation, and a wide range of symptoms including irritability, fever, and vomiting. In general, those infants diagnosed before six months of age follow a rapidly progressive fatal course. In older children or adults the disease is less severe and generally asymptomatic. The disorder is characterized by the finding of decreased levels of alkaline phosphatase in the bone, intestines, liver, and kidney. The patient's serum phosphorus and calcium levels are usually normal; however, phosphoethanolamine, thought to be a substrate of alkaline phosphatase, is present in increased amounts in the urine and serum.

Roentgenographic manifestations of the disorder in children are poorly ossified and underdeveloped bones; the similarity to rickets is evident (Figs. 3.26 and 3.27).

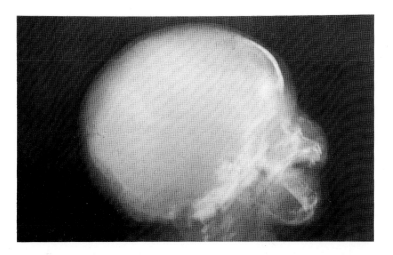

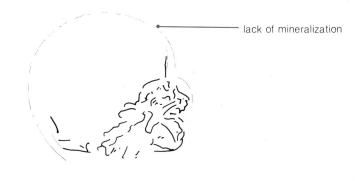

Fig. 3.26 Hypophosphatasia: roentgenogram of the skull in a newborn baby shows poor mineralization of the vault of the skull.

lack of mineralization

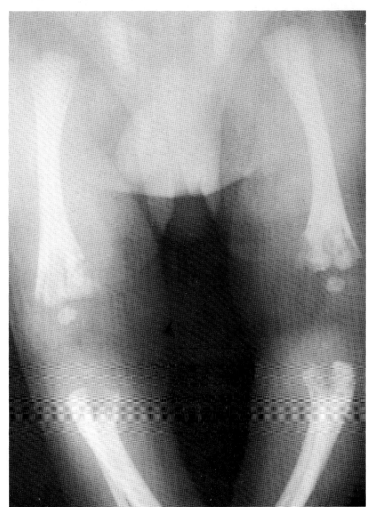

Fig. 3.27 Hypophosphatasia: the lower limbs in a newborn child show marked irregularity of the growth plate, with streaks of radiodensity into the metaphysis. This appearance is indicative of poor endochondral ossification.

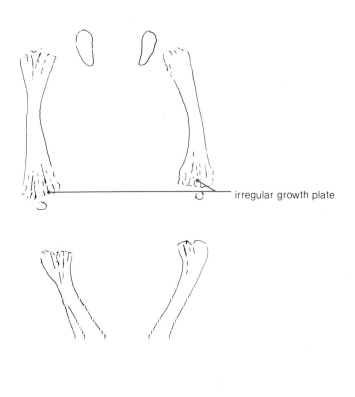

irregular growth plate

Histologic study of the affected tissue reveals increased osteoid and irregular epiphyseal cartilage with lengthened chondrocyte columns (Figs. 3.28 to 3.30).

Hypophosphatasia may not present clinically until the fourth, fifth, and sixth decades of life, although there is often a childhood history of a rickets-like disorder. Edentia, short stature, and deformity of the extremities, including bowing, are not uncommon clinical findings. Roentgenographic features include pseudofractures and osteopenia. The histopathologic examination of bone from these patients reveals an osteomalacic picture, with increased quantities of nonmineralized bone. Unlike other osteomalacic states, however, hypophosphatasia is characterized by a paucity of osteoblasts.

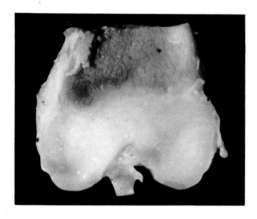

Fig. 3.28 Hypophosphatasia: section through the lower femoral epiphysis and metaphysis shows the irregularity of the growth plate.

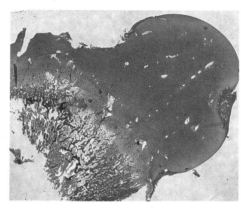

Fig. 3.29 Hypophosphatasia: low power photomicrograph of the upper femoral growth plate (*left*). The marked irregularity of the cartilage and the tongue of irregular

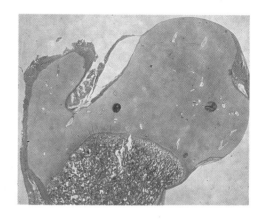

cartilage extending to the metaphyseal region are evident. For contrast, a normal upper femoral epiphysis in a patient of the same age is shown (*right*).

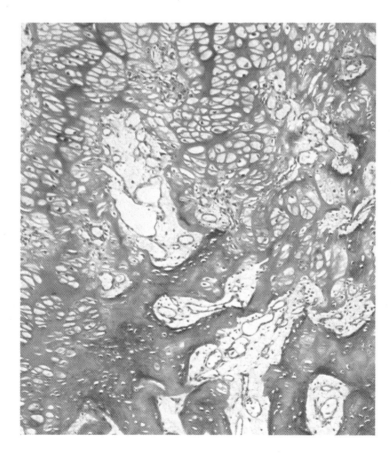

Fig. 3.30 Hypophosphatasia: photomicrograph of the metaphysis of the upper end of the femur taken at a somewhat higher magnification than in Fig. 3.29. Note the irregularity of the cartilage tongues extending into the metaphysis, with a lack of columnization and organized endochondral ossification. In patients with hypophosphatasia the epiphyseal growth cartilage fails to calcify, and, in the absence of calcification, normal endochondral ossification cannot take place.

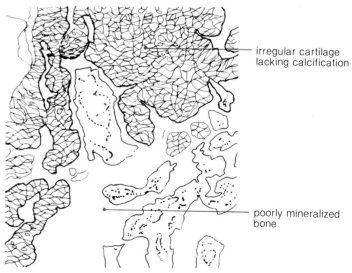

irregular cartilage lacking calcification

poorly mineralized bone

HYPERPHOSPHATASIA

Juvenile Paget's disease

Hyperphosphatasia is a rare autosomal recessive disorder characterized clinically by short stature and defective bone maturation. Patients with this disorder have elevated blood levels of serum alkaline phosphatase and acid phosphatase of bone origin, and an elevated urinary hydroxyproline level.

On roentgenographic examination, a thickened skull with "cotton ball" radiodensities is seen. Long bones show an increase in width, bowing, and loss of normal corticomedullary differentiation (Figs. 3.31 and 3.32).

Morphologic studies reveal that both the cortical and trabecular bone consist of immature fibrous (or woven) bone with abundant osteoblasts and osteoclasts and prominent osteoid seams (Fig. 3.33). The marrow space is replaced by a well vascularized fibrous connective tissue network. Using polarized light, one may observe a mosaic pattern of the bone matrix.

Hyperphosphatasia is distinguished clinically from Paget's disease by its early onset and the generalized symmetrical bone involvement.

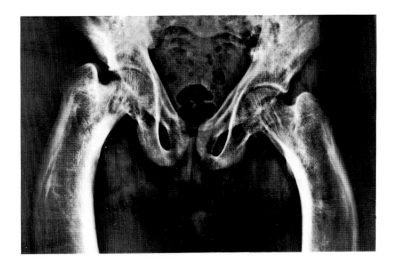

Fig. 3.32 Roentgenogram of the pelvis and upper femurs in the patient seen in Fig. 3.31 demonstrates marked thickening of the shafts of the femurs, with bowing of the femur and a dense irregular cortex.

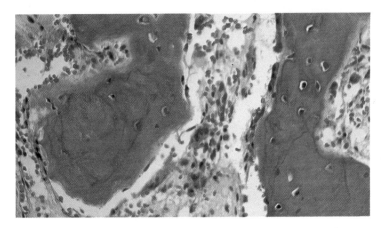

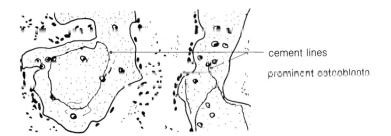

Fig. 3.33 Hyperphosphatasia: photomicrograph of bone biopsy from the patient shown in Figs. 3.31 and 3.32. The bone is somewhat immature, with large irregular cells. Note prominent cement lines and many osteoblasts on bone surface.

cement lines

prominent osteoblasts

Fig. 3.31 Roentgenogram of the skull in an 11-year-old patient with hyperphosphatasia. Note the marked thickening of the calvarium and the "cotton ball" radiodensities throughout.

FLUOROSIS

Fluoride has been shown to stimulate bone production, although its effect is dependent on the duration and degree of exposure. In general, one must consider on the one hand industrial or endemic exposure to fluoride, and, on the other hand, therapeutically induced effects associated with the treatment of osteoporosis with fluoride.

In populations with exposure to high fluoride content in water (in excess of 24 parts per 1,000,000), or in those people exposed to industrial fluoride contamination, the most dramatic roentgenographic change is marked coarsening and thickening of bony trabeculae, particularly involving the axial skeleton. Eventually significantly increased bone density occurs. There may be periosteal new bone formation and marked spinal osteophytosis. The propensity for bone formation in this condition is evident even in the calcification of muscle, ligament, and tendon attachments. These individuals may also have mottled enamel of the teeth, and anemia. Debilitating arthrosis may develop in patients in whom bone formation is particularly prominent in and around joints.

A histologic examination of the sclerotic bone reveals it to be predominantly lamellar when viewed under polarized light. There are increased osteocytes, and there may be prominent cement lines. A marked increase in the diameters of the cortical haversian systems gives a spongy appearance to the cortex.

In recent years fluoride has been used to stimulate bone production in osteoporotic patients. Although the specific mechanism is not understood, fluoride in doses of approximately 1 mg per kg of body weight per day produces a marked increase in osteoblastic activity, including the formation of osteoid. Although mineralization takes place, it is often irregular. A microscopic examination of the tissue produced in this way reveals increased cellularity and irregular arrangements of osteocytes. Peculiar basophilic densities are seen around the newly formed and irregular osteocytes (Fig. 3.34).

When used in conjunction with supplemental calcium and vitamin D, sodium fluoride has been shown by histomorphometric analysis to increase bone mass in osteoporotic patients. (However, it is not clear whether this bone has increased mechanical strength.) It should be noted that, in patients treated with sodium fluoride therapy for osteoporosis for over five years, calcification of ligaments and tendons as well as osteophytosis similar to that seen in patients with industrial fluorosis have been reported.

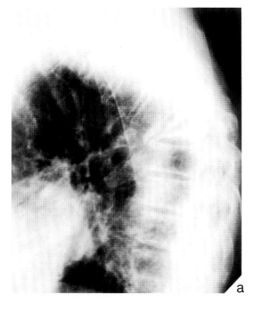

a

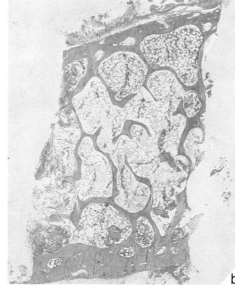

b

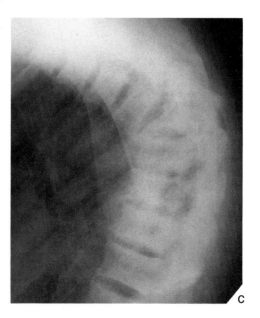

c

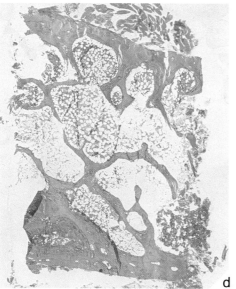

d

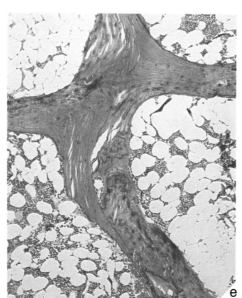

e

Fig. 3.34 The effect of sodium fluoride on osteoporotic bone. Roentgenogram of an osteoporotic spine (a) shows collapse of thoracic vertebrae with marked osteopenia. Transilial biopsy from same patient reveals osteoporosis (trabecular bone volume of 18.7%) (b). This section shows normal lamellar bone with little cellular activity. After several years of treatment with sodium fluoride, calcium carbonate, and vitamin D, spinal roentgenogram shows increased radiodensity (c). An increased trabecular bone volume of 30.5% is calculated from the transcortical ilial biopsy (d). Note dramatic histologic changes (e) characterized by distinct new lamellar bone on existing trabeculae. This lamellar pattern reveals increased osteocytes with pericellular basophilia. Note also increased osteoid and osteoclastic activity.

3.14

PAGET'S DISEASE

Patients with Paget's disease have disordered bone architecture that results from a disturbance in the rate of bone tissue breakdown by osteoclasts and bone tissue formation by osteoblasts (Figs. 3.35 to 3.37). Virtually any bone in the body may be involved, but the most common sites of disease are the lumbar spine, pelvis, skull, femur, and tibia.

The incidence of the condition varies with genetic background; common in northern Europeans, it is very rare in blacks and Asians. The incidence of Paget's disease in two large autopsy series in northern Europe was between 3 and 4 per cent of all individuals over the age of 40. In these autopsy series, the disease was most often limited to involvement of one or two bones, and usually it was part of the vertebral column and/or sacrum. Most of these individuals in whom the disease was discovered at autopsy would not have been diagnosed during life. Certainly the widespread bone involvement as described by Paget represents only a small portion of the total number of affected individuals.

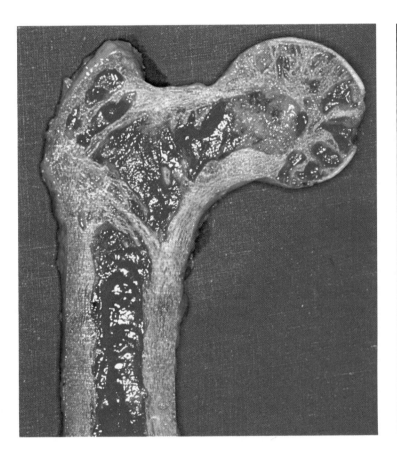

Fig. 3.35 Proximal end of femur involved by Paget's disease shows loss of normal cancellous architecture and replacement by coarse, thick bundles of trabecular bone. The cortical bone is irregularly thickened, pink, and has a coarse granular appearance in contrast to the smooth, ivory appearance of normal cortical bone.

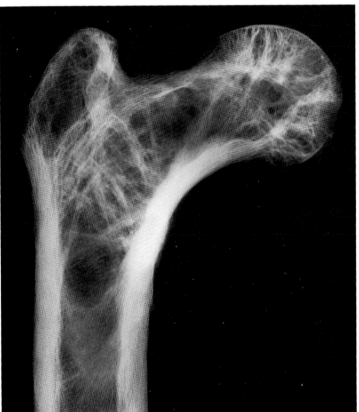

Fig. 3.36 Roentgenogram of the specimen shown in Fig. 3.35.

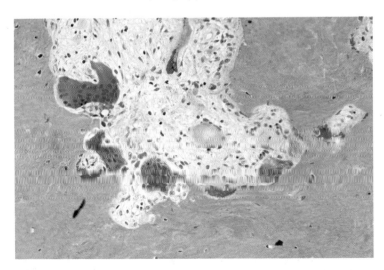

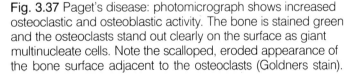

Fig. 3.37 Paget's disease: photomicrograph shows increased osteoclastic and osteoblastic activity. The bone is stained green and the osteoclasts stand out clearly on the surface as giant multinucleate cells. Note the scalloped, eroded appearance of the bone surface adjacent to the osteoclasts (Goldners stain).

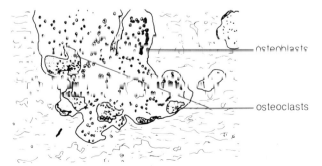

3.15

The complaints that bring the patient to the physician are pain or symptoms of one of the complications of Paget's disease (fracture, arthritis, heart failure, and tumor). The pain tends to be constant, aching, and diffuse in nature.

Radiologic Features. The radiologic appearance of the disease is variable and reflects the underlying morphologic changes. In the earliest stages of the disease, best typified radiographically in the skull, there is a striking radiolucent appearance without any thickening of the bone, a presentation known as osteoporosis circumscripta (Fig. 3.38). In the later stages of the disease the density of the bone increases and the bone thickens (Figs. 3.39 to 3.41). The radiologic examination of the vertebral bodies may reveal either uniformly increased radiodensity or,

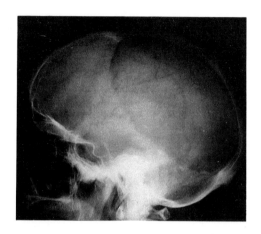

Fig. 3.38 Clinical roentgenogram of a skull. Note large circular lytic defect involving posterior half of the skull. One can also see some patchy osteoblastic reaction in the bone around the defect. This lesion, osteoporosis circumscripta, is a common radiologic presentation of Paget's disease.

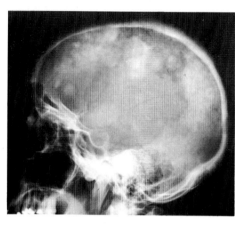

Fig 3.39 Clinical roentgenogram of the skull in the later stages of Paget's disease. Marked sclerosis appears in the bone, the diploetic architecture is lost, and the bone becomes extremely thick, on occasion becoming several times thicker than normal.

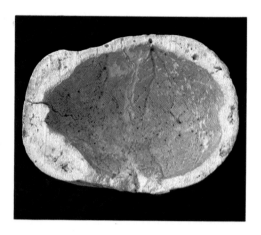

Fig. 3.40 A striking example of late, severe Paget's disease in which the thickening of the skull, the loss of diploetic architecture, and the granular pumice-like appearance of the bone can be seen.

Fig. 3.41 Paget's disease: close-up of the cut surface of a skull with large blood-filled lakes that may be present in pagetoid bone.

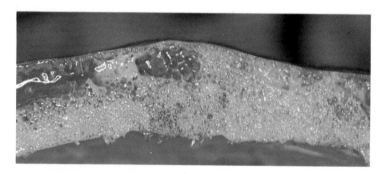

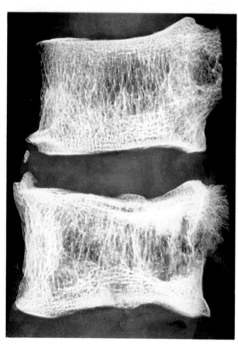

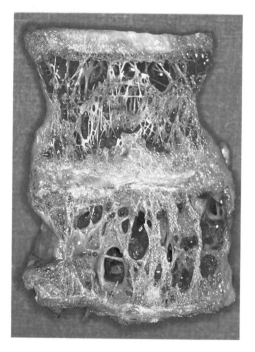

Fig 3.42 Careful examination of the vertebral bodies at autopsy may reveal isolated involvement by Paget's disease. This occurrence is probably most easily demonstrated by the radiologic examination of a slice taken through the vertebrae (*left*). The thickening of the trabeculae and the rather typical sclerosis around the edge of the vertebral body (giving rise to a picture-frame appearance) can be seen. In the gross specimen (*right*) the coarse appearance of the cancellous bone is apparent after the bone marrow has been carefully washed away with water. However, these changes could be easily missed in routine examination.

more commonly, a "picture frame" appearance (Figs. 3.42 and 3.43). In the pelvis it is common to find combinations of increased radiodensity, lytic areas, honeycombed sections, and striated appearances. In a long bone the process usually evolves at one or the other end, occasionally both, and spreads towards the center. The junction between the normal and the diseased bone is demarcated as an advancing wedge of rarefaction (Fig. 3.44). The surface irregularity involves not only the periosteal surface, but the endosteal surface as well. In the final stages of the disease, the distinctions between cortical and cancellous bone become largely obliterated.

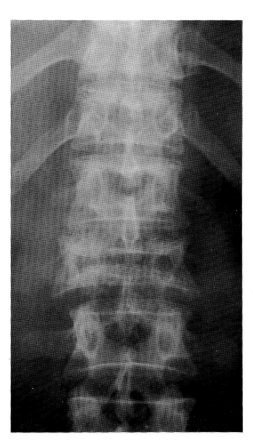

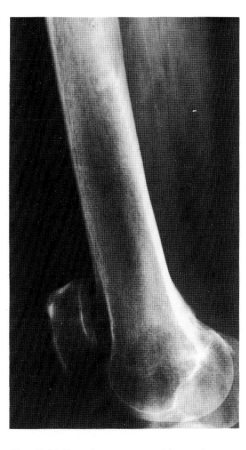

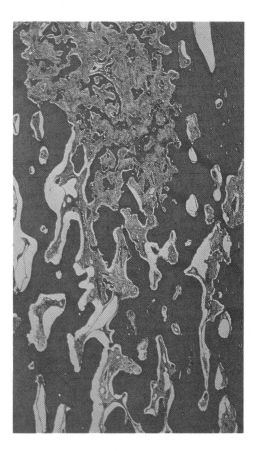

Fig. 3.43 Clinical roentgenogram of the spine shows a solitary focus of pagetoid bone. There is a loss of height of the vertebra, some increase in the width of the vertebra, and a typical picture-frame appearance.

Fig. 3.44 Roentgenogram of femur involved by Paget's disease (*left*). The cortex of the posterior femur in the proximal portion is irregularly thickened and more porotic than that in the distal part. At the junction between the involved upper bone and the normal lower bone, note a flame-shaped advancing edge. Histologic section of the advancing edge (*right*). Note the involved fibrotic and pagetoid bone eroding the normal bone cortex.

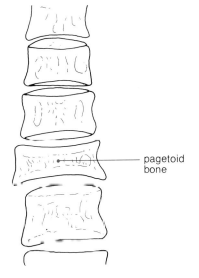

pagetoid bone

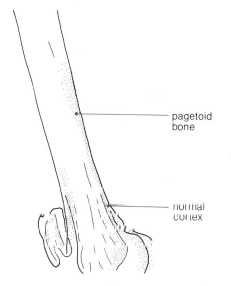

pagetoid bone

normal cortex

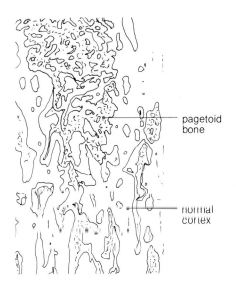

pagetoid bone

normal cortex

Microscopic Appearance. The microscopic picture depends upon the state of the disease process in the bone from which the specimen was taken. The dynamic course of the disease can be divided into three phases that are continuous. The osteolytic phase is characterized by an extremely vascular fibrous tissue that fills the marrow spaces (Fig. 3.45). The bone shows active osteoclastic resorption. In cancellous bone, the trabeculae are slender and sparse; in cortical bone, large resorption cavities are seen. Concurrent with the osteoclastic activity, appositional new bone formation by prominent osteoblasts may be found. Frequently, both events are found on the same trabecula. Inflammatory cells are lacking. The histologic picture is one of frenetic cellular activity, which may be confused with that of hyperparathyroidism.

This mainly destructive phase is followed closely by an osteoblastic phase or combined phase in which new bone formation predominates over reabsorption (Fig. 3.46). Massive trabecular plates are built up to a density that is neither cortical nor cancellous in its architecture. This process of bone formation proceeds without apparent regard for architectural structure, giving rise to the mosaic pattern, the essential feature of which is a marked increase in the number of cement lines.

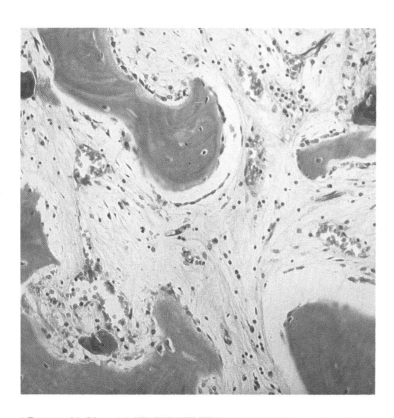

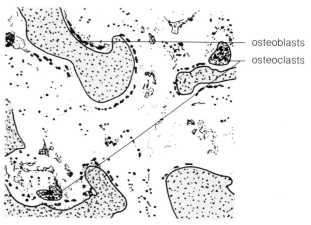

Fig. 3.45 Histologic features of the early stage of Paget's disease. Some fibrous replacement of the fatty marrow, which may be confined only to the surfaces of the bone, can be seen. Marked increased osteoclastic resorption of the bone is present. In this early stage the mosaic pattern is not evident. The histologic appearance is indistinguishable from that seen in association with hyperparathyroidism, and before a histologic diagnosis is made, careful clinical correlation is necessary.

osteoblasts
osteoclasts

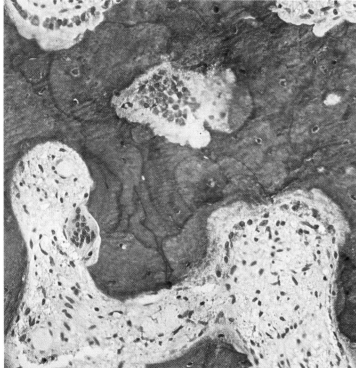

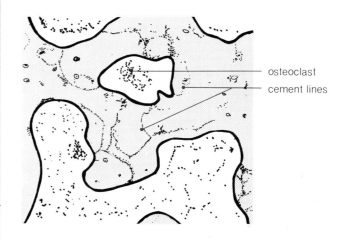

Fig. 3.46 Histologic features of more advanced Paget's disease. Not only is there marked osteoclastic reaction, with the osteoclasts frequently being very large and having many nuclei, but also increased osteoblastic reaction is seen. In the bone matrix of well prepared specimens, numerous irregular cement lines are observed. These changes are well seen in this undecalcified section.

osteoclast
cement lines

A final "burnt out" phase is generally described, although the clinician must accept this as a relative term. Cellular activity is less intense and vascularity may diminish, but it appears that the general turnover rate may still be well in excess of that of normal bone. The microscopic picture in these areas is that of heavily trabeculated bone showing a prominent mosaic pattern. With the aid of polarized light microscopy, studies of the orientation of the collagen in bone reveal the discordant nature of the new structure (Fig. 3.47).

Laboratory Features. The elevation of the patient's serum alkaline phosphatase activity to as much as 20 or 30 times the normal rate (in association with the increased osteoblastic activity) has been recorded. The acid phosphatase level, too, tends to be at its upper limit or slightly above normal. Regional blood flow studies have demonstrated increased vascularity, which was observed to be 20 times the normal in some instances.

The patient's serum calcium and phosphorus levels are ordinarily within normal limits in Paget's disease. However, hypercalcemia is an occasional complication following prolonged bed rest in a patient with extensive involvement.

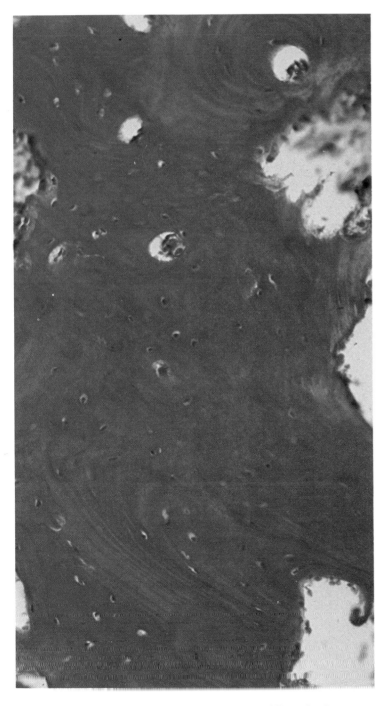
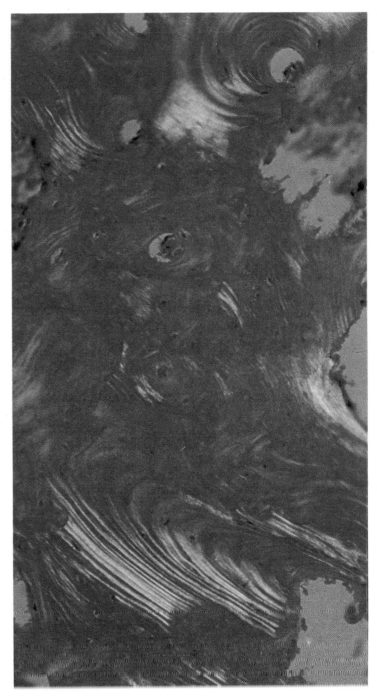

Fig. 3.47 Histologic features of the late stages of Paget's disease. The section on the left shows that the osteoblastic and osteoclastic reaction may be much less evident, and it can be difficult to appreciate the mosaic pattern either because the tissue has been overdecalcified or because the staining is not adequate to show the basophilic lines clearly. However, when the same histologic field is examined by polarized light with a first order red filter (*right*), the disorganized pattern of the bone structure is clearly demonstrated.

Clinical Assessment. In patients with Paget's disease, small incomplete cortical fractures may be numerous, particularly in weight-bearing bones. Progressive bowing of the femur and wedging of the vertebrae are the result of repeated microfractures. Occasionally these incomplete cortical fractures progress to complete transverse fractures.

Sarcoma is said to develop in 1 to 2 per cent of the patients with widespread Paget's involvement (Figs. 3.48 and 3.49). (However, if one considers the nondiagnosed cases, the overall incidence of sarcoma in Paget's disease is very much lower.) Sarcoma is not only a complication of widespread disease; it may, rarely, be engrafted on monostotic Paget's disease. The sarcoma that develops is not typical of osteogenic sarcoma, but usually shows a mixed pattern of osteosarcoma, fibrosarcoma, chondrosarcoma, and giant cell sarcoma; i.e., a mixed mesenchymal pattern. Occasionally a benign conventional giant cell tumor pattern may be seen.

The clinical evaluation of patients with Paget's disease

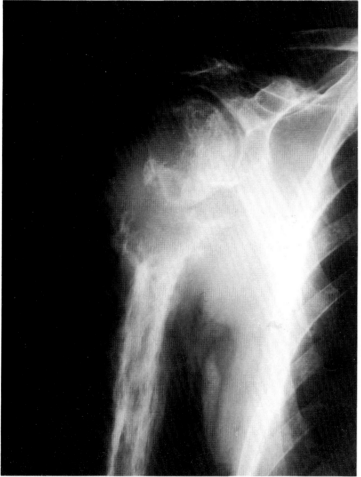

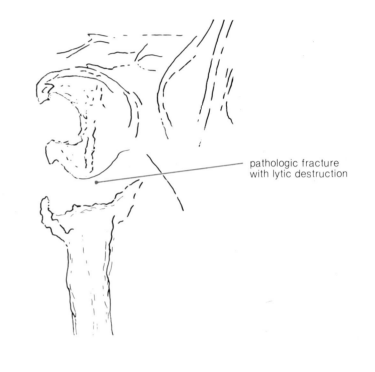

Fig. 3.48 Clinical roentgenogram of a patient with widespread Paget's disease of the skeleton shows, in addition, at the proximal end of the humerus, a destructive lytic lesion.

pathologic fracture with lytic destruction

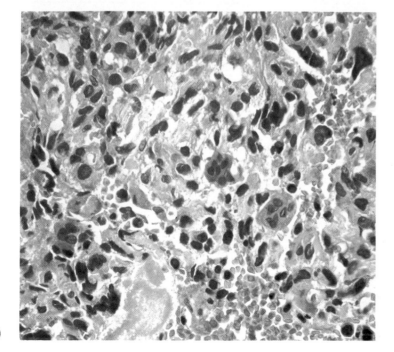

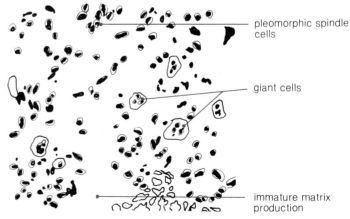

Fig. 3.49 High power view of a biopsy from the patient in Fig. 3.48 shows a pleomorphic spindle cell tumor with many giant cells, which is typical of the histologic appearance of Paget's sarcoma.

pleomorphic spindle cells

giant cells

immature matrix production

reveals a high incidence of arthritis in the joints adjacent to involved bones (Figs. 3.50 to 3.53). The arthritis that is most commonly seen in the hip joint is characterized on radiologic examination by concentric joint narrowing. This narrowing results from an accelerated rate of endochondral ossification in the calcified cartilage and the articular cartilage (consequent upon the increased vascularity and turnover of the subchondral bone). Bone deformity resulting from accelerated bone modeling also contributes to the arthritic process.

The cause of Paget's disease remains unknown. However, electron microscopic observations made on the osteoclasts of patients with Paget's disease have demonstrated the presence of specific intranuclear inclusions composed of microcylinders. These structures suggest an analogy with the virus material of the measles group, and studies with indirect immunofluorescence and immunoperoxidase techniques have lent further support to the hypothesis of a viral etiology in Paget's disease of the bone.

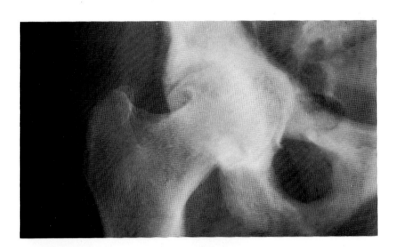

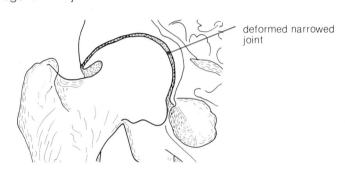

Fig. 3.50 Clinical roentgenogram of a patient with Paget's disease. In the hip joint there is marked concentric narrowing, indicative of degenerative joint disease.

deformed narrowed joint

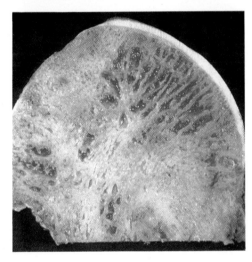

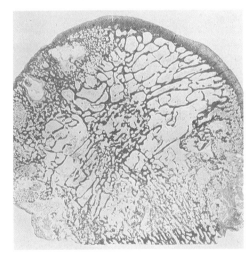

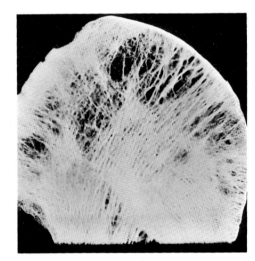

Fig. 3.51 A slice through a resected femoral head shows extensive involvement by Paget's disease and erosion of the cartilage on the medial side.

Fig. 3.52 Histologic section (*left*) of the femoral head shown in Fig. 3.51 and a roentgenogram (*right*) of a slice of the specimen. The pagetoid bone is seen to

have a fine and disorganized trabecular pattern, which contrasts markedly with the normal cancellous bone that remains in some areas.

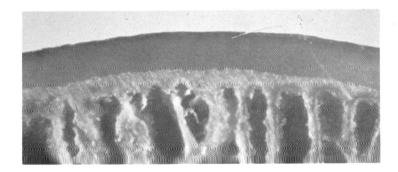

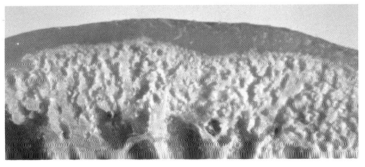

Fig. 3.53 Close-up of the articular surface. In the left illustration there is normal cancellous bone, subchondral end plate, and articular cartilage. In the right illustration one sees pagetoid bone, which has an irregular subchondral bone end plate with marked

thinning of the overlying cartilage. It may well be that the accelerated remodeling of the affected subchondral bone has resulted in accelerated endochondral ossification of the overlying cartilage, which produces the evident thinning.

Osteopetrosis

Osteopetrosis is a rare disorder characterized by a marked increased density of the skeleton. The bones are usually short and frequently show a modeling defect apparent in the loss of the normal metaphyseal flare. The disease is frequently complicated by multiple fractures and by anemia. Two forms of the disorder have been recognized: a severe form that usually causes death in utero or early childhood and that would appear to be inherited as an autosomal recessive condition, and a less severe form in which the patients live into adult life and that appears to be inherited as an autosomal dominant characteristic. The condition should be differentiated on roentgenographic examination from other causes of increased bone sclerosis, particularly widespread osteoblastic metastases, chronic fluorosis, myelosclerosis, and idiopathic osteosclerosis.

In severely affected patients, the radiologic examination of the skeleton may reveal a uniform opacity of the skeletal tissue with loss of any cortical medullary differen-

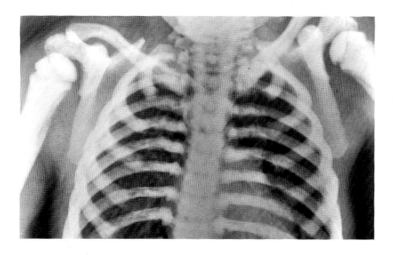

Fig. 3.54 Roentgenogram of the upper body of a child with osteopetrosis. The marked increase in density of all the bones is apparent.

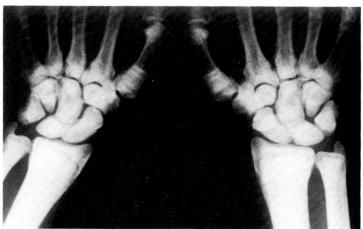

Fig. 3.55 Clinical roentgenogram of the hands of an adult patient with osteopetrosis. The proximal end of the thumb clearly shows alternating stripes of dense involved bone with more lytic and apparently normal bone distally.

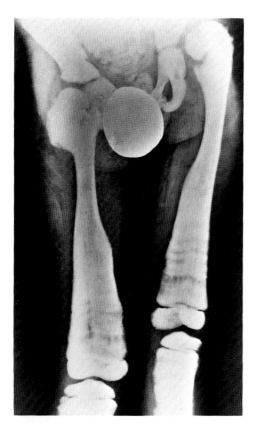

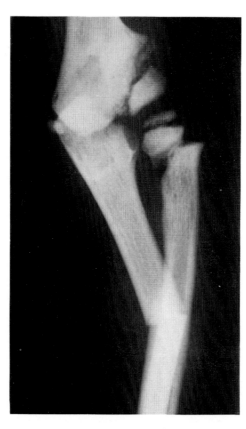

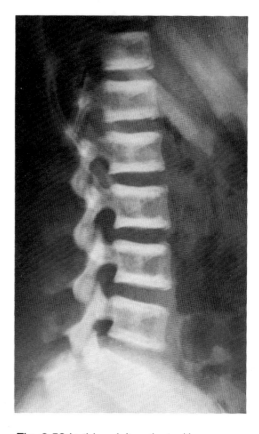

Fig. 3.56 Roentgenograms of the legs in a child with osteopetrosis show a lack of metaphyseal remodeling, which gives rise to an Erlenmeyer flask deformity. The normal cortical medullary differentiation is not seen, and the bones are strikingly dense.

Fig. 3.57 Multiple fractures of the forearm and elbow are demonstrated in this young patient with osteopetrosis.

Fig. 3.58 In this adult patient with osteopetrosis, a roentgenogram of the spine shows marked increased density of the proximal and distal thirds of the vertebral bodies, giving a sandwich-like appearance.

tiation (Figs. 3.54 to 3.57). However, in less severely affected patients it is not unusual to find, particularly in the pelvis and the peripheral bones, alternating areas of affected bone and apparently normal bone, which results in a peculiar striped appearance in the tissue. In the vertebral bodies a more lytic stripe is often seen horizontally, which gives the vertebrae a sandwich-like appearance (Fig. 3.58).

On gross examination the bones usually show widening in the region of the metaphysis and the diaphysis, the characteristic Erlenmeyer flask deformity (Figs. 3.59 to 3.61). The bone may be readily appreciated to have an increased weight, and it may weigh two or three times more than a normal bone, despite the fact that the affected bones are usually somewhat smaller than normal. On sectioning, these bones may be observed to be very dense, with a complete loss of the normal architecture of cancellous and cortical bone.

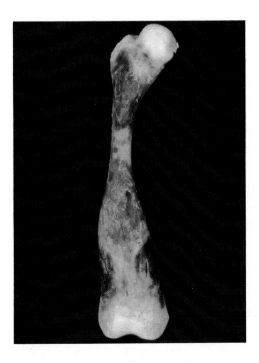
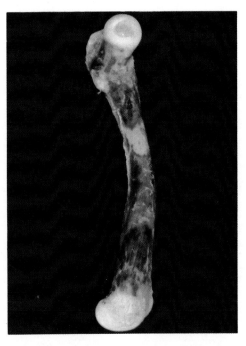
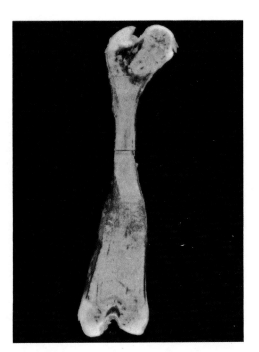

Fig. 3.59 Gross appearances of a femur removed from a child with osteopetrosis seen in frontal (*left*), lateral (*center*), and cut section (*right*). Note the characteristic Erlenmeyer flask deformity of the distal end of the femur, the exaggerated anterior bowing, subperiosteal hemorrhage, and uniform density of the bone on cut section.

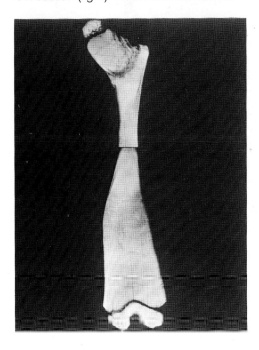
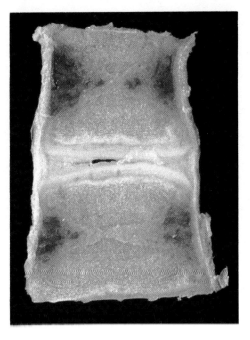
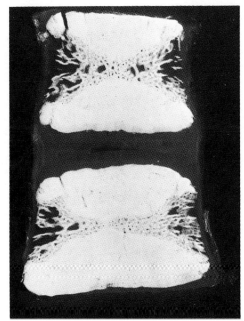

Fig. 3.60 Roentgenogram of a slice of the bone illustrated in Fig. 3.59 shows the tremendous density of the osseous tissue. The vertical striae represent vascular markings within the bone.

Fig. 3.61 Osteopetrosis: gross appearance of two resected vertebral bodies in frontal section (*left*) and a roentgenogram of these vertebrae (*right*).

3.23

Histologic sections show extremely irregular bone tissue, nearly all of which contains within it a cartilage core (Fig. 3.62). It appears as though the primary spongiosa, which normally forms in the metaphysis during development and which is remodeled to the adult form of bone, had forever remained unmodeled. Although it has often been said that there is a paucity of osteoclasts in this condition, osteoclasts are often abundant. However, electron microscopic studies have demonstrated that these osteoclasts lack ruffled borders and, although in proximity to the bone, they do not show the morphologic features that are normally present in the osteoclast that is resorbing (Fig. 3.63). In other words, although osteoclasts are present in the tissue, they do not appear to be functioning. One possible cause of or explanation for these morphologic findings may lie in the observation that, in osteopetrosis, the enzyme collagenase does not appear to be present in the bone.

Recent experimental work has reported the restoration of normal bone and cartilage resorption in osteopetrotic mice and rats following the transplantation of normal bone and spleen cells. This procedure has also been tried in a few humans with some promise of success.

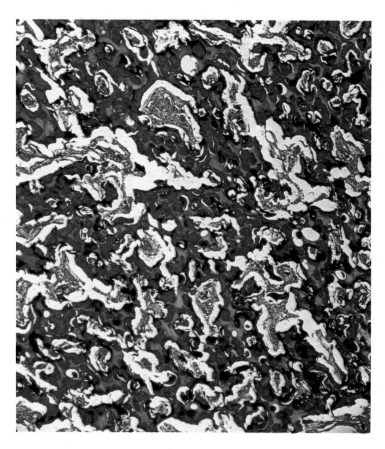

Fig. 3.62 Osteopetrosis: histologic section of bone removed from the metaphyseal end of the femur in a 10-year-old child shows a complete disorganization of the osseous tissue. Close inspection will show that most of the bone contains within it a core of calcified cartilage. A similar appearance is seen in the tissue of adults with osteopetrosis, and it would appear to represent a failure of the primary spongiosa to remodel.

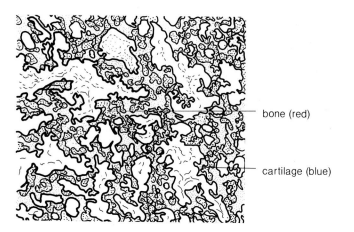

bone (red)

cartilage (blue)

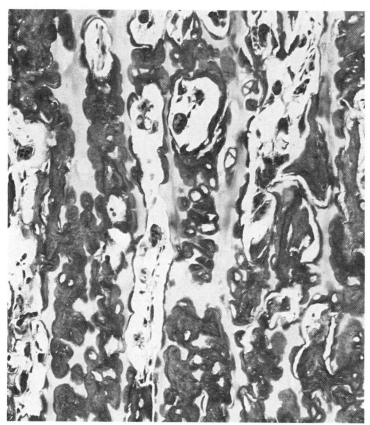

Fig. 3.63 Histologic section taken from a young child with osteopetrosis shows numerous osteoclasts in the tissue, though these osteoclasts do not seem to be resorbing bone.

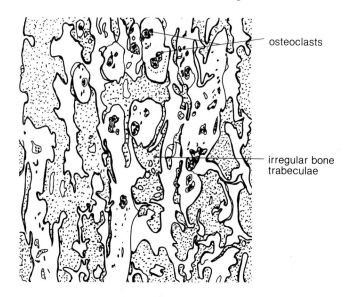

osteoclasts

irregular bone trabeculae

CAMURATI-ENGELMANN DISEASE

Camurati-Engelmann disease is a skeletal abnormality, the clinical features of which are painful legs, a waddling gait, and wasting muscles. The disease is usually hereditary, and it is thought to be autosomal dominant in transmission. Camurati-Engelmann disease begins early in life, usually before the age of 10 years. Sporadically, however, cases have been reported in the literature in which the patient's age at diagnosis has been as late as the fifth decade of life.

The disease is diagnosed primarily by a roentgenographic examination, in which symmetric sclerosis and, often, fusiform enlargement of the diaphysis of the long bones, especially the femur and tibia, may be noted (Figs. 3.64 and 3.65). There may also be changes in the skull, but rarely in the pelvis, mandible, clavicle, ribs, metacarpals, phalanges, and spine.

The disorder is characterized histologically by a thickened cortex, the increased width of which results mainly from increased endosteal new bone formation (Fig. 3.66). However, periosteal new bone formation is sometimes observed. In children the enlargement of the cortex of the bone produces a narrowed medullary cavity, which, if severe, may lead to extramedullary hematopoiesis sufficient to cause hepatosplenomegaly.

The serum chemistries in patients with Camurati-Engelmann disease are usually normal, although an increase in the level of alkaline phosphatase (of bone origin) may be observed. The disorder is of obscure etiology, but the pain may be relieved by the administration of steroids.

In 1962 Van Buchen and his associates reported seven cases of a disease that was similar in many ways to Camurati-Engelmann disease, but different in that there was prominent skull involvement and a suggestion of autosomal recessive transmission (hyperostosis corticalis generalista). Other obscure entities with diaphyseal cortical bone thickening include hyperostosis generalista with pachyderma, in which the metaphysis and epiphysis, as well as the diaphysis, are significantly involved. This disorder has been reported to occur in puberty, with eventual synostosis and ossification of the joint capsule. There is little histologic information by which to separate these entities.

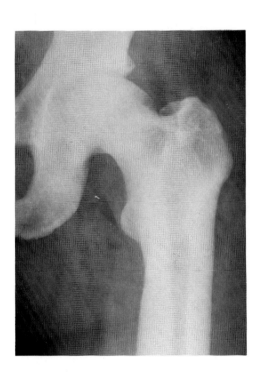

Fig. 3.64 Roentgenogram of a 49-year-old man with a 3-year history of bone pain. Note the markedly thickened, dense cortex, which is more clearly defined than the thickened but pumice-like bone of Paget's disease. In this patient the serum calcium and phosphate levels were within normal limits, although the alkaline phosphatase level was persistently elevated (up to 1600 mU/ml).

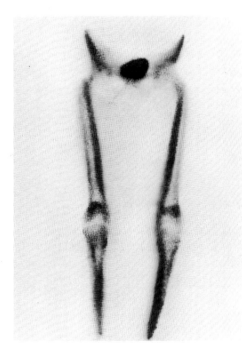

Fig. 3.65 Bone scan demonstrates increased diaphyseal uptake over the femurs and tibias bilaterally.

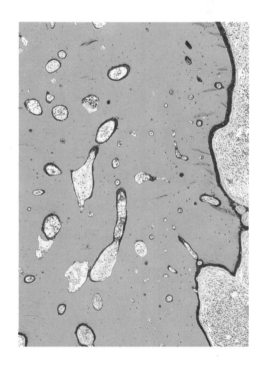

Fig. 3.66 Photomicrograph of a cortical biopsy from a patient with Camurati-Engelmann disease. The bone surfaces are covered by a thin layer of osteoid, indicating increased bone formation. The endosteal portion (top) appears to be hypercellular with respect to osteocytes. The bone is lamellar in type and does not show an increase in the cement lines, thus differentiating this disease from Paget's disease.

HYPERTROPHIC PULMONARY OSTEOARTHROPATHY

Marie-Bamberger syndrome

Hypertrophic pulmonary osteoarthropathy refers to symmetrical periosteal new bone formation in the diaphysis of the bones of the appendicular skeleton. This condition is seen in association with neoplastic and non-neoplastic diseases of the lung and, less commonly, other organs. The classic presentation of this disorder is in an adult, with complaints of arthralgia and/or aching bone pain, with or without clubbing of the fingers and toes.

A striking roentgenographic feature of hypertrophic pulmonary osteoarthropathy is the symmetric "onion skin periostitis" of the shafts of long bones, especially of the tibia and fibula, which is confined to the diaphyses but progresses proximally (Fig. 3.67). Densities in the sites of insertions of ligaments and tendons have also been noted.

Although the joints do not show significant roentgenographic change, patients may have painful effusions that are characteristically noninflammatory. The arthralgia is usually relieved by aspirin. The patient's level of serum alkaline phosphatase (of bone origin) may be elevated.

On histologic examination one may note marked periosteal new bone formation. The outer layer of the periosteum may show a mononuclear cell infiltrate. No endosteal bone deposition is seen (Fig. 3.68).

The etiology of pulmonary osteoarthropathy remains obscure despite numerous attempts to define an ectopic hormonal secretion or a vascular abnormality. Treatment should be directed at the underlying disease.

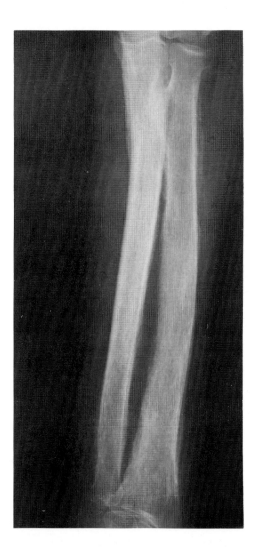

Fig. 3.67 Roentgenogram of the forearm in a patient with carcinoma of the lung shows periosteal bone formation on both the radius and the ulna. In this patient all the long bones demonstrated dramatic periosteal new bone.

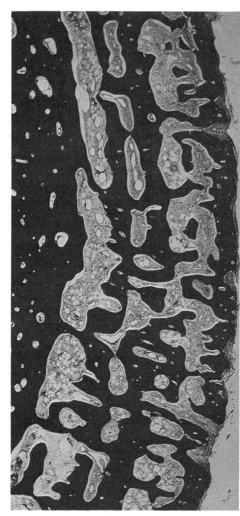

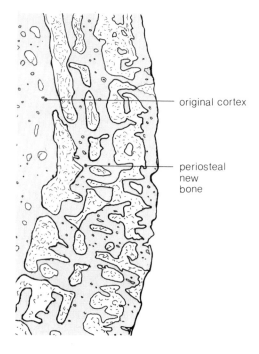

Fig. 3.68 Photomicrograph of a biopsy of cortical bone from a patient with pulmonary osteoarthropathy. Note the three layers of new periosteal bone.

original cortex

periosteal new bone

4 Injury and Repair

When considering the effects of injury, the most important questions are:

1. What happens to the cell, to the extracellular matrix, and to tissue after injury?
2. How much injury can be sustained?
3. How does the body deal with injured cells and tissue, and effect repair?

These questions have formed the basis of pathology research for over 100 years, and the results of these investigations are reviewed in depth in a number of texts devoted to general pathology. In this chapter we will briefly review the processes associated with injury and repair—especially repair of connective tissue—for the sake of those readers who are not pathologists, because without some basic understanding of these processes it is difficult to appreciate the alteration of cellular activity in disease states.

EFFECTS OF INJURY

The cell is a complex structure in which the basic processes of energy conversion, protein synthesis, and other vital activities are constantly occurring (Fig. 4.1). It exists in an ever-changing environment, and its ability to adapt to new conditions determines its continued functional activity. Injury occurs when conditions in the local environment are such that the cell is unable to maintain its physiologic equilibrium.

The nature of the injurious agent and the duration of its application determine what happens to the cell. If the injury results in only transient alterations in either the intracellular or extracellular regulatory mechanisms, the cell may revert to its normal basal state with cessation of the adverse conditions. A more severe injury may result in more permanent adaptive changes, e.g., hyperplasia or atrophy. When the insult causes irreversible changes in the cell, cell death (necrosis) occurs.

Injury may result from physical agents (mechanical trauma, extremes in temperature, or ionizing radiation), chemicals (either acting locally by corrosive action, or systemically by their effect upon cell organelles), or biologic agents (bacteria, viruses, fungi, or other organisms). Regardless of the injurious agent, two effects may be expected: (1) a local effect at the site of injury, and (2) a general effect on the body as a whole. (Shock following severe hemorrhage in association with an open fracture is an example of the generalized effect of injury.)

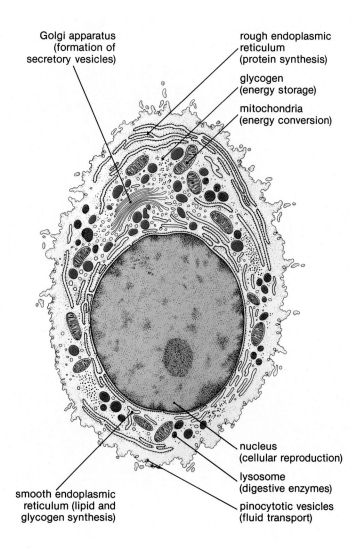

Golgi apparatus (formation of secretory vesicles)

rough endoplasmic reticulum (protein synthesis)

glycogen (energy storage)

mitochondria (energy conversion)

nucleus (cellular reproduction)

lysosome (digestive enzymes)

smooth endoplasmic reticulum (lipid and glycogen synthesis)

pinocytotic vesicles (fluid transport)

Fig. 4.1 Diagram of a cell showing the basic cytoplasmic organelles and their function.

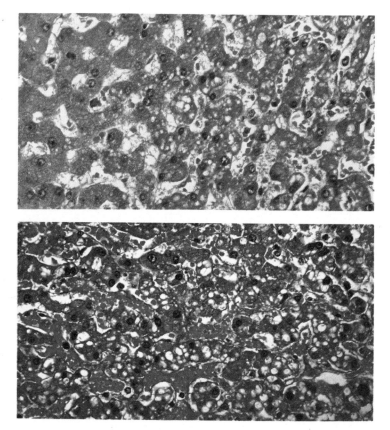

Fig. 4.2 Cellular changes due to hypoxia are well-demonstrated in these photomicrographs of the centrilobular part of the liver. (Upper) On the left can be seen normal liver tissue, while on the right some vacuolization is apparent within the cytoplasm and there is swelling of the cellular outline. (Lower) In this photomicrograph of tissue adjacent to the central veins, congestion of the liver sinuses is readily apparent, with marked vacuolization, inclusions of proteinaceous material, and some shrinkage and darkening of nuclei also in evidence. This appearance is characteristic and indicative of chronic anoxic conditions.

In addition to the types of injurious agents (physical, chemical, or biologic), there are other considerations that affect the degree of injury. Among these is the intensity of application of an injurious agent, which may eventually result in irreversible cellular damage. Another consideration is the site of injury. For example, anoxia rapidly produces irreversible damage to brain cells and cardiac muscle, whereas connective tissue can usually withstand anoxia for considerable periods of time. Furthermore, the effects of injury are influenced by an individual's general health, including his nutritional state and the presence or absence of drugs in the body.

Because of the varying types of injury and the widely differing susceptibility of various body tissues, it is difficult to generalize about the morphologic effects of injury. However, we do know that mechanical injury usually causes cell disruption; freezing depresses cellular metabolic activity and ultimately leads to the formation of destructive intracytoplasmic ice crystals; and heat increases rates of metabolism, enzyme inactivation, and protein coagulation, and, at extreme temperatures, may even cause tissue charring. The effects of ionizing radiation are felt mostly by the nucleus, where they cause chromosome breakage and gene mutation. Chemicals act by interfering with metabolic processes in the cell, especially by the inactivation of enzymes, but also by the denaturation of cellular protein. Finally, many biologic agents manufacture toxins that cause cellular metabolic disturbances.

HISTOLOGIC OBSERVATIONS

The most commonly observed microscopic change associated with altered cell homeostasis is a change in cell volume. This results from an inability to regulate electrolyte and fluid metabolism due to altered function of both the mitochondria and the cell membrane. In sublethal injury, e.g., hypoxia, alterations in lipoprotein synthesis and secretion may result in the accumulation in cells and tissues of both lipid droplets and amorphous eosinophilic material (Fig. 4.2).

A fundamental characteristic of living cells is their ability to sense and to adapt to changes in the environment. This ability to adjust enables cells to survive in the face of situations that might otherwise prove lethal. Such cellular adaptations, which include atrophy, hypertrophy, and hyperplasia, are commonly observed in the course of many disease processes (Fig. 4.3).

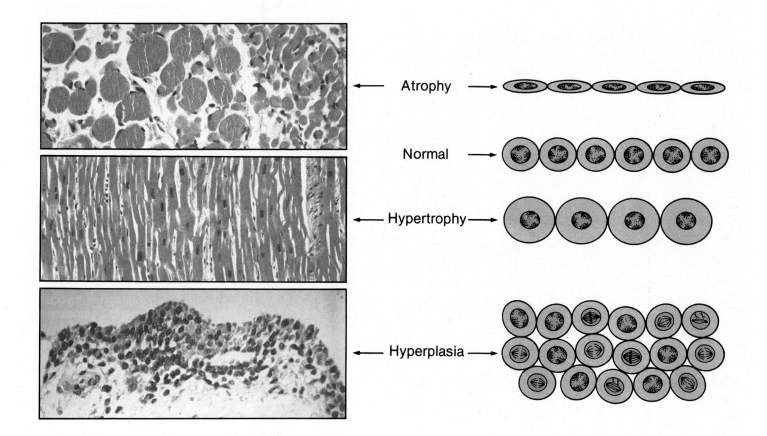

Fig. 4.3 Diagrammatic representation and photomicrographs of atrophy, hypertrophy, and hyperplasia. *(Upper)* Cellular atrophy: On the right side of this photomicrograph of skeletal muscle tissue can be seen small, atrophied fibers, in marked contrast to the normal muscle fibers seen at left. *(Center)* Cellular hypertrophy: On the right side of this photomicrograph of myocardial muscle can be seen fibers with increased diameter and nuclei of increased size, characteristic of hypertrophic cells.

In hypertrophic myocardial cells, the nuclei also have a characteristic squared appearance. *(Lower)* Cellular hyperplasia: Normally, the synovial lining is only one cell thick; however, in this photomicrograph of the synovial lining from a patient with chronic osteoarthritis, one can readily see a marked proliferation of synoviocytes, characteristic of a hyperplastic condition. Note the mitotic structure in the synovial lining on the upper left.

4.3

Atrophy. Atrophy refers to a decrease in the size and activity of cells, and is particularly striking clinically when it occurs in the musculoskeletal or central nervous systems. It is seen as an adaptation to diminished use, or as a result of a reduction in blood supply, poor nutrition, or a decrease in normal hormonal stimulation. Cellular atrophy is usually accompanied by a corresponding shrinkage of the affected organ. In parenchymal organs, atrophy may result solely from a decrease in cell size. However, in the later stages of disease, the decrease in cell size may also be accompanied by an actual loss of cells. In connective tissue, visible atrophy results from a loss of extracellular matrix, which in turn reflects an alteration in cellular activity. In bone, this altered activity gives rise to osteoporosis.

Hypertrophy. Hypertrophy refers to an increase in cell size that results from an augmentation of the intracellular organelles, especially the endoplasmic reticulum; as a result, there is generally enhanced protein synthesis. Frequently, hypertrophy is a compensatory reaction, as in the heart muscles of patients with increased cardiac workload. In muscles, hypertrophy results from an increased number of myofibrils. In connective tissue such as bone, hypertrophy is evident as an additional amount of extracellular matrix.

Hyperplasia. Hyperplasia, an increase in the number of cells, is commonly seen in the synovium of patients with arthritis. The accelerated breakdown of the joint constituents (cartilage and bone) that occurs in all forms of arthritis results in enhanced phagocytosis by the synovium. This increased activity is associated with the augmentation of the synovial lining cells, which results in an increase not only in the thickness of the synovial lining, but also in the absolute area of the synovium which is frequently thrown up into papillary projections that extend into the joint cavity.

Necrosis. Necrosis (cell death) is usually recognized microscopically by changes in the nucleus. These changes include swelling of the nucleus, which is followed by condensation of the nuclear chromatin (pyknosis), and finally the dissolution of the nucleus (karyolysis) (Fig. 4.4).

The gross and microscopic appearance of necrotic tissue depends on the organ involved, and the type and extent of injury. In tissue necrosis associated with sudden and complete cessation of the blood supply (an infarct),

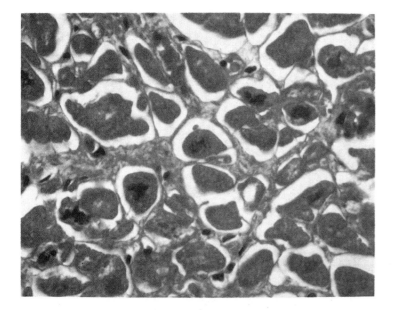

Fig. 4.4 High power photomicrograph of necrotizing myocardium demonstrates a number of dense, shrunken, and fragmented nuclei, characteristic of cellular necrosis.

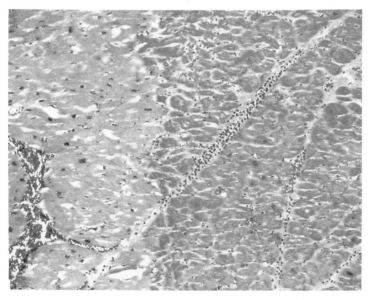

Fig. 4.5 On the right side of this photomicrograph of myocardial tissue there are fibers with granular, eosinophilic cytoplasm devoid of nuclei. In addition, one can clearly see acute inflammatory infiltration between the muscle fibers and along the course of the myocardial capillaries. All of these features are characteristic of necrotic tissue. By contrast, note the pale cytoplasm and intact nuclei seen in the normal, viable tissue on the left.

the affected tissue usually has an opaque appearance and a firm consistency, like a boiled egg. Microscopic examination of infarcted tissue usually reveals maintenance of structural anatomy, with preservation of the ghostlike outlines of the cells (Fig. 4.5). Conversely, in most bacterial injuries the cells are totally broken down, resulting in a soft area of necrotic material in which no visible cellular structural elements are recognizable microscopically (Fig. 4.6).

Calcification. Dead tissue that does not undergo rapid absorption frequently becomes calcified. This type of calcification, which is not related to a disturbance in calcium homeostasis, is called dystrophic calcification. Calcification is common in areas of infarction and also in caseous necrosis, as occurs in patients with tuberculosis. Of particular interest to orthopaedic surgeons is the calcification that is common in areas of necrotic connective tissue, e.g., in necrotic tendons or ligaments (Fig. 4.7).

RESPONSE TO INJURY

The collective responses of the body to both local and systemic injury are considered under the term "the inflammatory reaction." These responses include the removal and/or sequestration of the necrotic tissue and the injurious agent, defense against further injury, and the replacement of injured cells and the restoration of tissue architecture by reparative tissue. It is important to realize that the inflammatory reaction is not confined to a local, acute cellular response; it involves the whole body's defenses, and it continues until a homeostatic state has been restored.

Following local injury, vascular dilatation and an increased blood flow occur in the injured area. White blood cells attach themselves to the vascular endothelium and cross the wall of the vessel to the extravascular space (Fig. 4.8). These observations, first made in the nineteenth

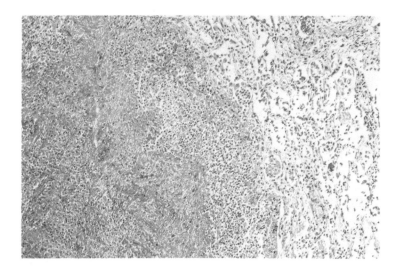

Fig. 4.6 Photomicrograph shows the cellular degradation within an abscess. Note that at the periphery of the abscess (at right) there is an infiltration of acute inflammatory cells as well as fibrin. However, toward the center of the abscess there is a complete loss of tissue architecture, with an accumulation of cellular debris and acute inflammatory cells.

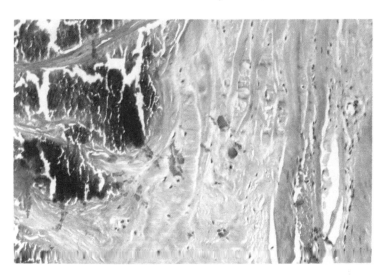

Fig. 4.7 Photomicrograph shows extensive calcification in the capsule of the shoulder joint. Such dystrophic calcification is a common complication of tissue necrosis following injury.

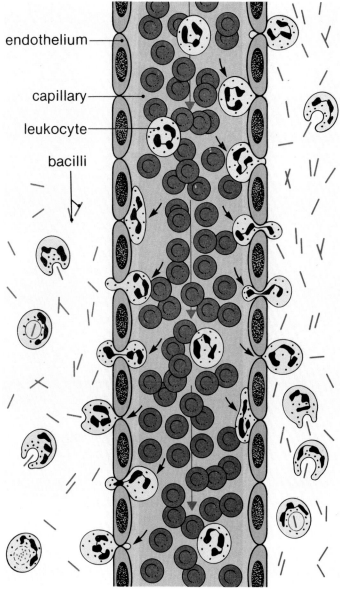

endothelium

capillary

leukocyte

bacilli

Fig. 4.8 Schematic diagram illustrates the migration of leukocytes across the vascular endothelium into the adjacent tissue. Once in the tissue, the leukocytes may encounter and engulf any existing microbes through the process of phagocytosis.

century by Julius Cohnheim, explain the four cardinal signs of inflammation:

1. Redness, caused by vasodilatation
2. Heat, the result of increased blood flow
3. Swelling, caused by exudation of fluids and cells into the extravascular spaces
4. Pain, the result of swelling on the nerve endings

Though Cohnheim described the migration of white blood cells through the vessel walls, it was Elie Metchnikoff who, a few years later, determined the function of these cells. He observed that they were capable of engulfing foreign matter, including bacteria, and he called this process phagocytosis (see Fig. 4.8). Since there were both large and small cells involved in phagocytic activity, he called the large cells macrophages and the small cells microphages (Fig. 4.9). (The microphages are now referred to as polymorphonuclear leukocytes or neutrophils.)

Swelling results from the accumulation of fluid in the injured tissue, and it is always present to a greater or lesser degree in the acute stage of inflammation. This excessive accumulation of fluid occurs because the vessels of the inflamed tissue become more permeable and allow plasma proteins to leak out into the extravascular space. This protein-rich fluid is called an exudate.

There are basically two reasons why fluids leak from the vessels in injured tissue: first, as a result of direct injury to the wall of the vessel, and second, because the vessels are rendered leaky by substances released or produced by the damaged tissue. These latter substances are referred to as the mediators of inflammation, and they are derived from both the blood (the blood-clotting system itself, platelets, and the components of the complement system) and the tissues (histamine, prostaglandins—particularly PGE and PGE2—and various lysosomal enzymes).

The migration (diapedesis) of leukocytes across the wall of the venule is an active rather than a passive phenomenon. Even after fluid exudation has passed its peak, leukocyte migration continues, presumably as a result of a persistent chemotactic effect of the injurious agent and the injured tissue.

The type of cell seen microscopically in the cellular infiltrate depends on the nature of the injury (e.g., bacteria will result in a marked neutrophilic infiltrate whereas a

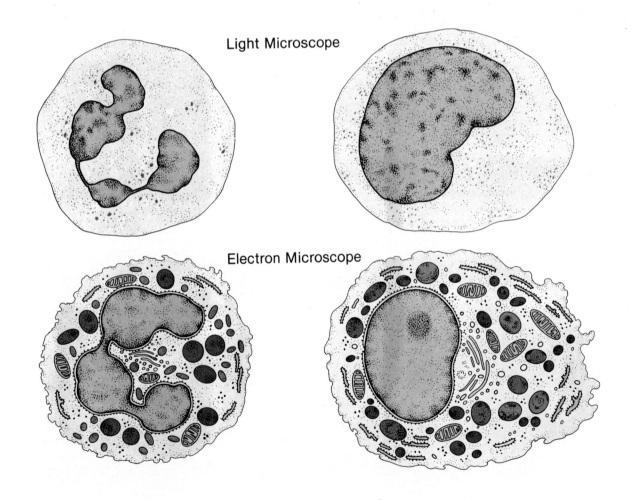

Light Microscope

Electron Microscope

Fig. 4.9 Diagrammatic representations of the light microscopic and electron microscopic characteristics of a polymorphonuclear (PMN) leukocyte (left) and a histiocyte (right).

mechanical injury will not) and the time elapsed since the injury. Within the first few hours, and up to a day or so, the predominant cells in the tissue exudate are polymorphonuclear leukocytes. However, after a period of 24 to 48 hours, more and more of the cells in the exudate are seen to be mononuclear—lymphocytes and macrophages. This biphasic response may be the result of the sequential action of specific chemical mediators.

Polymorphonuclear and mononuclear phagocytes migrate into the damaged tissues, and then ingest and digest unwanted bacteria and necrotic cells (see Fig. 4.8). These cells are equipped for this task by having large numbers of granules within their cytoplasm, including large dense granules (lysosomes) that contain various enzymes such as acid phosphatase, an antibacterial substance called lysozyme, and peroxidase (Fig. 4.10).

The acute inflammatory reaction may either subside, as is usually the case, or it may persist in the presence of continuing cell injury and become chronic. On histologic examination, chronic inflammation is distinguished from acute inflammation by the marked increase in the number of mononuclear cells present in the lesional area. These mononuclear cells include macrophages, lymphocytes, and plasma cells (Figs. 4.11 and 4.12).

Chronic inflammation occurs as a result of many types of infection, including tuberculosis, syphilis, and fungal infections. In certain diseases (e.g., rheumatoid arthritis and systemic lupus erythematosis), inflammation is due to immunologic disturbances. Chronic inflammation is also seen in response to the introduction of foreign bodies, e.g., around suture material or in particulate debris generated by total joint replacement procedures.

The inflammatory reaction serves as a defense against further tissue damage, a means by which the injurious agent is removed or rendered innocuous, and a means by which necrotic tissue is either removed or sequestered. The last component of the inflammatory reaction to be considered here is the healing phase (repair).

The damaged area may eventually be restored with tissue similar to the original via regeneration, or replaced by fibrous connective tissue (scar tissue), but usually by a combination of these two processes. Various tissues of the body differ in their ability to regenerate. In general, the skin, the epithelium of the gastrointestinal tract and the respiratory tract, and bone all regenerate well, though the anatomy may not be restored to normal. However, the more specialized and differentiated tissues are more limited in their regenerative power.

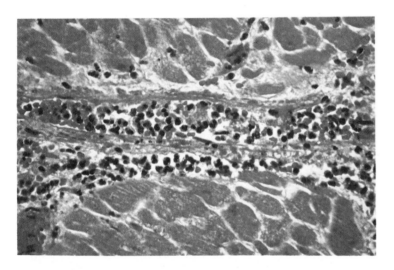

Fig. 4.10 This photomicrograph illustrates what takes place during an acute inflammatory reaction brought on by tissue necrosis (in this case, specifically, by myocardial infarction). A small capillary is seen congested with blood and with many more PMNs than would normally be expected. These PMNs have infiltrated through the vessel wall by diapedesis and are now seen in the perivascular tissue.

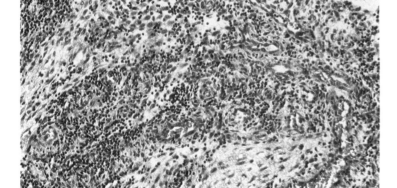

Fig. 4.11 In this photomicrograph, one can discern that a chronic inflammatory reaction has taken place by the extensive infiltration of mononuclear cells.

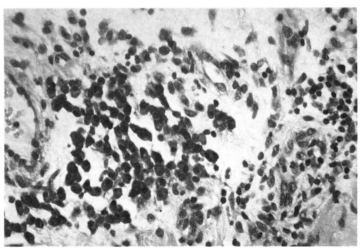

Fig. 4.12 In this high power photomicrograph, one can see a chronic inflammatory infiltrate within the perivascular tissue, which exhibits the characteristics of lymphocytes and plasma cells.

In the medical and surgical management of injured tissues, an important objective is the prevention of delayed healing or excessive scarring. The clinician should take every opportunity to promote regulated healing. These therapeutic measures include wound debridement, adequate administration of antibiotics, use of nonreactive suture material, and good operative technique. The avoidance of drugs or at least care in the use of drugs that suppress the inflammatory reaction (e.g., cortisone) is important, and the assurance of adequate intake of those substances necessary for wound healing (protein and vitamin C) is essential.

During most of the inflammatory response to injury, the exudative and reparative events take place side by side, though the exudative features predominate in the early stages of the process, and the reparative features become more prominent after the removal or neutralization of injurious agents and the removal of necrotic tissue by the macrophages. In the reparative stage, the most characteristic histologic finding is the proliferation of fibroblasts that produce the structural extracellular matrix, composed of collagen, proteoglycan, and other noncollagenous proteins (Fig. 4.13). These substances give body and strength to the new tissue.

REPAIR OF CONNECTIVE TISSUES FOLLOWING TRAUMA

Surgical Wound Healing. In the case of a surgical wound, all tissue in the path of the knife blade (including the epithelium, fibrous connective tissues, blood vessels, nerves, fat, etc.) is injured either reversibly or irreversibly. When the wound edges have been apposed and the sutures applied, a thin clot fills the space between the apposed wound edges, and mediators of inflammation induce an acute inflammatory reaction. However, in the absence of bacterial contamination, the leukocytic infiltrate is not marked. The macrophages rapidly mobilize to remove red blood cells, fibrin, and damaged cellular tissue. Meanwhile, the fibroblasts on either side of the wound hypertrophy and migrate together with capillary sprouts, and within a few days circulation is reestablished across the margins of the wound.

As the fibroblasts begin to lay down collagen, the cellular inflammatory infiltrate diminishes. The epithelial cells at the surface begin to undergo mitosis and to migrate over the vascularized granulation tissue. In the case of a nonlinear wound, as the epithelial cells migrate over the granulation tissue, they extend beneath the fibrin clot (scab) that closes off the surface of the wound.

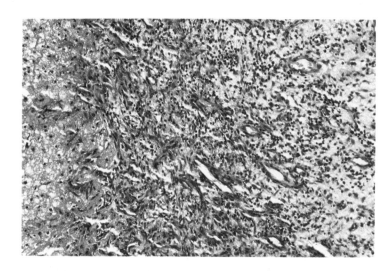

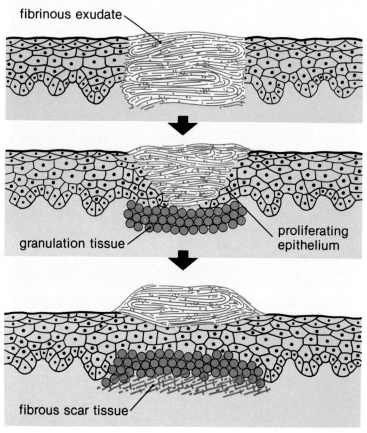

Fig. 4.13 Photomicrograph of granulation tissue in an early stage of repair. Note the fibrin clot on the left, and the proliferating fibroblasts and capillaries interspersed with chronic inflammatory cells toward the right.

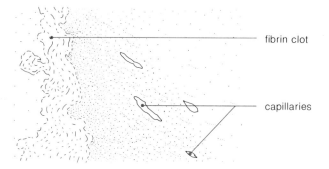

Fig. 4.14 Schematic diagram illustrates the healing process in epithelial tissue following ulceration. The wound is first filled with a fibrinous exudate composed of acute inflammatory cells. Gradually, this is replaced by granulation tissue, with proliferating epithelium extending from the margins of the wound, over the granulation tissue, and beneath the residual fibrin on the surface. As the epithelium completely re-covers the wound, the dried-up layer of fibrin forms a scab which eventually falls off.

When the epithelium is firmly reestablished underneath the scab, the scab usually sloughs off (Fig. 4.14).

The suture material that has been used to appose the wound edges frequently causes a foreign-body giant-cell reaction (Fig. 4.15), and may also act as a track along which bacteria may travel. With infection, healing will be delayed until the infection has been overcome. Healing may also be delayed if there is poor circulation in the area or if the patient is severely debilitated.

Muscles. Muscle tissue, contrary to what is often believed, regenerates well, but the restoration of normal structure and function depends very much on the type of injury that the muscle has sustained. In severe infections, the muscle fibers may be extensively destroyed. However, the sarcolemmal sheaths usually remain intact, and rapid regeneration of muscle cells within the sheaths occurs, so that the function of the muscle may be completely restored (Fig. 4.16).

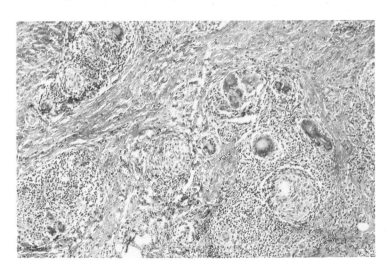

Fig. 4.15 The introduction of foreign matter in tissue frequently results in a chronic inflammatory reaction, with proliferating macrophages digesting the foreign material. The photomicrograph at left shows giant cells and chronic

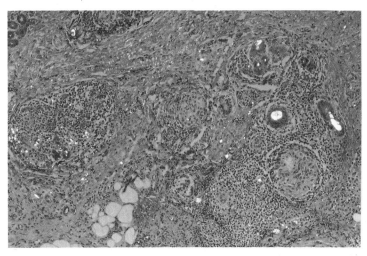

inflammatory cells, giving the appearance of a granulomatous inflammation. However, under polarized light *(right)*, one can clearly see the fragments of suture material which gave rise to this reaction.

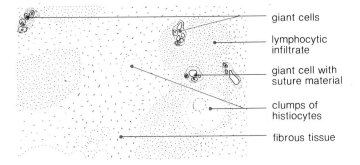

- giant cells
- lymphocytic infiltrate
- giant cell with suture material
- clumps of histiocytes
- fibrous tissue

Fig. 4.16 Photomicrograph shows the appearance of a regenerating muscle fiber. Note the basophilic cytoplasm and the centrally located nuclei.

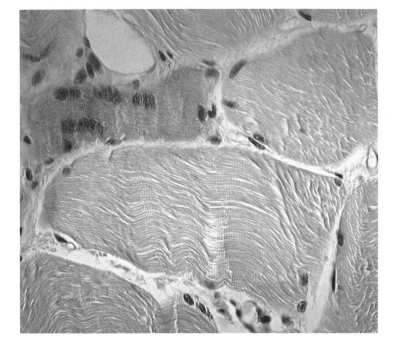

Following the transection of a muscle, muscle fibers may regenerate either by growing from undamaged stumps or by growth of new independent fibers. The nuclei for both of these processes are derived from the satellite or reserve cells found in the endomysium. It should be noted that, at the same time that the muscle fibers are regenerating and growing, there is also an ingrowth into the damaged muscle of capillaries and fibroblasts, with accompanying production of collagen; this scarring usually overrides and prevents muscle fiber regeneration (Fig. 4.17). However, in muscle regeneration and healing, much depends upon the alignment of the supportive structures by meticulous surgical restoration.

Tendons. Tendons may heal either as a result of proliferation of the tenoblasts from the cut ends of the tendon, or, more likely, as a result of vascular ingrowth and fibroblasts derived from the surrounding tissues that were injured at the same time as the tendon. Because the surrounding tissues contribute so much to the healing of a tendon, adhesions are very common. To avoid this com-

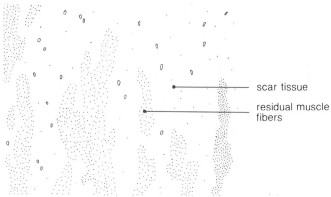

Fig. 4.17 Photomicrograph of damaged myocardial tissue shows extensive fibrous scarring, with only a few muscle fibers enmeshed in the dense scar tissue. This scarring blocks any potential there may be for regeneration and restoration of the muscle tissue.

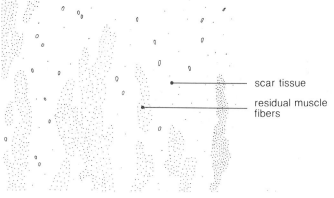

scar tissue

residual muscle fibers

Fig. 4.18 Following nerve damage, the proximal stump of the damaged nerve demonstrates proliferation of Schwann cells and, eventually, of axons. Unless the nerve fascicles are meticulously approximated, adequate restoration of the nerve fibers will not occur. This photomicrograph shows the proximal stump to the right, and a tangled mass of proliferating (regenerative) Schwann cells and axons to the left.

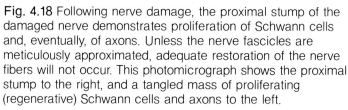

Fig. 4.19 In the development of a bone fracture, the propagation of cracks is likely to follow the cement lines. In a hypermetabolic bone disease such as Paget's disease, shown in this photomicrograph, the cement lines increase in number, significantly weakening the bone structure.

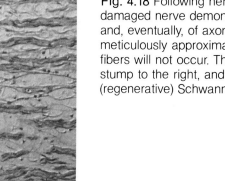

plication, the repair of tendons requires meticulous atraumatic technique.

Peripheral Nerves. When a nerve fiber is divided, the peripheral portion rapidly undergoes myelin degeneration and axonal fragmentation. The lipid debris is removed by macrophages mobilized from the surrounding tissues. In the central stump, the nerve fibers retract, and the axons adjacent to the cut degenerate. However, within 24 hours of section, new axonal sprouts from the central stump can usually be demonstrated, together with a proliferation of Schwann cells from both the central and peripheral stumps (Fig. 4.18). With careful microsurgical approximation of the nerve, function may be achieved. The most important feature of nerve regeneration is the maintenance of the neurotubules along which the new axonal sprouts may pass.

Bone. Fracture of the bone results from mechanical injury. The force required to produce a fracture in bone depends upon the strength of the bone itself. (Many fractures seen in hospital practice are in elderly people, and most fractures of the femoral neck and of the wrist have occurred as the result of osteoporosis and weakening of bones. Fractures may also result from weakening of the bone due to local disease such as tumor or infection.)

The gross appearance of a fracture depends upon the microstructure of the bone tissue. Bone is a composite material, and it is also anisotropic (see Chapter 1). Bone's most important features, in terms of fracture propagation, are its numerous weak interfaces (cement lines) and the osteocytic lacunae and canaliculi dispersed throughout its structure. The osteocytic lacunae can act as sites of crack initiation, and the cement lines that are aligned predominantly in a longitudinal direction in the cortical bone provide the major planes of fracture propagation (Fig. 4.19). In diseases in which the microstructure of bone is markedly disturbed, as for example in osteopetrosis or Paget's disease (see Chapter 3), the patterns of fracture (usually transverse in a long bone) reflect the disturbance in microarchitecture.

The direction in which a load is applied will also determine the direction of the fracture. In general, tensile loads cause flat fractures, whereas compressive loads result in oblique fractures and, usually, greater damage to the bone. Bending forces cause fractures that have the combined features of both tensile and compressive fractures, and torsional loads usually result in helical fractures (Fig. 4.20).

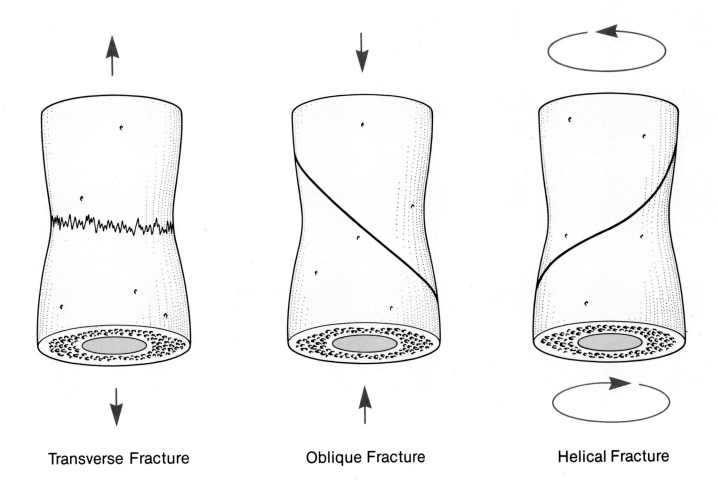

Transverse Fracture   Oblique Fracture   Helical Fracture

Fig. 4.20 The following diagrams illustrate three different kinds of fractures, and how they are caused. *(Left)* Transverse fracture, caused by traction (pulling force). *(Center)* Oblique fracture, caused by compression. *(Right)* Helical fracture, caused by torsion.

Repeated stress to the bone, as occurs in long-distance running and walking, may result in the development of stress (or fatigue) fractures in which the accumulation of microfractures eventually results in a complete fracture through the bone cortex (Fig. 4.21). Such a lesion will occur without a history of significant mechanical trauma and, as a result, the nature of the lesion may be misinterpreted by the clinician, radiologist, or pathologist as a neoplasm.

Repeated trauma at ligamentous and tendinous insertions may result in an avulsion fracture at these sites.

In young adolescents, these types of injury are most likely to occur in and around the pelvis, particularly at the origins of the adductor muscles along the inferior pubic ramus adjacent to the symphysis pubis; the lower head of the rectus femoris just above the acetabulum; and the origins of the hamstring muscles at the ischial tuberosity, as well as the insertions of the gluteus at the greater trochanter and the psoas at the lesser trochanter. Repeated trauma at the insertion of the adductor muscles of the thigh may result in a bony spur on the lower medial aspect of the femur, often referred to as a rider's spur

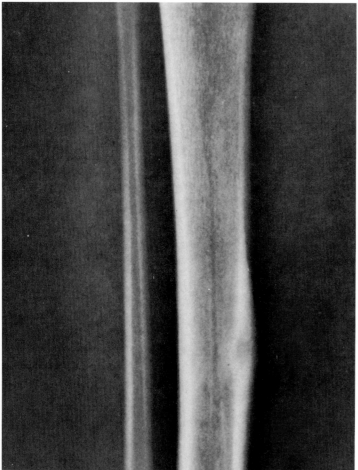

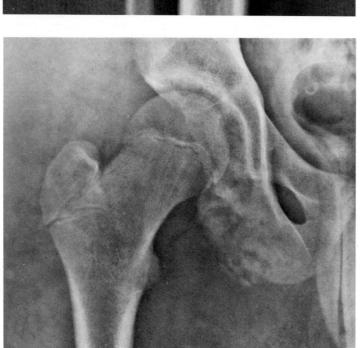

Fig. 4.21 Clinical roentgenogram of a stress fracture of the leg. A patient with this type of fracture usually does not have a history of trauma, and presents clinically with pain and swelling in the affected parts following strenuous physical activity. The periosteal elevation combined with a lack of displacement or obvious fracture line through the bone may lead to this fracture being misdiagnosed radiographically as a tumor. Even if a biopsy is obtained, the hypercellular appearance of the callus may lead the pathologist to believe that this is a cellular bone-forming neoplasm or, as in this case, an osteoid osteoma.

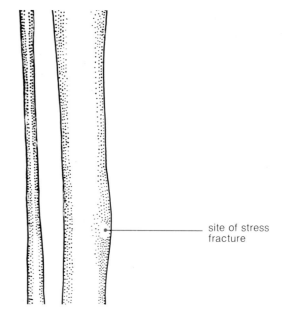

site of stress fracture

Fig. 4.22 Clinical roentgenogram shows an avulsion fracture in the pelvis. Note the fragmentation due to avulsion injury of the ischial tuberosity. This fracture, like the stress fracture in Fig. 4.21, may well lead to misdiagnosis as a tumor.

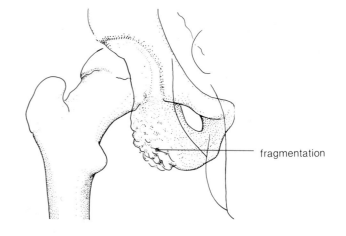

fragmentation

because it is commonly seen in people who ride horses. At these sites, the nature of the lesion may be mistaken for a malignant tumor (Fig. 4.22).

In children around the ages of 10 and 11, avulsion fractures are also seen at the tibial tubercle, where the effects of the injury and eventual repair result in a lesion known as Osgood-Schlatter disease (Fig. 4.23).

Fortunately, the healing of bone is one of the great successes of nature. Under favorable conditions, bone can be regenerated and remodeled to function optimally. The single most important factor in the primary healing of a fracture is complete immobilization of the fractured ends. In nature, this immobilization is achieved through the production of immature bone and cartilage matrix under the periosteum as well as in the soft tissues around the broken ends of the bone. This repair tissue is referred to as the fracture callus (Fig. 4.24).

The amount of callus produced depends upon a number of factors, including the degree of instability and the vascularity of the injured bone. In unstable fractures, the amount of callus is usually increased, and the callus often contains much cartilage tissue (Fig. 4.25). In poorly

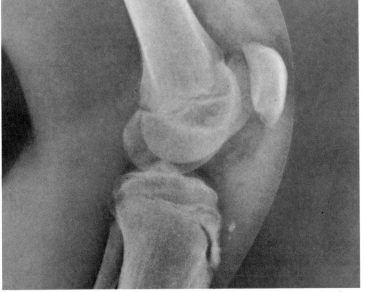

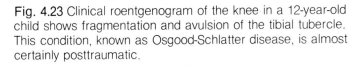

Fig. 4.23 Clinical roentgenogram of the knee in a 12-year-old child shows fragmentation and avulsion of the tibial tubercle. This condition, known as Osgood-Schlatter disease, is almost certainly posttraumatic.

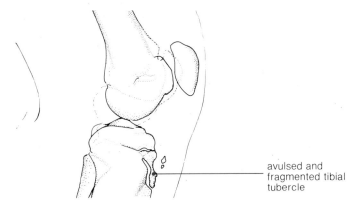

avulsed and fragmented tibial tubercle

Fig. 4.24 Low power photomicrograph shows reparative new bone that has formed in the soft tissue and periosteum which surrounds a fractured rib. Restoration of bone cortex and medulla depends on complete immobilization of the fracture site, which is naturally accomplished through the formation of external callus. However, where a fracture is treated by rigid internal fixation, external callus may not be evident.

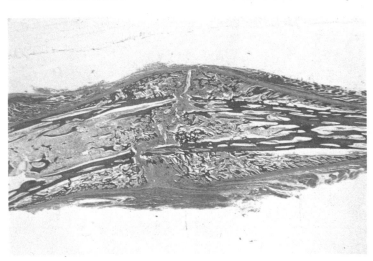

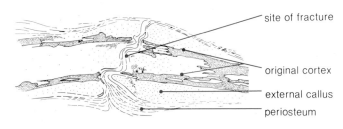

site of fracture

original cortex

external callus

periosteum

Fig. 4.25 A normal fracture callus contains variable amounts of bone, cartilage, and fibrous tissue. However, where a fracture is unstable or where a fracture site is poorly vascularized, an abundance of cartilage will be found, as seen in this photomicrograph.

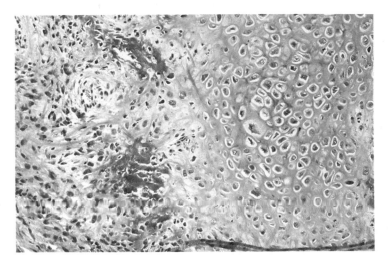

vascularized areas of the skeleton (e.g., the midshaft of the tibia), callus formation may be scant; consequently, healing may be delayed, sometimes indefinitely. This delay gives rise to chronic nonunion of the fracture site (Fig. 4.26).

When a fracture occurs, the amount of injury sustained by the tissues depends on the direction and magnitude of the force applied. The bone fragments may be displaced. The fracture line may be single (a simple fracture), or the

bone may be broken into many fragments (a comminuted fracture). If the skin over the fractured bone is also broken, it is considered a compound fracture, and infection is a common complication. In some cases, soft tissue may become interposed between the fractured ends of the bone, causing healing to be significantly delayed. For all these reasons, the histologic appearance of the reparative tissue surrounding a fracture may vary greatly.

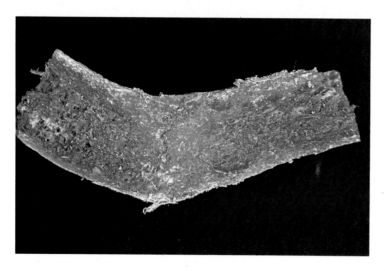

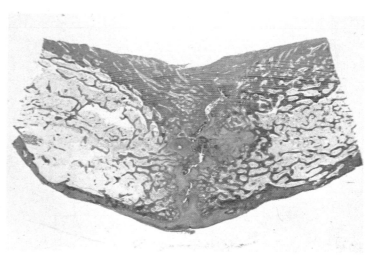

Fig. 4.26 In a poorly vascularized or extremely unstable fracture, healing may be delayed and, on occasions, may not even occur at all. In such a case, a false joint or pseudarthrosis

will be formed. *(Left)* Gross specimen of a false joint. *(Right)* Histologic appearance of a false joint.

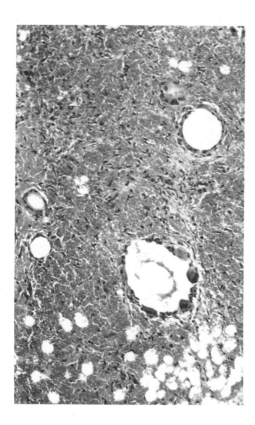

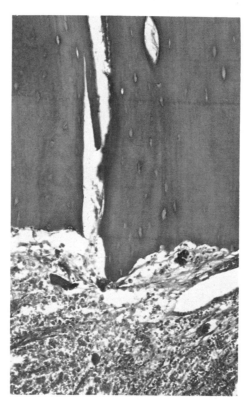

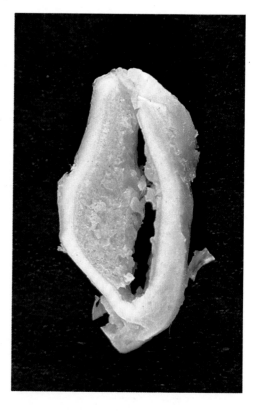

Fig. 4.27 Photomicrograph of tissue obtained from the area around a fracture site shows extensive hemorrhage and a large fat cyst surrounded by giant cells, characteristic of fat necrosis.

Fig. 4.28 Photomicrograph of the broken end of a bone taken one week after the fracture demonstrates both hemorrhage and bone necrosis. Note that the osteocytic lacunae in the bone are completely empty.

Fig. 4.29 Following injury, the blood supply may be so compromised as to cause complete necrosis of the affected tissue. In this gross specimen, complete osteonecrosis of the carpal lunate bone has occurred. The necrotic bone is recognized by its opaque-yellow appearance.

Tissue obtained within a few days of injury usually shows areas of hemorrhage and acute tissue damage (Fig. 4.27). The bone on either side of the fracture tissue undergoes necrosis, the extent of which depends on the local anatomy (Fig. 4.28). Fractures of the femoral neck, of some of the carpal and tarsal bones, and of the patella frequently demonstrate widespread bone necrosis because the local vascular supply is so severely compromised (Fig. 4.29). In a comminuted fracture, the separate bone fragments are likely to undergo necrosis, and if the necrosis is extensive it will delay healing.

Microscopic examination of tissue from a two-week-old fracture callus reveals markedly cellular tissue, usually hypervascular, that produces irregular islands and trabeculae of immature bone and cartilage matrix (Figs. 4.30 and 4.31). The hypercellularity and disordered organization may produce a pseudosarcomatous appearance in the tissue (Figs. 4.32 and 4.33). Since a biopsy

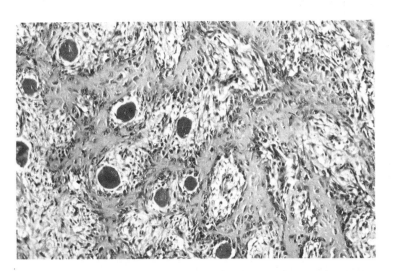

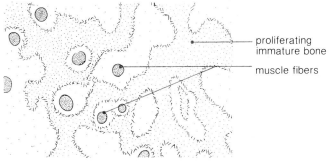

Fig. 4.30 Photomicrograph of a fracture callus obtained from the soft tissue around a two-week-old fracture demonstrates proliferating trabeculae of immature cellular bone growing around and between muscle fibers. This histologic finding could be misdiagnosed as an infiltrating bone-forming tumor.

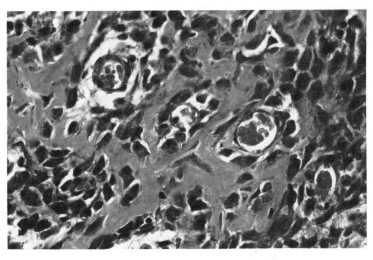

Fig. 4.31 Higher power photomicrograph demonstrates the immature and cellular appearance of a fracture callus.

Fig. 4.32 Lower power photomicrograph demonstrates the hypercellular, proliferative appearance of callus, which in this case shows only minimal bone matrix formation. The pseudosarcomatous appearance of this tissue may result in misdiagnosis.

Fig. 4.33 Photomicrograph of a fracture callus taken from the area around a ten-day-old fracture. Note the proliferating cartilage and immature bone to the left, and the degenerate muscle fibers to the right.

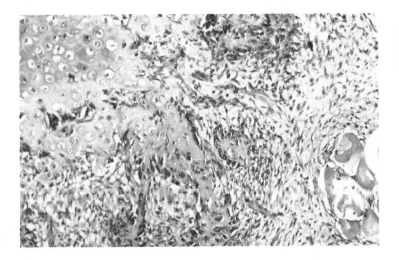

is not likely to be taken unless the clinician has failed to recognize the traumatic origin of the patient's complaints, the pseudosarcomatous appearance of the callus may easily lead to errors in interpretation by the pathologist. Such errors are most likely to occur in diagnosing patients with stress fractures, from whom a history of injury is not usually forthcoming. Since stress fractures are common in young people following strenuous exercise (the same age group in which osteosarcomas are most often seen), recognition of the true nature of the problem is important and, on occasion, is among the most difficult problems in differential diagnosis for the pathologist (Fig. 4.34).

Once the callus is sufficient to immobilize the fracture site, repair occurs between the cortical and medullary bones. When this has been achieved, the callus is remodeled and eventually disappears. Very little callus is produced when a fracture is treated with rigid internal or external surgical fixation, and primary healing of the bone proceeds without the abundant external callus seen in association with unstable fractures.

Cartilage. The healing of cartilage is adversely affected by two factors: its avascularity and its low cell-to-matrix ratio. Nevertheless, it is essential to recognize that cartilage cells can indeed proliferate, and that in arthritis, where the cartilage is damaged, cartilage regeneration with both cartilage cell proliferation (Fig. 4.35) and cartilage matrix production (Fig. 4.36) is a regular feature.

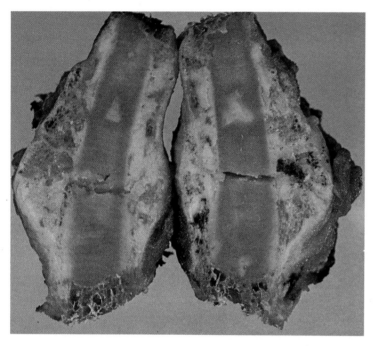

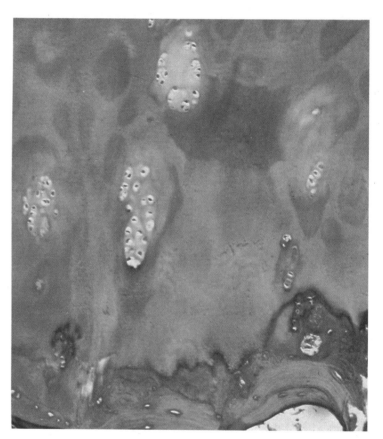

Fig. 4.35 Following injury to cartilage tissue resulting in cell death, proliferation of groups or clones of reparative chondrocytes may appear, as seen in this photomicrograph.

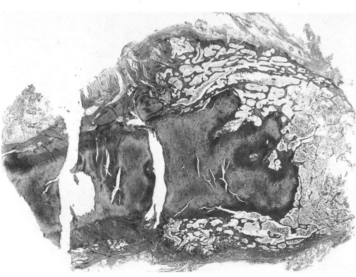

Fig. 4.34 A segment of the costochondral junction was resected from a patient who presented with a swelling in the region *(upper)*. Roentgenographic examination revealed extreme density, which was interpreted by both the clinician and the radiologist as a form of neoplasm. However, the histologic preparation of the resected specimen *(lower)* shows a fracture through the calcified costal cartilage, surrounded by a mass of firm tissue. This is the histologic picture expected of a fracture callus.

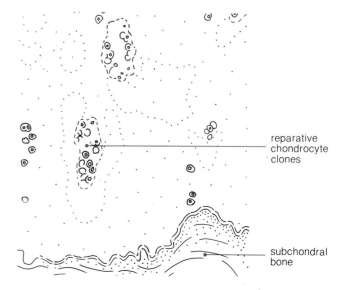

reparative chondrocyte clones

subchondral bone

The ability of cartilage cells to produce an adequate matrix and to restore functional tissue probably depends upon their mechanical environment. Following an injury to the articular surface, as may occur in an athletic injury, continued irritation will probably result in a worsening of the condition.

The Menisci of the Knee. The menisci are composed mainly of collagen, although some proteoglycan is also present. From examination of carefully oriented sections,

it has been shown that the principal orientation of the collagen fibers in the menisci is circumferential. The few, small, radially disposed fibers that do occur exist primarily on the tibial surface. The circumferential orientation of most of the collagen fibers appears designed to withstand the circumferential tension within the meniscus during normal loading. The radially disposed fibers probably act as ties to resist any longitudinal splitting of the menisci that may result from undue compression (Fig. 4.37).

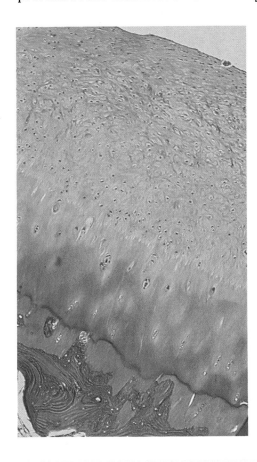 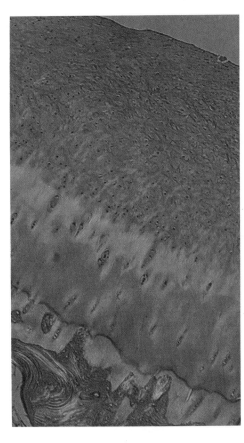

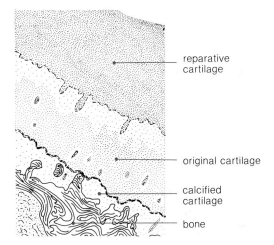

Fig. 4.36 Following cartilage damage, there may be regeneration of both cartilage cells and matrix. The photomicrograph at left shows normal cartilage in the center, covered by a thick layer of reparative cartilage. Viewed under polarized light *(right)* one can appreciate the alteration in the collagen structure of the matrix. The concept of articular cartilage repair is an important consideration in the management of patients with arthritis.

reparative cartilage

original cartilage

calcified cartilage

bone

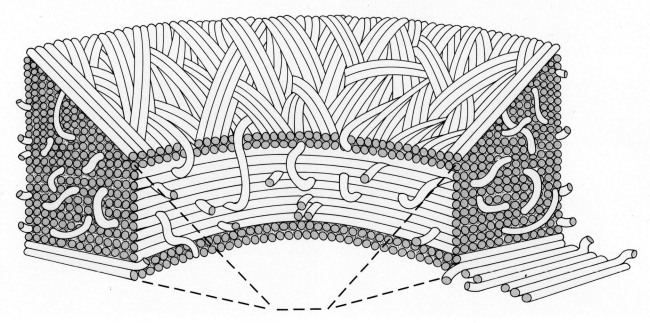

Fig. 4.37 Diagrammatic representation of the distribution of collagen fibers in the meniscus of a knee. Collagen is orientated throughout the connective tissues in such a way as to maximally resist the forces which are brought to bear on these tissues. The majority of the fibers are circumferentially arranged; a few radially arranged fibers, particularly on the tibial surface, resist lateral spread of the meniscus. In the case of a meniscus tension is generated between the anterior and posterior attachments.

The menisci of young individuals are usually white, have a translucent quality, and are supple on palpation. The menisci in older individuals lose their translucency, become more opaque and yellow in color, and feel less supple (Fig. 4.38).

Lacerations of the meniscus lead to symptoms that require surgical treatment in two groups of patients: young active patients in whom injury is frequently related to athletic activity, and older individuals in whom degeneration leads to laceration. Most lacerations occur in the posterior horn of the meniscus and, more commonly, in the medial meniscus. They usually occur as clefts that run along the circumferentially directed collagen fibers (Fig.

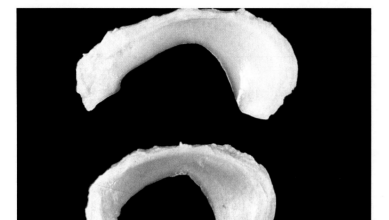

Fig. 4.38 Gross photographs of menisci obtained from a young *(upper)* and an old *(lower)* patient. In contrast to the meniscus from the young patient which has a bluish-white color and is supple, the meniscus from the old patient has a characteristically yellowish color and feels stiffer on palpation.

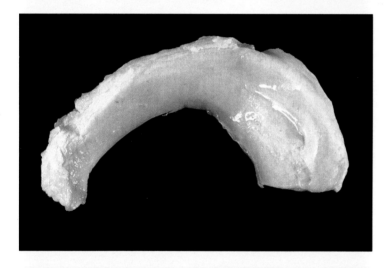

Fig. 4.39 Gross photograph of a medial meniscus with an early tear in the posterior horn. Characteristically, these tears occur as clefts in the substance of the meniscus and run in the direction of the collagen fibers.

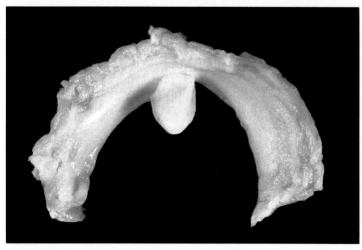

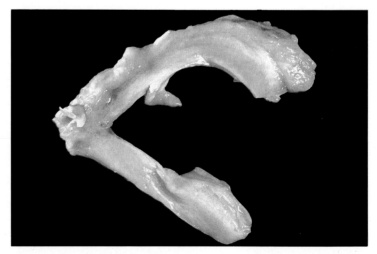

Fig. 4.40 Occasionally, a tear, such as that shown in Fig. 4.39, will extend onto the medial margin and form a tag which extends into the joint space. Such a tag may become smoothed off at its margins, as seen in this specimen.

Fig. 4.41 Extension of the meniscal tear along the length of the meniscus may result in a bucket-handle tear, as demonstrated in this photograph.

4.39). Such a cleft may extend in time to the medial margin of the meniscus and create a tag, which eventually may become quite smooth (Fig. 4.40). Extension of the tear may lead to the bucket-handle deformity (Fig. 4.41). On occasion, the meniscus shows peripheral detachment, again usually posteriorly.

The advent of arthroscopy and arthrography have assisted in the clinical diagnosis of tears in the menisci. They help localize tears and, where injury is limited in scope, have facilitated partial meniscectomies.

In histologic sections of torn menisci, evidence of both injury and repair may be seen, with the findings likely to be time-dependent (Fig. 4.42). It is difficult to determine whether histologic changes of degeneration seen at the time of meniscectomy are the result of or contribute to the tear (Fig. 4.43). The presence of a horizontal cleavage in the posterior horn of the meniscus is found at autopsy in over 50 per cent of older individuals.

SUMMARY

Following injury, effects occur locally in both the cells and the tissue, and also systemically. The response of the body to injury (the inflammatory response) is effected mainly through the vascular system. The purpose of the inflammatory response is to restore the body's status quo. In the case of minor injuries that frequently befall all of us, the status quo is indeed restored. But in the case of more severe injury, a new status quo that may result in some disability is likely to occur.

Trauma plays a contributory role in a number of diseases of the skeletal system including osteoarthritis, slipped capital femoral epiphysis, congenital pseudarthrosis, myositis ossificans, interdigital (Morton's) neuroma of the foot, etc. However, in many of these disease states predisposing conditions may exist, all of which are not clearly understood at this time.

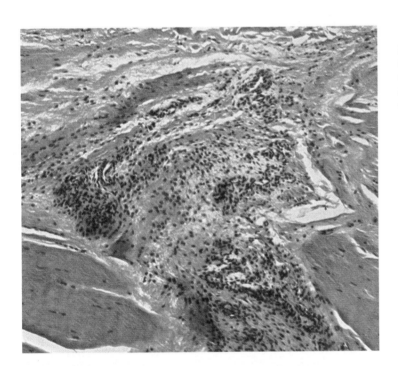

Fig. 4.42 Photomicrograph of an area of laceration in a meniscus. On both the right and left side one can see intact collagen fibers, while in the center a defect filled with granulation tissue is evident. Repair is much more likely to be seen in the peripheral third of the substance of the meniscus where the tissue is vascularized.

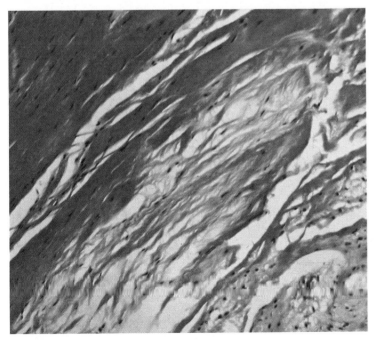

Fig. 4.43 Photomicrograph of meniscal tissue shows foci of normal-appearing collagen in the upper left; splitting of the collagen fibers, which appear to be frayed and open, in the middle; and some myxomatous tissue, possibly the result of degenerative changes, in the lower right.

5 Diseases Resulting from the Deposition of Metabolic Products and Hematologic Disorders

DISEASES RESULTING FROM THE DEPOSITION OF METABOLIC PRODUCTS

EXAMINATION OF SYNOVIAL FLUID FOR CRYSTALS

An important diagnostic procedure in the clinical diagnosis of crystal synovitis is the examination of synovial fluid for crystals, and the recognition of these crystals by the use of polarized light microscopy.

In order to perform this examination, one must have a polarizing microscope with a compensating first order red filter. With the red filter in position, the crystals in the synovial fluid should be aligned so that their long axis is parallel to the line that is drawn on the compensating filter, which is the axis of slow vibration (Fig. 5.1). Sodium urate crystals are generally needle-shaped and show strong negative birefringence; that is, they appear bright

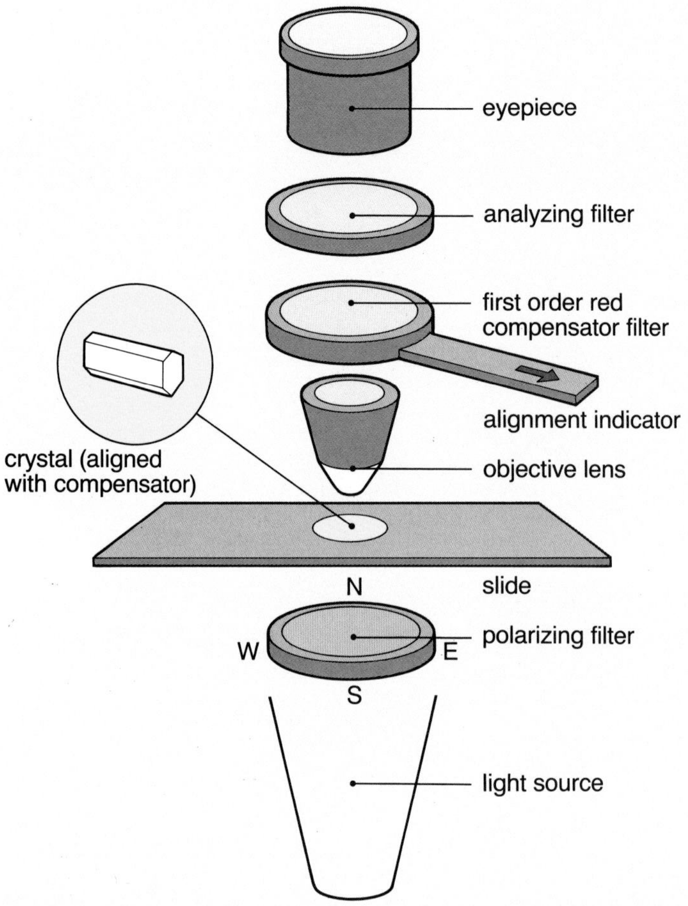

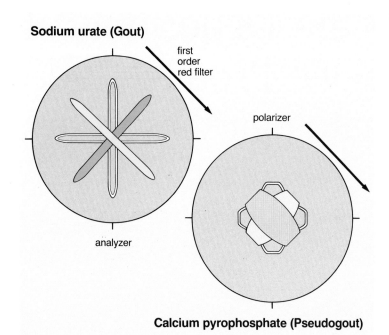

eyepiece

analyzing filter

first order red compensator filter

alignment indicator

crystal (aligned with compensator)

objective lens

slide

N

polarizing filter

W   E

S

light source

Fig. 5.1 The light is first passed through a polarizing filter that is usually oriented east-west. The polarizing filter will lie somewhere between the light source and the object being examined. The analyzing filter will lie between the object being examined and the observer, and usually the analyzer is oriented north-south. Generally, a refractile body will show maximum refraction when the axis of the body is oriented at 45 degrees to the axis of the polarizing filter and the analyzing filter. When the axis of the body being examined is either parallel to or at right angles to the orientation marks on the polarizing filter, it does not refract, and these points are called the extinction points. The use of a first order red compensator filter allows the observer to distinguish between positive and negative birefringence.

Sodium urate (Gout)

first order red filter

polarizer

analyzer

Calcium pyrophosphate (Pseudogout)

Fig. 5.2 In this illustration the effect of rotating a crystal of calcium pyrophosphate dihydrate or sodium urate through 90 degrees is seen. With the crystal lying at 45 degrees to the orientation line on the polarizing filter, and parallel to the orientation line on the first order red compensator filter, the calcium pyrophosphate dihydrate crystal appears faintly blue. This appearance is described as weak positive birefringence. However, when the crystal is observed perpendicular to the orientation line, rather than parallel to the orientation line, it will appear pale yellow. In the case of sodium urate, when the crystal is parallel to the orientation line it appears bright yellow, and we speak of this appearance as strong negative birefringence. When the crystal is perpendicular to the orientation line of the first order compensator filter, it appears bright blue.

yellow when aligned parallel with the line on the compensating filter. Calcium pyrophosphate dihydrate crystals are usually rhomboidal crystals, and they show a weak positive birefringence, which is to say that when their long axis is aligned with the line on the compensating filter, they appear blue and much less bright than urate crystals (Fig. 5.2).

There are two important facts to note: (1) When a crystal is oriented at 90 degrees to the line on the compensating filter, it will appear the opposite color to which it appears when parallel; and (2) the shape of the crystal may be misleading, because pyrophosphate crystals are occasionally needle-shaped, and urate crystals may be broken up into short squared-off fragments (Figs. 5.3 and 5.4).

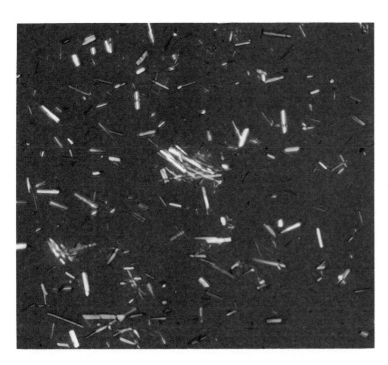

Fig. 5.3 (*left*) Multiple short pieces of crystalline material are seen in aspirated fluid. Despite their shape, these are sodium urate crystals.

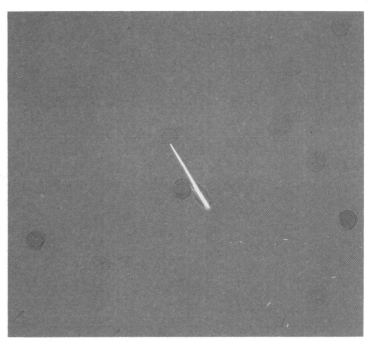

Fig. 5.3 (*right*) Needle-shaped crystal in a synovial fluid sample. When this crystal was aligned with the indicator on the compensating filter, it appeared bright yellow and so was identified as a sodium urate crystal.

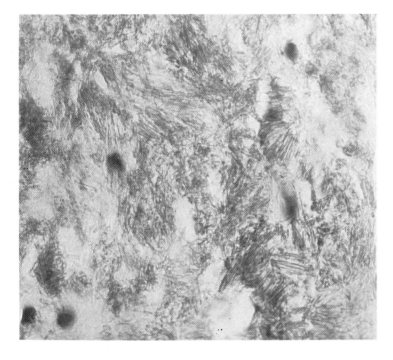

Fig. 5.4 (*left*) Tissue removed from a patient with calcium pyrophosphate dihydrate deposition disease. The crystals are needle-shaped rather than rhomboidal; however they are only weakly birefringent.

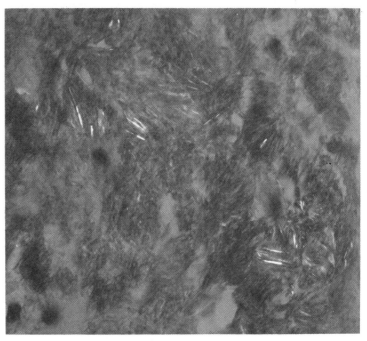

Fig. 5.4 (*right*) Same field viewed under polarized light.

GOUT

Gout occurs either as an inherited or an acquired disease, usually in men. Patients with gout present with hyperuricemia and acute attacks of crystal-induced inflammation in the joints and in the kidneys. Primary gout is an inherited error of metabolism that results from an enzymatic defect in purine synthesis and/or in the renal excretion of uric acid. However, hyperuricemia occurs most often as a condition secondary to disorders that increase the production or decrease the excretion of uric acid. These disorders include the myeloproliferative disorders, in which there is an increased turnover of nucleic acid, and various forms of chronic renal disease. In patients with cancer, in whom the breakdown of cells and the turnover of nucleoprotein is abnormally rapid, hyperuricemia is commonly observed. The prolonged presence of hyperuricemia eventually leads to the deposition of monosodium urate crystals in both the joints and the visceral tissue, but especially in the kidneys, in which precipitates of urates and subsequent stone formation are seen in nearly all patients with gout.

Gout may be divided into three clinical stages: acute gouty arthritis, an intermediate stage called intercritical gout, and the chronic stage in which diffuse deposits are seen (chronic tophaceous gout). Acute gouty arthritis is usually monoarticular, with a particular predilection for the lower extremities. The first metatarsal phalangeal joint (the great toe) is the most common site of initial involvement. Acute gout is characterized by the rapid onset of severe pain and swelling, often accompanied by a low-grade fever and leukocytosis. Between attacks of acute gout, the patient may have long periods in which he is

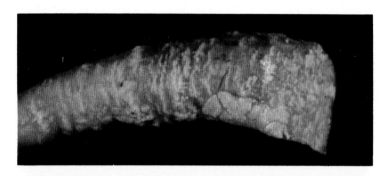

Fig. 5.5 Segment of a tendon with extensive tophaceous gout deposits.

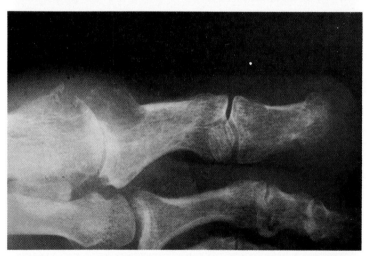

Fig. 5.6 Roentgenogram of the great toe shows involvement of the first metatarsal phalangeal joint. Overlying the joint there is soft tissue swelling, and at the joint margin a clearcut bony erosion with a characteristic overhanging edge. There is no porosis of the surrounding bone, as would be seen in a patient with rheumatoid arthritis.

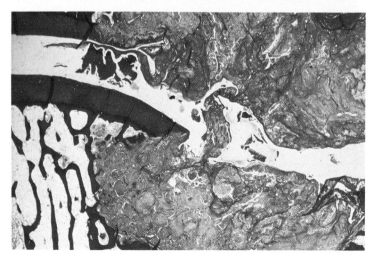

Fig. 5.7 Low power photomicrograph of a portion of the joint shown in Fig. 5.6. The erosion of the bone and articular cartilage by an amorphous material is evident.

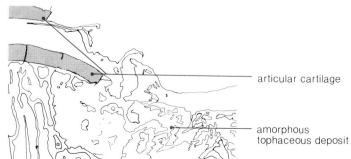

articular cartilage

amorphous tophaceous deposit

clinically asymptomatic, even though the hyperuricemia persists. Eventually the state of chronic tophaceous gout occurs, in which the deposition of monosodium urate crystals occurs throughout the body, but particularly in the kidneys and para-articular regions (Fig. 5.5). Although the reason for the deposition of crystals is not understood, the process is known to be accelerated by the presence of a low pH, as seen in the joint spaces.

The roentgenographic features of gout include the swelling of the soft tissues and the subsequent erosion of the joint space, giving rise to the classic punched-out lesion. Radiologic examinations in these patients reveal little reactive sclerosis and, in contrast to films from patients with rheumatoid arthritis, no regional osteoporosis (Fig. 5.6).

In patients with acute gouty synovitis, the microscopic examination of the synovial fluid reveals an inflammatory exudate, which may seem to be evidence of an infection. However, further examination by polarized light using a first order red filter reveals crystals with a strong negative birefringence, characteristically found in polymorphonuclear leukocytes. The chalky tophi seen in the chronic phase of the disease consist of large deposits of crystals surrounded by fibrous tissue and rimmed by both mononuclear cells and giant cells (Figs. 5.7 to 5.10). (It should be noted that preservation of the crystals for identification with polarized light microscopy requires alcohol fixation to prevent their dissolution in the aqueous solutions used in routine formalin processing procedures, and staining by the de Galantha method.)

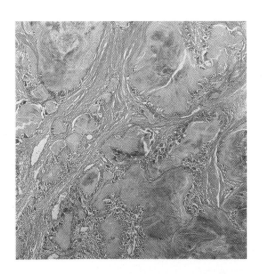
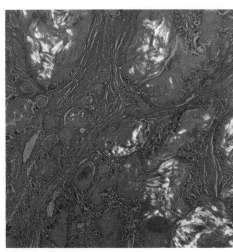

Fig 5.8 Low power photomicrograph of a tophaceous deposit (*left*). A bluish amorphous material is seen surrounded by bundles of dense collagenized tissue and inflammatory cells. The same field examined by polarized light (*right*). The birefringence of the crystalline material is evident. (Preservation of the crystals requires fixation in alcohol.)

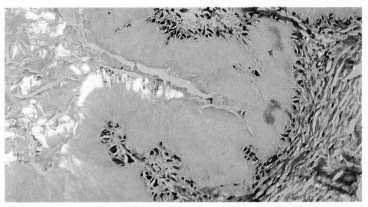

Fig. 5.9 Photomicrograph at somewhat higher power shows a detail of the field shown in Fig. 5.8. Surrounding the amorphous crystalline deposit is a thin layer of mononuclear and giant cells, with an occasional sprinkling of chronic inflammatory cells.

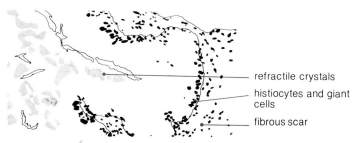

refractile crystals

histiocytes and giant cells

fibrous scar

Fig. 5.10 Photomicrograph of another section of tophaceous gout fixed in alcohol. This section has been stained by de Galantha's method for the demonstration of monosodium urate crystals.

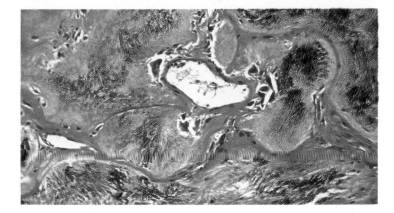

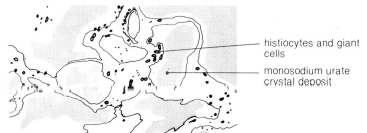

histiocytes and giant cells

monosodium urate crystal deposit

CHONDROCALCINOSIS

Pseudogout, calcium pyrophosphate dihydrate (CPPD) crystal deposition disease

Disease resulting from the deposition of calcium pyrophosphate has been recognized only recently. Initially the term chondrocalcinosis was introduced to describe a familial condition with typical radiologic changes. The term pseudogout came into use later because of the gout-like symptoms with which many of the patients present. Since the disease may clinically mimic many conditions, including rheumatoid arthritis, osteoarthritis, neuropathic arthritis, and ankylosing spondylitis, the terms chondrocalcinosis or calcium pyrophosphate dihydrate (CPPD) deposition disease are more appropriate.

The disease may be seen as a hereditary condition, occasionally as a sporadic condition, or associated with some other metabolic condition such as hyperparathyroidism, hypothyroidism, gout, or hemochromatosis. (It is probable that patients with the sporadic condition would show a familial history if they were more carefully investigated.) Reports in the literature on the incidence of this disease vary considerably. Because most affected individuals are asymptomatic, the incidence of chondrocalcinosis found at autopsy is much higher than that found in clinical stages. (The average incidence at autopsy in elderly people is believed to be at least 5 per cent, if not more.) Presumably the majority of patients with findings of chondrocalcinosis at autopsy were not diagnosed as having the condition during life.

Assessment of Patients. The most common clinical presentation of chondrocalcinosis is similar to that of a patient with osteoarthritis. About 50 per cent of the

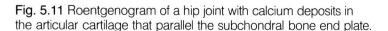

Fig. 5.11 Roentgenogram of a hip joint with calcium deposits in the articular cartilage that parallel the subchondral bone end plate.

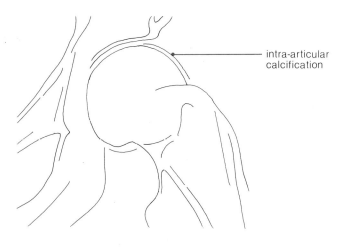

intra-articular calcification

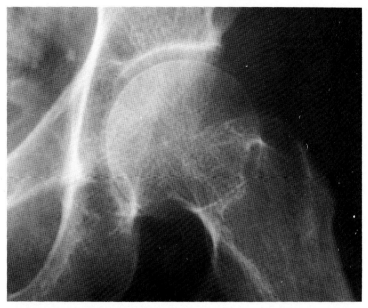

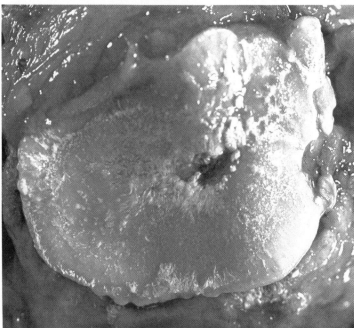

Fig. 5.12 A degenerated patella with extensive deposits of chalky-white material both on the surface and in the deeper portions of the cartilage, as well as in the synovium.

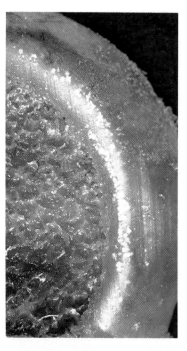
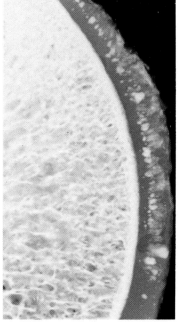

Fig. 5.13 In this cut surface of a femoral head, chalky-white deposits of calcium pyrophosphate dihydrate can be seen in the depths of the cartilage (*left*). Roentgenogram of the specimen clearly demonstrates the calcific nature of the deposit (*right*).

noticeably affected patients present with a progressive degeneration that often affects several joints. In order of frequency of involvement, the joints most likely to be affected are the knees, ankles, wrists, elbows, hips, and shoulders. Rarely will the metacarpals or metatarsals be involved. The initial manifestation of the disease is likely to occur in the patient's third or fourth decade of life.

The group of patients described as having pseudogout account for about 25 per cent of the patients presenting with chondrocalcinosis. Like gout, pseudogout has an acute onset with marked inflammatory changes and swelling. However, its severity is likely to be less than that of gout, and often there are cluster attacks; that is, a single joint will first be affected, and then satellite joints around it will become involved. Pseudogout, like gout, may be provoked by an associated illness or by trauma (including surgery), and the examination of the blood may on occasion show hyperuricemia further complicating the diagnosis.

The other three clinical presentations that may occur are multiple symmetrical involvement of the joints in a rheumatoid-like fashion, rapidly degenerating joint conditions similar to Charcot's joints, and stiffening of the spine (usually a familial condition).

On roentgenographic examination the calcium deposits are characteristically seen in fibrocartilage, but they may also appear in hyaline cartilage. The deposits are punctate or linear, and when they occur in hyaline cartilage, they usually parallel the subchondral bone end plate (Figs. 5.11 to 5.16).

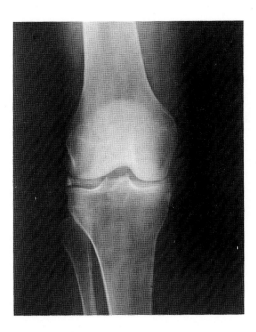

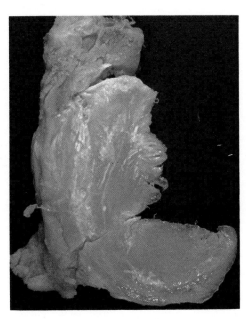

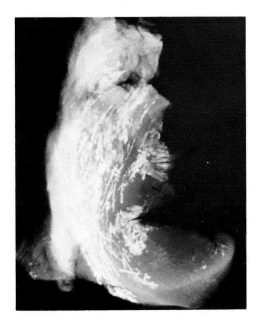

Fig. 5.14 Roentgenogram of a knee joint in an elderly individual with extensive calcification of the menisci.

Fig. 5.15 Gross appearance of a meniscus with extensive calcium pyrophosphate dihydrate deposition (*left*) and a roentgenogram of this specimen (*right*).

Fig. 5.16 Detail of gross specimen shown in Fig. 5.15.

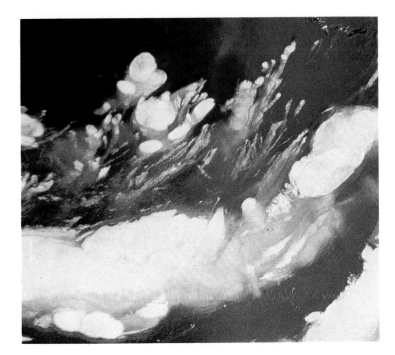

Punctate calcification may also be seen in the synovial tissue (Figs. 5.17 and 5.18). In addition to the large joints, the intervertebral disc and symphysis pubis are often affected. Chondrocalcinosis may be associated roentgenographically with joint space narrowing and sclerosis similar to that seen in patients with degenerative joint disease, but different in its distribution. The radiocarpal compartment of the wrist, the glenohumeral joint, and the elbow are commonly involved.

Gross examination reveals chalky white deposits that, on microscopic studies, may be either crystalline or amorphous in appearance, and surrounded by a chronic inflammatory and giant cell reaction (Fig. 5.19, *upper*). The crystals are distinguished from gout crystals by their shape (rhomboidal) and their weak, positive birefringence (Fig. 5.19, *lower*).

Most investigators who have studied this condition are of the opinion that, at least in the articular form of chondrocalcinosis, the crystal deposition has a chondrocytic origin. Unlike gout and ochronosis, the immediate changes take place in relationship to the cartilage lacunae, which become enlarged and coalescent. The adjacent matrix is replaced by chondromucoid material from which the cells ultimately disappear. The characteristic calcified punctate lesions come about through the deposition of crystals in these chondromucoid pools. It is thought that the deposits are finally released into the joint, where they produce an inflammatory reaction.

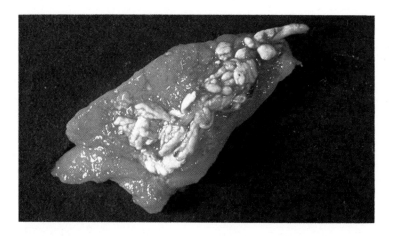

Fig. 5.17 Synovial tissue with extensive calcific deposits immediately at the surface.

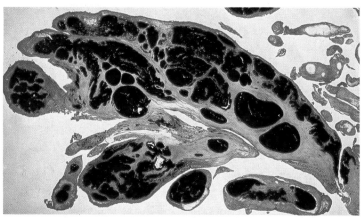

Fig. 5.18 Histologic preparation of the tissue shown in Fig. 5.17, which has been stained with a von Kossa stain to demonstrate the calcium deposits.

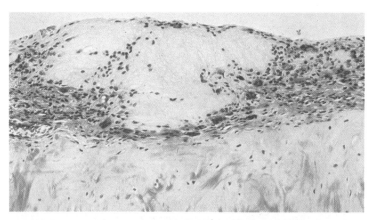

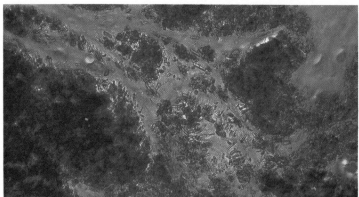

Fig. 5.19 (upper) This photomicrograph shows a deposit of calcium pyrophosphate dihydrate on an articular surface. The deposit is surrounded by mononuclear histiocytes and giant cells, which gives the lesion an appearance very similar to that seen in patients with gout.

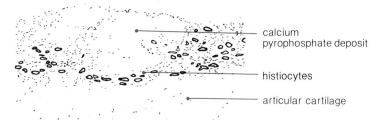

calcium pyrophosphate deposit

histiocytes

articular cartilage

Fig. 5.19 (lower) High power photomicrograph of calcium pyrophosphate dihydrate crystals photographed with polarized light. Note the short rhomboidal shape of the crystals (which distinguishes them from the long needle-shaped crystals of gout) and their weak birefringence.

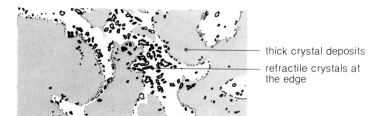

thick crystal deposits

refractile crystals at the edge

OXALOSIS

Calcium oxalate crystals may be deposited in the connective tissues, including bone and cartilage, in either of two conditions. In primary (familial) oxalosis there occurs excessive biosynthesis of oxalate, with subsequent crystal deposition. However, more commonly patients are affected by secondary oxalosis, in which the setting is usually that of chronic renal failure.

The roentgenographic appearance of patients with oxalosis depends on the severity of the disease process. However, in general, radiodense areas in the metaphyseal region of the long bones have been associated with this condition. Histologic examination reveals that the crystals from both primary and secondary oxalosis may be deposited in mineralized bone, articular cartilage, and bone marrow. The identification of the crystals is achieved by the use of polarized light microscopy, which reveals highly refractile needle-shaped crystals that form star-like clusters (Figs. 5.20 and 5.21). Positive identification of the crystals depends on chemical analysis, x-ray diffraction, or electron diffraction. (The latter technique offers an exact method of identification of extremely small quantities of calcium oxalate in bone biopsy specimens.)

The microscopic examination of specimens from patients with oxalosis may reveal either no cellular response, a mononuclear cell reaction, or a giant cell reaction similar to that seen in patients with other crystal deposition disorders. (Osteoclastic resorption of bone may be noted, but this finding, as well as those of osteomalacia, may be expected in the setting of chronic renal failure.)

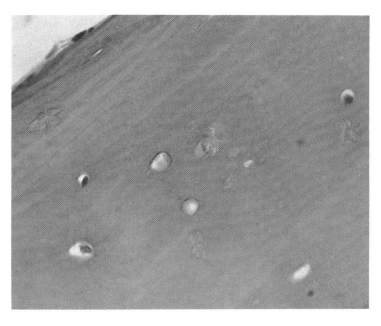
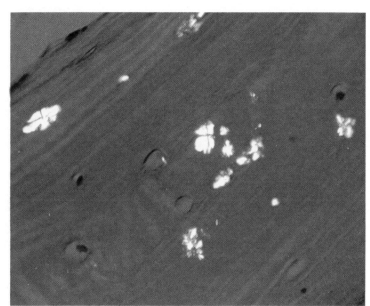

Fig. 5.20 Oxalosis: Photomicrographs of lamellar bone. Within the matrix of the bone and adjacent to the cells can be seen some indistinct deposits (*left*). On examination with polarized light (*right*), these deposits become evident as brightly refractile star-like clusters of crystallized material.

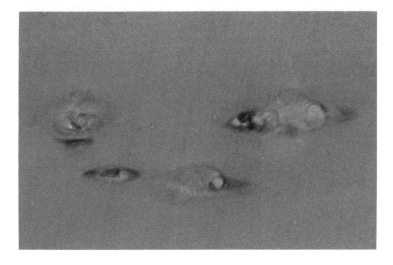
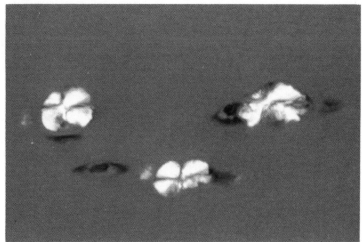

Fig. 5.21 Oxalosis: Photomicrograph of cartilage. Deposits of greyish yellow material can be seen within the chondrocytic lacunae (*left*), with the same field photographed using polarized light (*right*).

OCHRONOSIS

The term ochronosis denotes a blackish pigmentation of connective tissue. The condition results from a rare hereditary disorder of tyrosine and phenylalanine degradation, in which the absence of the enzyme homogentisic acid oxidase leads to the accumulation of homogentisic acid and its oxidation products.

The presence of homogentisic acid in the urine, known as alkaptonuria, causes darkness of the urine on exposure to air, and this discoloration may be the only abnormality in children affected by ochronosis (Fig. 5.22). However, in time the widespread deposition of dark oxidative products occurs in virtually all structures in the body that contain collagen, including the sclerae and the skin. The predominant deposition of homogentisic acid in cartilage (including the intervertebral discs and articular cartilage) results in brittleness and consequent breakdown of the cartilage, which in turn leads to spondylosis and arthropathy, in which the spine and large joints are most severely involved.

The roentgenographic examination of patients with ochronosis reveals the calcification of the intervertebral

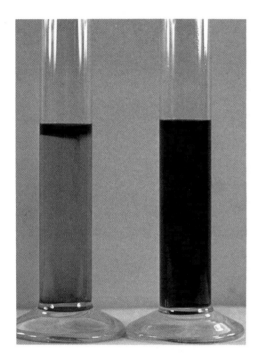

Fig. 5.22 In the flask on the left is urine from a patient with ochronosis that has been left to stand for 15 minutes. Some darkening, owing to oxidation of homogentisic acid, is apparent at the surface. After two hours the specimen is entirely black (flask on the right).

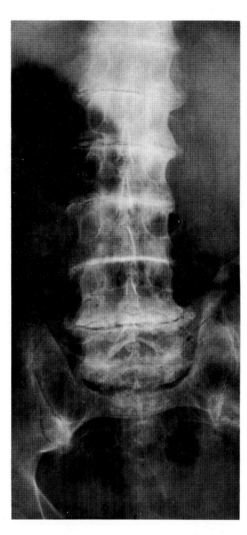

Fig. 5.23 Roentgenogram of the vertebral column in a patient with ochronosis. There is marked narrowing of the intervertebral disc spaces, together with some calcium deposition.

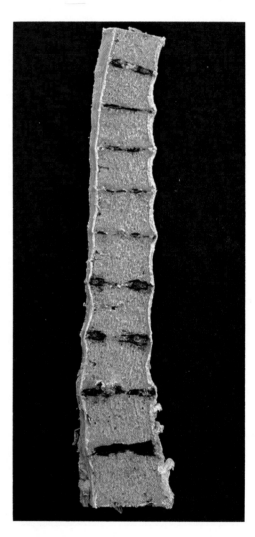

Fig. 5.24 Section obtained at necropsy through the spine of a patient with ochronosis. Note the black discoloration of the intervertebral discs and the pronounced narrowing of the disc spaces.

discs with narrowing of the disc spaces. The arthropathy may be indistinguishable on roentgenograms from "osteoarthritis" with osteophytosis and subchondral sclerosis (Figs. 5.23 to 5.25).

Gross examination of the affected tissues reveals a blackish to bluish-black discoloration, often with concomitant degenerative joint changes, e.g., the eburnation of the articular surfaces (Fig. 5.26). Histologic features of ochronosis include the intracellular accumulation of blackish pigment, as well as irregular fragments of pigmented cartilage that may be embedded in the synovium, a phenomenon that suggests a secondary destructive arthropathy (Fig. 5.27). Study of the condition's ultrastructural pathology reveals the widening and fragmentation of collagen fibers in association with the deposition of the pigment.

The precise mechanism of the tissue injury is not yet understood, but the disruption of collagen crosslinking by metabolic products of homogentisic acid is a probable explanation.

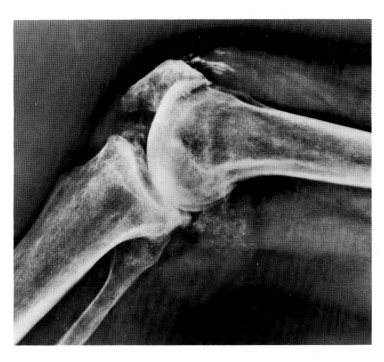

Fig. 5.25 Roentgenogram of the lateral aspect of the knee in a patient with ochronosis. Note the joint space narrowing together with irregular calcified material in the joint space, both in the suprapatellar space and in the popliteal space.

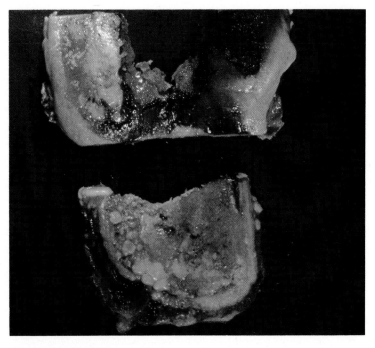

Fig. 5.26 Pieces of the articular surface of a femoral condyle removed at surgery show severe degenerative arthritis and marked black pigmentation of the cartilage. (On occasion dark cartilage will be seen in patients with chronic hemarthrosis. However, in these patients the cartilage usually has a greenish cast, not the intense black seen in patients with ochronosis.)

Fig. 5.27 Photomicrograph of the synovial membrane from a patient with ochronosis shows irregular fragments of pigmented cartilage within the synovial tissue. In addition, there is some fibrosis and mild chronic inflammation of the synovium.

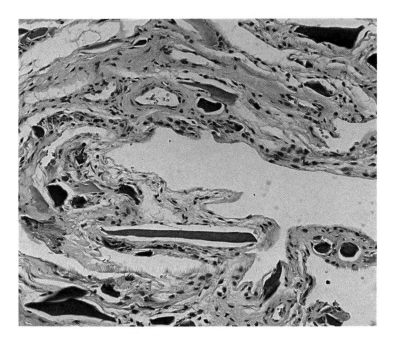

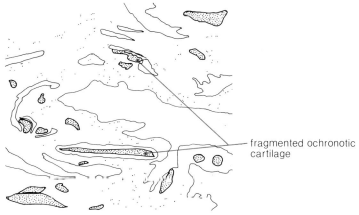

fragmented ochronotic cartilage

AMYLOIDOSIS

Amyloid, a twisted β-pleated fibrillary protein, is seen histologically as glassy eosinophilic deposits. It may be seen in bone and/or juxta-articular tissues, either as a manifestation of the primary form of amyloidosis, or as a secondary amyloidosis resulting from multiple myeloma, rheumatoid arthritis, or some other chronic disease.

Involvement of the skeleton is not uncommon, but it is rarely observed clinically. Clinically evident quantities of amyloid may be seen in the joints, or as diffuse marrow deposits, or, in the rarest form, as localized destructive lesions (tumors). Generally, multiple joints (e.g., the wrists, shoulders, elbows, and hips) are involved bilaterally.

Roentgenograms may reveal juxta-articular osteoporosis, extensive swelling of the soft tissues, multiple well defined subchondral cysts, pressure erosions from synovial hypertrophy, and relative preservation of the joint

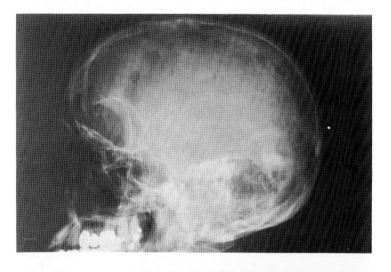

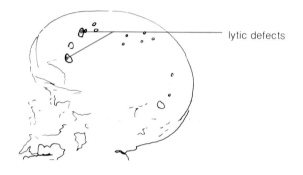

Fig. 5.28 Roentgenogram of the skull in a patient with generalized primary amyloidosis shows osteoporosis and multiple lytic areas, which suggest the presence of a myeloma.

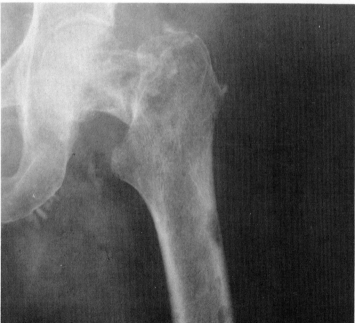

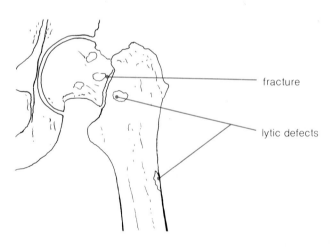

Fig. 5.29 Roentgenogram of a portion of the pelvis and the right hip in the same patient illustrated in Fig. 5.28. Again multiple lytic lesions can be seen in the neck and shaft of the femur, and, in addition, a fracture has occurred through the femoral neck.

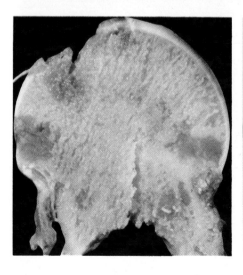
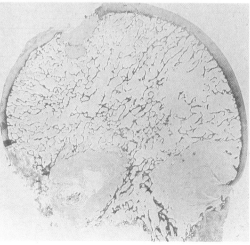

Fig. 5.30 Cut surface of the femoral head removed from the patient with the pathologic fracture shown in Fig. 5.29 (left). The lytic areas are represented by sites of bone destruction filled by a glassy pink tissue. Histologic section (right) demonstrates that glassy areas are acellular deposits of amyloid.

space. Patients with diffuse marrow disease show a predominantly axial distribution of amyloid, and they may have painful compression fractures that mimic myelomas. The localized lytic form of amyloidosis affects the long bones, skull (Fig. 5.28), and ribs, and is usually manifest roentgenographically as one or more well marginated lytic lesions. Patients often have aching pain and pathologic fractures (Figs. 5.29 and 5.30).

Amyloid deposits in the wrist may result in carpal tunnel syndrome, which, on occasion, may be the presenting symptom of amyloidosis (Fig. 5.31).

Histologic sections stained with Congo red have a characteristic apple-green birefringence when examined under polarized light (Figs. 5.32 and 5.33). It may be difficult to recognize amyloid deposits when they occur in connective tissue matrix, because collagen produces a similar apple-green color when examined under polarized light.

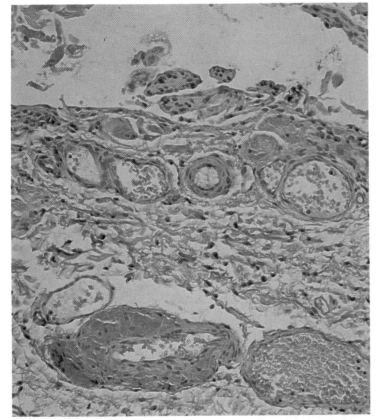

Fig. 5.31 Tissue removed from the transverse carpal ligament in a patient with carpal tunnel syndrome. The amyloid deposit in the vessel wall has been stained by Congo red stain.

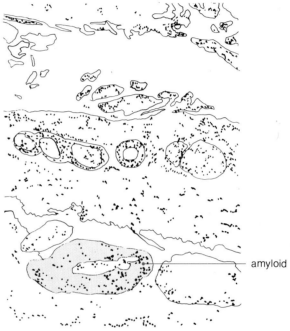

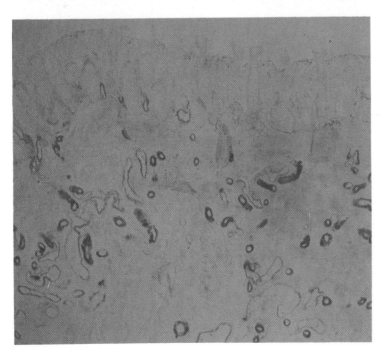

Fig. 5.32 Low power microscopic view of a rectal biopsy stained with Congo red. The amyloid deposits are seen within the vessel walls.

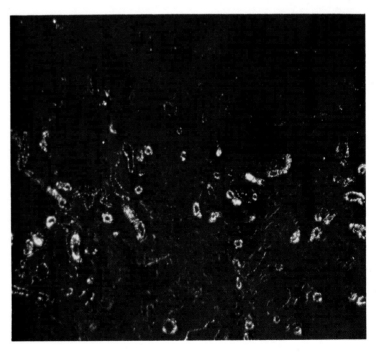

Fig. 5.33 When the same field is examined using polarized light, the amyloid deposits are birefringent and apple green.

HEMOCHROMATOSIS

Conditions that cause excessive iron accumulation, such as massive oral iron intake or severe chronic anemia requiring protracted courses of transfusion therapy, may lead to damage of the visceral organs, particularly of the liver and heart. In cases in which a pathogenic mechanism is not apparent the condition is called idiopathic hemochromatosis. More commonly, an excessive course of iron can be identified, and the condition is called secondary hemochromatosis.

The brown discoloration of the synovial tissue classically seen in patients with this disorder may be confused by the orthopaedic surgeon with local iron deposition from extravasated blood, as seen in patients with rheumatoid synovitis, pigmented villonodular synovitis, or hemophilic arthropathy.

In general the bone and joint changes in hemochromatosis are nonspecific and are best characterized as a noninflammatory arthropathy with involvement of the metacarpophalangeal joints or joints such as the shoulder and elbows (a distribution that is atypical for classic osteoarthritis) (Fig. 5.34). There may be regional osteoporosis as well as peculiar cysts and erosions around the affected joints. Of interest is the associated high incidence of chondrocalcinosis in patients with this condition, which is usually attributed to iron interference with enzymatic degradation of pyrophosphates. Treatment should be directed at the underlying disorder that is causing the accumulation of iron.

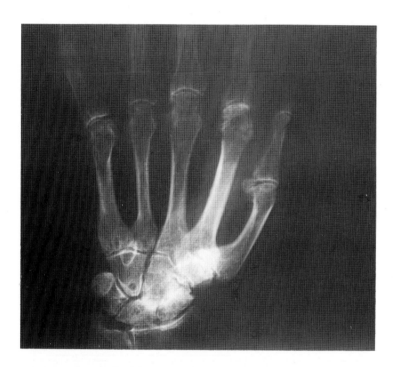

Fig. 5.34 Roentgenogram of the hand of a patient suffering from hemochromatosis. Note the joint narrowing and periarticular erosions in many of the joints, particularly the first and second metacarpophalangeal joints. These changes, though nonspecific, are characteristic of hemochromatosis. (The histology of the synovium in hemochromatosis is similar to that seen in hemosiderosis. See Fig. 5.57.)

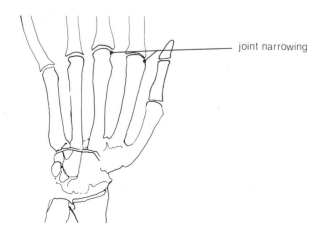

— joint narrowing

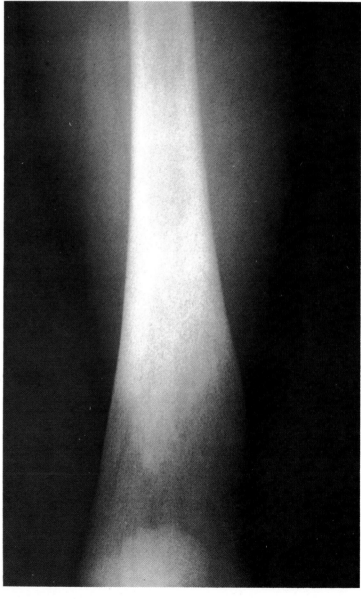

Fig. 5.35 Roentgenogram of the femur in a child with Gaucher's disease shows flaring of the metaphysis and distal diaphysis, together with decreased density of the bone. (The distal growth plate appears at the bottom of the frame.)

GAUCHER'S DISEASE

The so-called "lipidoses" encompass a wide variety of disorders in which congenital enzyme deficiencies lead to the accumulation of complex lipid compounds. By far the most common of these disorders is Gaucher's disease, an inborn error of metabolism of the glucosyl ceramides (glucocerebrosides). These compounds accumulate in cells of the reticuloendothelial system, including the liver, spleen, lymph nodes, and bone marrow, as a result of a deficiency in the activity of glucosylceramide β-glucosidase. Splenomegaly may be dramatic. The disease occurs frequently in Ashkenazic Jews.

Most patients have a chronic form of the disease that has a rather benign, moderate course. Some patients, however, may have many complications and, in rare cases, an acute neuropathic form of the disease is seen in which most individuals die before age three years.

Although the clinical course varies, those patients who present with the disease in infancy or childhood generally have a poor prognosis.

The long bones show irregular thinning of the cortices, which gives a trabeculated appearance. Frequently the lower end of the femur, the upper end of tibia, and the upper end of humerus expand, which produces the "Erlenmeyer flask" deformity (Fig. 5.35).

Skeletal alterations in Gaucher's disease result from the massive infiltration of the marrow space by typical large histiocytes that usually measure 40 to 80 μm in diameter and have a characteristic crumpled or wrinkled appearance of the cytoplasm (Figs. 5.36 to 5.38). The tissue stains positively with PAS stain. Secondary morphologic changes induced by infiltrating Gaucher's cells include infarction of bone, especially the femoral head. Secondary infection may be a problem following biopsy.

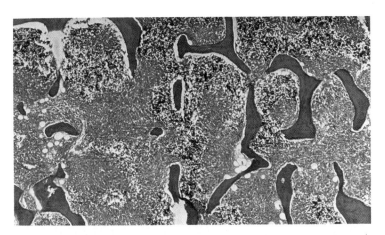

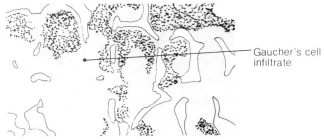

Fig. 5.36 Gaucher's disease: photomicrograph shows replacement of the bone marrow by sheets of large pink cells. Some residual normal marrow is seen at the top of the frame.

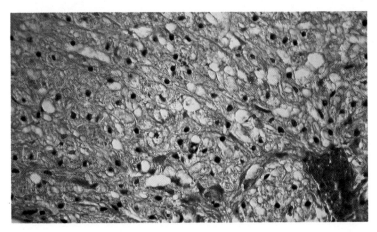

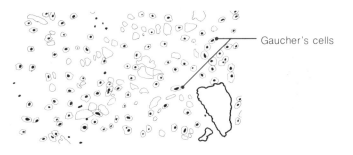

Fig. 5.37 Photomicrograph of the Gaucher's cells at a higher power. The characteristic crumpled appearance of the cytoplasm should be noted.

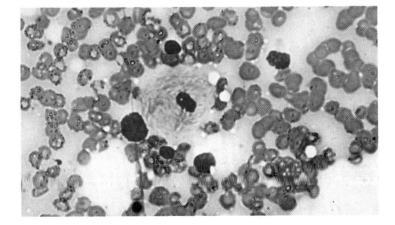

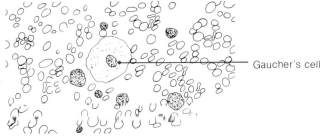

Fig. 5.38 Photomicrograph of a Gaucher's cell seen here in a bone marrow aspirate. The size of the cell can be appreciated from the surrounding hematopoietic cells.

XANTHOMATOSIS
Chester-Erdheim disease of bone

Xanthomatosis refers to the tumor-like accumulation of lipid-laden histiocytes (foam cells, xanthoma cells) in the body. These tumor nodules may be noted in a broad range of clinical settings, including both familial and acquired disorders (such as biliary cirrhosis, pancreatitis, and diabetes mellitus) that result in hypercholesterolemia and/or hyperlipoproteinemia.

The most common presentation of xanthomatosis in the connective tissue is that of yellow nodular tumors in the Achilles tendon or the extensor tendons of fingers. Patients so affected often have bilateral involvement of other sites, including subcutaneous tissue. They also

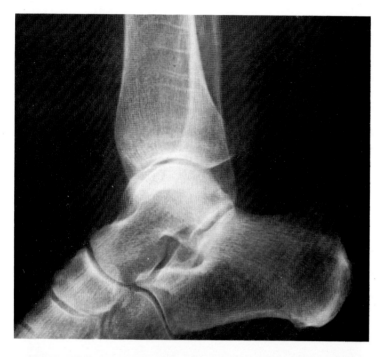

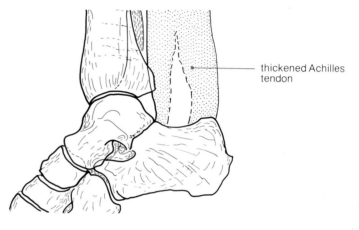

Fig. 5.39 Roentgenogram of the heel in a 25-year-old woman who had bilateral thickening of the Achilles tendon owing to xanthomas. She also had xanthomas of the patellar tendon and xantholasmas of the skin. The patient had hypercholesterolemia. Several members of the family suffered from the same condition.

thickened Achilles tendon

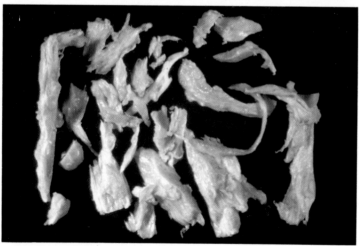

Fig. 5.40 Tissue removed from the thickened heel cord shown in Fig. 5.39.

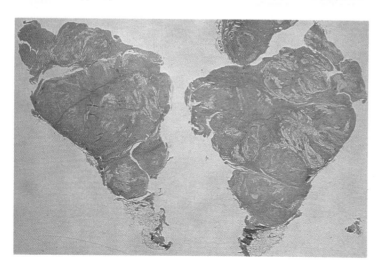

Fig. 5.41 Lower power photomicrograph of tissue shown in Fig. 5.40 shows extensive fatty replacement and cyst formation.

5.16

have hypercholesterolemia, manifested as Type II hyperbetalipoproteinemia on lipoprotein electrophoresis.

The involvement of the skeleton is decidely rare (Figs. 5.39 to 5.44). On roentgen examination the bone lesions show a patchy sclerotic change with coarsened trabeculae, often with focal lytic destruction. The cortical bone may be thinned by endosteal erosion, and ischemic necrosis may follow. Curettage has revealed yellow fragmented tissue with replacement of the marrow elements by foamy histiocytes. These cells have been found to contain intracytoplasmic cholesterol, phospholipids, and/or triglycerides. The amount of inflammation and fibrosis is variable.

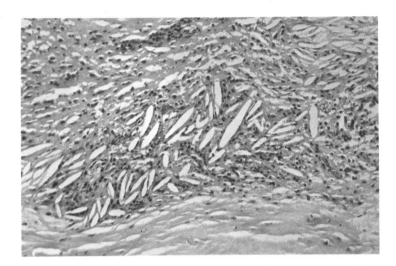

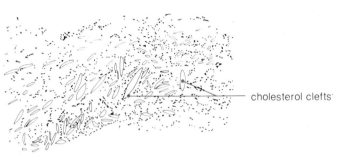

Fig. 5.42 Photomicrograph at a higher power of cyst seen in Fig. 5.41 shows lipid-filled foamy histiocytes and cholesterol clefts in the wall of the cyst.

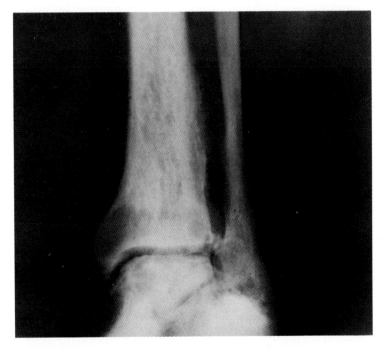

Fig. 5.43 Roentgenogram of the lower leg in a patient with lipogranulomatosis of the bone (Chester-Erdheim disease). Note the patchy sclerosis with coarsening of the trabeculae.

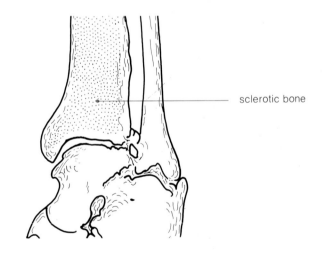

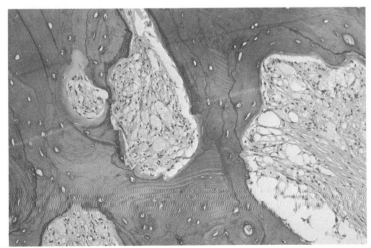

Fig. 5.44 Photomicrograph of a biopsy obtained from the patient shown in Fig. 5.43. In addition to thickening of the bone trabeculae, there is replacement of the fatty marrow by foamy histiocytes, fibroblasts, and occasional inflammatory cells.

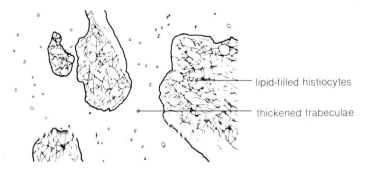

5.17

SKELETAL MANIFESTATIONS OF HEMATOLOGIC DISEASES

Hematologic diseases such as the hemoglobinopathies, hemolytic anemias, or bleeding diatheses may lead to severe bone and joint disease. The skeletal changes result from: secondary erythroid hyperplasia following chronic states of anemia (as seen in patients with thalassemia and sickle cell disease); vascular thrombosis with subsequent infarction, and often infection (as seen in patients with sickle cell disease); and joint destruction secondary to chronic synovial bloody effusions (as seen in patients with hemophilia).

The severity of skeletal disease depends, to a certain extent, on the age of the patient. Children are dramatically affected because of the effect of blood disorders on the growing skeleton. Interestingly, in patients in whom chronic hematologic disease is manifested in infancy, the hands and feet show marked skeletal alterations, whereas in slightly older children the skull may be the predominant site of involvement. In the mature skeleton of an adult the most dramatic changes usually occur in the pelvis and in the spine.

THALASSEMIA MAJOR
The osseous alterations observed in patients with thalassemia major result from secondary erythroid hyperplasia subsequent to chronic anemia. Changes are

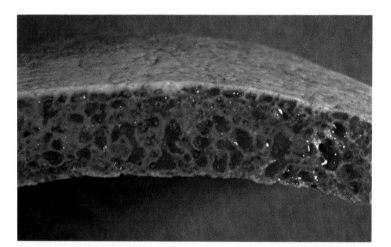

Fig. 5.45 Thalassemia: section through the skull shows marked thinning of the cortices and an open porotic cancellous bone. The mahogany brown color results from extensive iron deposition in the marrow.

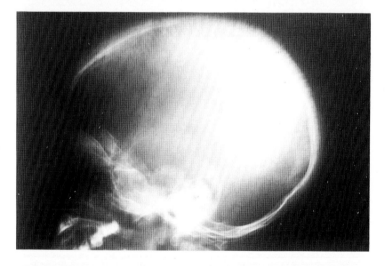

Fig. 5.46 Roentgenogram of the skull of a patient with thalassemia major shows characteristic "hair on end" appearance.

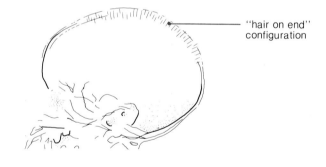

"hair on end" configuration

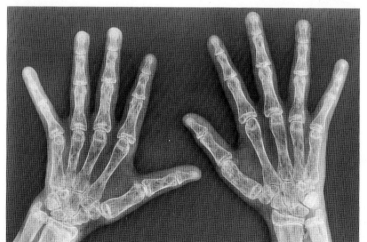

Fig. 5.47 Roentgenogram of the hands in a patient with thalassemia shows severe osteoporosis with a "honeycomb" and cystic cancellous pattern.

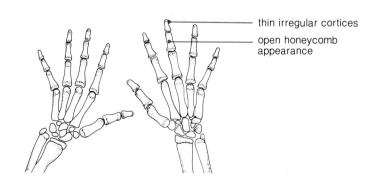

thin irregular cortices

open honeycomb appearance

manifested in the skull, long bones, and metacarpals and metatarsals. Generally, as the patient matures, one finds less involvement of the peripheral skeleton. (Although osseous changes may be observed in patients with thalassemia minor, they are usually less severe.)

On roentgenographic examination the long bones show medullary widening with cortical thinning, often involving the humerus and femur with the development of "saber shins". Involvement of the spine is usually manifested as kyphosis or scoliosis. One may see a dramatic widening of the diploetic space of the skull, with thinning and displacement of the outer table and subsequent rearrangement of the trabeculae, producing a "hair on end" appearance (Figs. 5.45 and 5.46). In the patients' hands and feet one may observe medullary

widening and cortical thinning of the metacarpals and metatarsals, which appears on roentgenographic films as a honeycomb pattern (Fig. 5.47). Involvement of the maxillary bones and sinuses may lead to a peculiar "rodent" facies.

Upon microscopic examination of tissue from severely affected patients, the marrow and erythroid components may be seen to be dramatically hyperplastic. The bones grossly appear to be dusky red, and roentgenograms of involved bones may reveal severe osteoporosis (Figs. 5.48 and 5.49). In histologic sections of bone, Perls' Prussian blue staining demonstrates iron deposition in the zones of mineralization and cement lines (Fig. 5.50).

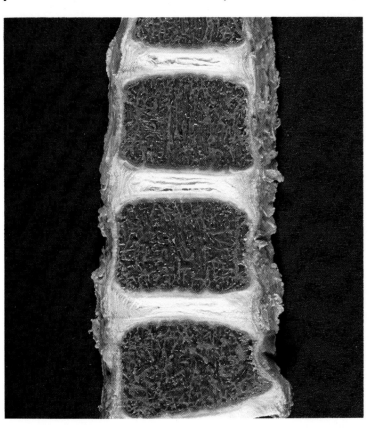

Fig. 5.48 Segment of the vertebral column from a young patient with thalassemia major. The bone marrow is mahogany brown.

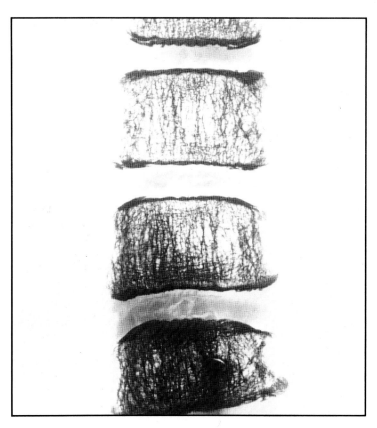

Fig. 5.49 Roentgenogram of the specimen shown in Fig. 5.48. reveals marked osteoporosis.

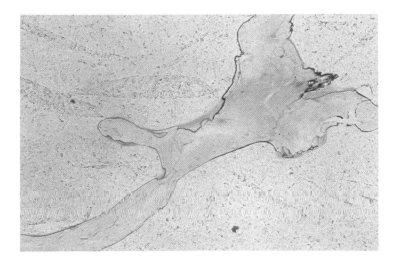

Fig. 5.50 Thalassemia: photomicrograph of a section of bone stained with Perls' stain for iron, which stains a Prussian blue color. It can be appreciated that, on the surface of the bone and also running through the cement lines, there is much iron deposition, as well as extensive deposits throughout the bone marrow.

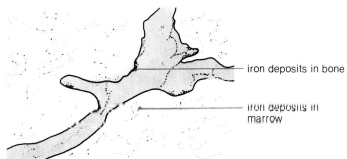

iron deposits in bone

iron deposits in marrow

SICKLE CELL DISEASE

The osseous and joint disorders seen in patients with sickle cell disease result from both erythroid hyperplasia (as seen in patients with thalassemia) and bone ischemia and infarction subsequent to thrombosis, or the decreased oxygen-carrying capacity of the "sickle" red blood cells. In patients with severe sickle cell disease one may observe medullary widening of the bones. Changes in the spine include kyphosis or scoliosis, and osteoporosis (Fig. 5.51). A "hair on end" appearance of the skull may be noted on roentgenographic studies of individuals with this condition, as well as in those of patients with thalassemia major. Characteristic roentgenographic changes may also be found in the hands and feet. In late childhood foci of avascular necrosis are common.

On microscopic examination the bones show a congested dusky red appearance, indicative of marked erythroid hyperplasia of the marrow (Fig. 5.52). The blood cells themselves are deformed and often crescent-shaped, an appearance giving rise to the term "sickle" cell (Fig. 5.53). Patients may develop profound osteoporosis on the basis of marrow impingement on adjacent trabecular bone structure. Infarction may be seen, and is usually attributed to vascular clogging by microthrombi. Osteomyelitis is the feared complication of chronic sickle cell disease, as it often leads to the amputation of the involved extremity (Fig. 5.54).

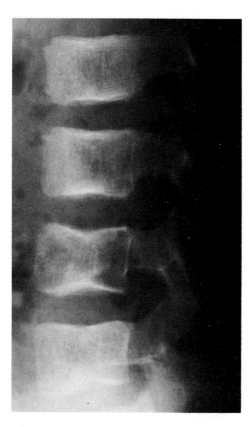

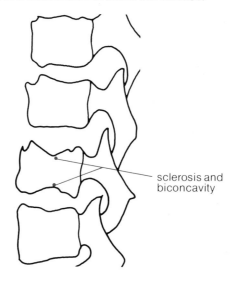

Fig. 5.51 A roentgenogram of the lumbar spine shows osteoporosis and sclerosis around the vertebral end plates, particularly noticeable in L4. In association with this increased density, collapse of the end plates occurs, giving rise to a biconcavity of the vertebral body. When this biconcavity is seen in a young patient, it is characteristic of sickle cell disease.

— sclerosis and biconcavity

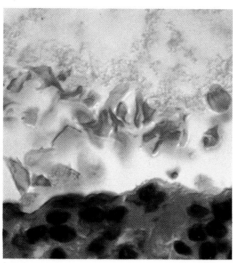

Fig. 5.53 Photomicrograph of "sickled" red cells within the lumen of a blood vessel. (Normarski differential interference contrast microscopy.)

Fig. 5.52 Histologic section of two vertebral bodies from a child with sickle cell disease. The marrow space is entirely filled with hematopoietic tissue and there is no fat evident. (Normally the marrow is 50 per cent fat and 50 per cent hematopoietic tissue.) Osteoporosis is also present.

Fig. 5.54 Section taken through the tibia from a patient with sickle cell disease who developed osteomyelitis. The specimen shows extensive necrosis, seen as an opaque yellow coloration of the bone towards the ankle joint, and between the necrotic bone and the living bone above there is a focus of infected tissue.

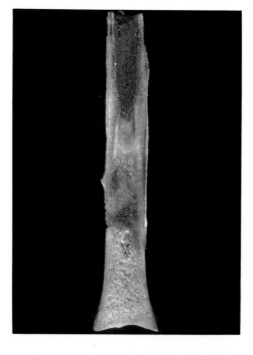

HEMOPHILIA

Hemorrhage into a joint space, observed clinically as a warm, painful, swollen joint, is one of the commonly observed clinical complications of hemophilia. These bloody joint effusions may be precipitated by even minor trauma or stress, and are seen typically in the knees, elbows, and ankles. Chronic, even subclinical, bloody effusions in joint spaces may lead to a destructive arthropathy that is characterized on roentgenographic studies by a narrow joint space, cartilage destruction, bone erosion, multiple juxta-articular cysts, and, if the lesion has progressed over a long period of time, osteophytes (Fig. 5.55). One may also note on roentgenograms a peculiar juxta-epiphyseal osteoporosis.

Hemophilia or other bleeding diatheses are characterized by copious iron deposition and a markedly hyperplastic synovial tissue (Figs. 5.56 and 5.57). The hyperplasia is often limited to the synovial lining cells, although reactive changes in the subsynovial capillary bed may be dramatic. The differential diagnosis would include rheumatoid arthritis and pigmented villonodular synovitis. However, in hemophilia-related destructive joint disease, one does not find the striking lymphoplasmacytic infiltrate that characterizes rheumatoid arthritis, nor does one observe the nodular proliferation of mononuclear and giant cells characteristic of pigmented villonodular synovitis. Bleeding into the periosteum may give rise to a large pseudotumor (Fig. 5.58).

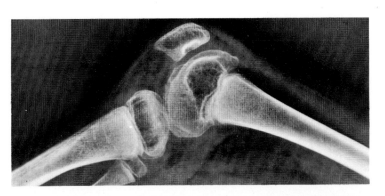

Fig. 5.55 Roentgenogram of a young patient with hemophilia. Note the presence of osteoporosis of the epiphyses, irregularity of the articular margins, and squaring off of the patella.

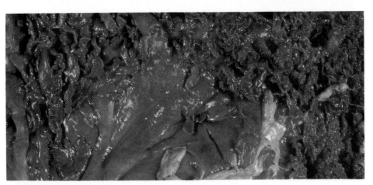

Fig. 5.56 Photograph of the synovium removed from the knee of a patient suffering from hemophilia. The staining of the synovium with hemosiderin is apparent as a mahogany color. Also apparent is the papillary proliferation of the synovium (compare Fig. 6.24).

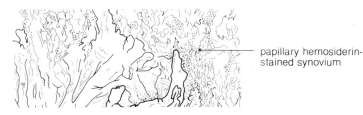

papillary hemosiderin-stained synovium

Fig. 5.57 Photomicrograph of a section of the synovium shown in Fig. 5.56. Note the marked proliferation of the synovial lining. In this section the hemosiderin deposits have been stained by Perls' Prussian blue stain.

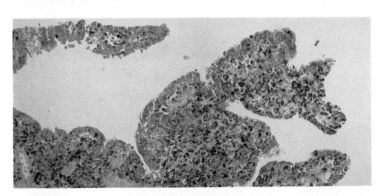

hemosiderin deposits
hypertrophic synovium

Fig. 5.58 Roentgenogram of a large pseudotumor subsequent to a subperiosteal hemorrhage in the distal femur of a hemophiliac.

MYELOSCLEROSIS AND MYELOFIBROSIS

Myeloproliferative syndromes may progress to a condition that is characterized clinically by marked anemia and morphologically by a fibrotic and partially obliterated marrow space (Fig. 5.59). This condition may be characterized on roentgenograms by profound bony sclerosis, which, in combination with the marrow fibrosis observed on histologic examination, accounts for the often "dry taps" when attempts are made to aspirate the marrow. In approximately one-half of all adult patients there is dramatic involvement of the spine, pelvis, ribs, sternum, proximal humerus, and femur (the common sites of adult hematopoiesis). The skull is rarely involved.

When examined microscopically, the marrow shows obliterative fibrosis in late stages, but, in early stages, one may note marked marrow hyperplasia with bizarre cell types, as well as an increase in reticulum fiber production (Fig. 5.60). The thickened bone can be found, when viewed with polarized light, to have a largely woven appearance (Fig. 5.61).

Neoplastic conditions of the marrow and lymphoid system frequently manifest local or generalized skeletal involvement. In most cases there are discrete tumors, but in some instances only a diffuse osteoporosis is noted. In patients with leukemia, it is not unusual to find widespread infarction of the bone and bone marrow at autopsy (Fig. 5.62).

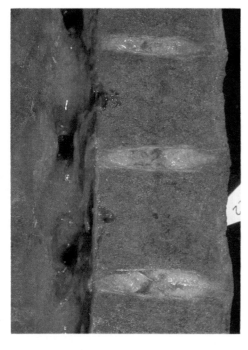
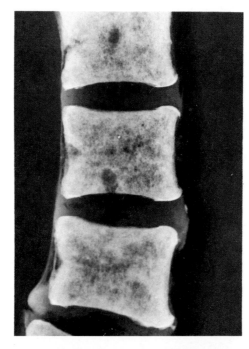

Fig. 5.59 A segment of the spine from a patient with myelofibrosis (*left*). The bone has a dense appearance, and the patient is noted to have severe disc degeneration. The considerable increase in bone density can be appreciated in a roentgenogram of the same specimen (*right*).

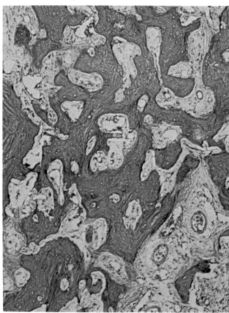

Fig. 5.60 Myelofibrosis: photomicrograph of a section of bone from the patient shown in Fig. 5.59. There is extensive new bone formation, as well as fibrosis of the marrow space with displacement of the hematopoietic tissue.

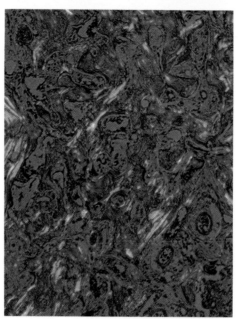

Fig. 5.61 Photomicrograph of a section of bone from a patient with myelofibrosis. The specimen, photographed with polarized light, shows that the extensive new bone formation has an immature or woven pattern.

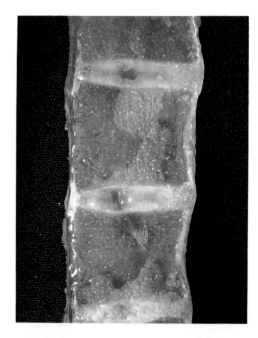

Fig. 5.62 A segment of the spine from a patient who died with leukemia. Within the vertebral bodies there are geographic areas of necrosis identified as yellow opacification of the bone and marrow.

6 Arthritis I

To be able to understand the nature of a disease, it is first necessary to have an understanding of the normal function and functional anatomy of the organ system under consideration. Therefore, before one considers the pathology of arthritis—the concern of the next three chapters—one must turn one's attention to the morphology and physiology of the joints.

The normal function of a joint depends principally upon three factors: the freedom of the articulating surfaces to move over each other, the ability of the joint to maintain stability during use, and a proper distribution of stress through the tissues comprising the joint so that these tissues are not damaged. These aspects of joint function are governed by the interdependent actions of the shape of the articulating surfaces of the joint (Fig. 6.1); by the integrity of the ligaments, muscles, and tendons that support the limb; and by the biologic cellular control of the mechanical properties of bone, cartilage, and the other tissues that comprise the joint (Fig. 6.2). Clinical arthritis is the result of a breakdown in these functions; that is to say, a loss of the freedom to move easily, a loss of stability, or an improper distribution of weight through the tissues. These changes in function result from changes in the shape or structure of the joint, in the mechanical properties of the tissues making up the joint, or in the integrity of the supportive tissues in the limb.

Articulating diarthrodial joints are formed of the expanded bone ends; the covering articular cartilage; the lining synovial membrane; and the surrounding ligaments, tendons, and muscles (Fig. 6.3). Dysfunction may begin in any of these structures, but by the time joint disease comes to the attention of a physician, most or all of these structures are involved. Because of this overall involvement it can be difficult for the pathologist to determine the etiology of any particular case of arthritis, especially in the late stages of disease in which the morbid anatomy of many kinds of arthritis tends to be similar to that of many others.

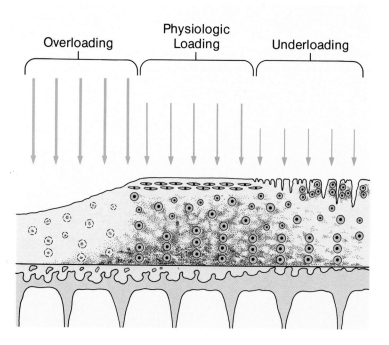

Fig. 6.1 The shape of the joint determines the freedom of the joint surfaces to articulate, the stability of the joint, and the distribution of stress on the tissues. A does not allow acceptable freedom of movement. B permits total freedom of movement, but is unstable. C allows freedom of movement and is stable; however, the shape is not optimal because it does not provide space between the articulating surfaces for lubrication or nutrition (i.e., it is completely congruent). Furthermore, when the joint is loaded, the stress is not equally distributed over the joint surfaces. D is the optimal shape for a joint because it is stable, it articulates easily, and there is some space between the joint surfaces so that the synovial fluid can move into the joint space to provide for the nutrition of the cartilage and the lubrication of the surfaces. This shape also distributes an increasing load equally, as the deformability of cartilage and bone allows the tissues to respond and conform to stresses imposed upon them.

Fig. 6.2 The continued optimal functional integrity of connective tissue depends on balanced rates of matrix production and breakdown by the cells. Healthy tissue *(center)* results from a physiologic range of stress that maintains optimal cell activity. If this range of stress is exceeded *(left)*, the result is cell injury and, eventually, necrosis. (In cartilage, this is called chondrolysis.) If the stress is inadequate *(right)*, disuse atrophy, i.e., lack of adequate matrix production by the cells, may occur. In cartilage, this is associated with increased water content and fibrillation of the collagen.

COMMONLY OBSERVED HISTOLOGIC CHANGES
SEEN IN ASSOCIATION WITH ARTHRITIS

In Chapter 1 the normal histology of cartilage, synovium, and bone is illustrated and discussed. Patients with arthritis are likely to exhibit changes in all three of these tissues. The changes observed may be divided into two categories: those that result from cell injury, and those that can be regarded as reparative or reactive changes. Although there may be characteristic patterns that define a particu-

lar form of arthritis, many similar histologic changes may be seen in the joints of patients with arthritis, regardless of the etiology.

Cartilage. An obvious sign of injury in the cartilage is the death of some or all of the cells. Although the former is not uncommon, the latter (total cellular necrosis) is not generally observed. (When total cellular necrosis does occur, it is usually referred to as chondrolysis. See Fig. 6.4.)

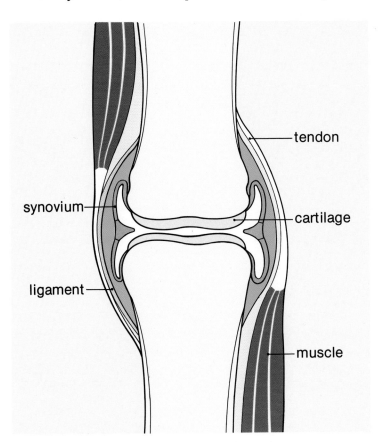

Fig. 6.3 A joint consists not only of the articular cartilage and synovial lining, but it is also a mechanical system that includes all the surrounding ligaments, tendons, and muscles.

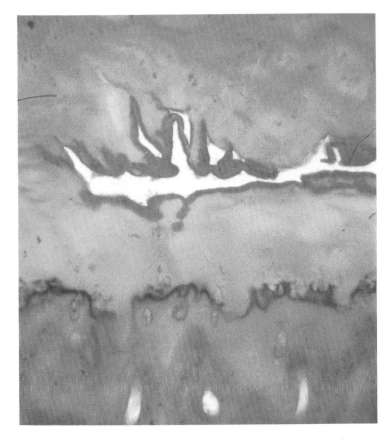

Fig. 6.4 Photomicrograph demonstrates total cartilage necrosis in a patient with idiopathic chondrolysis. Note also the horizontal cleft resulting from failure of the cartilage matrix to resist shear forces within its substance.

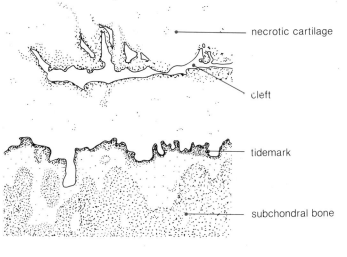

Injury is more often recognized in the matrix, in which two distinctive features may be observed: first, a loss of the normal basophilic staining associated with changes in the proteoglycan content of the matrix (Fig. 6.5), and second, splitting of the matrix, usually vertically (Figs. 6.6 and 6.7) but sometimes horizontally (Fig. 6.8), resulting from breakage in the collagen fibers. This splitting of the cartilage, which may be confined to the superficial layer or extend (from the surface) into the deep part of the cartilage, is referred to as fibrillation.

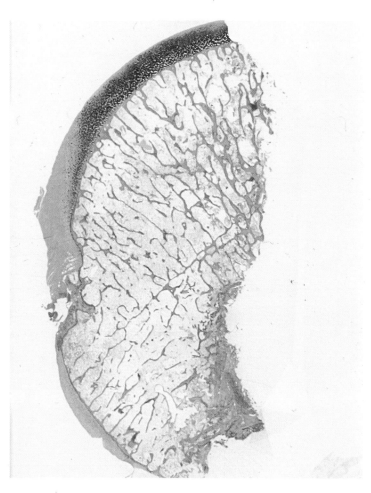

Fig. 6.5 Section through a femoral head shows the difference in basophilic staining of the cartilage (between the cartilage of the superior surface and the cartilage around the fovea and the inferomedial surface). The degree of basophilic staining correlates with the sulfated glycosaminoglycan content of the cartilage. (Hematoxylin and eosin stain, low power.)

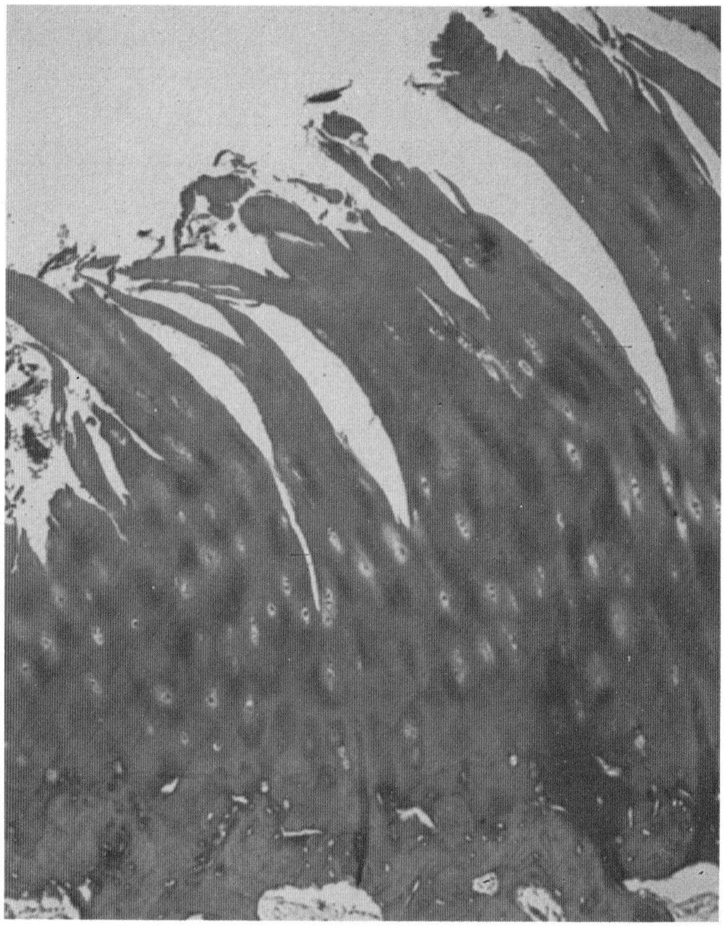

Fig. 6.6 Low power photomicrograph of the articular surface of a joint obtained from a patient with osteoarthritis. The articular cartilage contains vertical clefts resulting from fraying and splitting of the collagen fibers at the surface of the cartilage.

Fig. 6.7 Photograph of the articular surface of the patella illustrates the splitting of the cartilage matrix (i.e., fibrillation, which results from mechanical breakdown of the collagen component of the matrix).

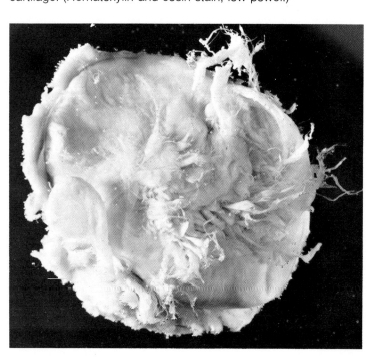

Cartilage repair is usually evident in one of two forms: either as the cloning of chondrocytes within the damaged cartilage (Fig. 6.9), or as a proliferation of new cartilage from the underlying bone or from the periphery of the joint. In the case of proliferating new cartilage, the tissue is usually more cellular, and it may differ both chemically and organizationally in its matrix constituents from normal articular cartilage (Fig. 6.10).

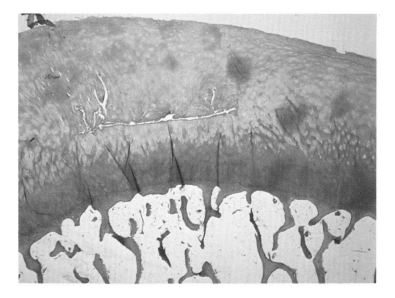

Fig. 6.8 Section through the articular cartilage of the patella demonstrates a horizontal failure with cleft formation in a patient with chondromalacia patellae. In patients with this condition, a soft blister on the surface of the cartilage may indicate structural failure within the substance of the cartilage.

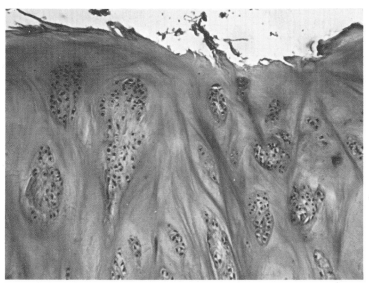

Fig. 6.9 Section through an area of fibrillated cartilage shows clones of proliferating chondrocytes within the matrix. This appearance is a common finding in damaged cartilage.

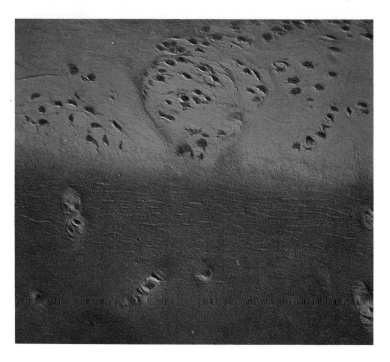

Fig. 6.10 In this photomicrograph a layer of proliferating new cartilage is seen lying directly over a layer of residual normal cartilage.

6.5

Bone. A loss of cartilage from the articular surface of the joint results in damage to the underlying bone. This change is seen in the form of superficial necrosis of the articulating bone surface (Fig. 6.11), as microfractures of individual trabeculae in the cancellous bone underlying the articular surface (Figs. 6.12 and 6.13), and as a cystic degeneration within the bone, possibly related to excessive pressure on the articular surface (Figs. 6.14 to 6.17).

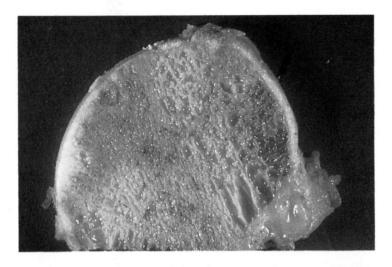

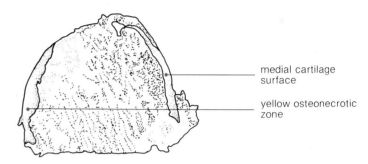

Fig. 6.11 A portion of the eburnated surface of an osteoarthritic joint demonstrates focal superficial bone and bone marrow necrosis, which is seen macroscopically as an opaque yellow area.

medial cartilage surface

yellow osteonecrotic zone

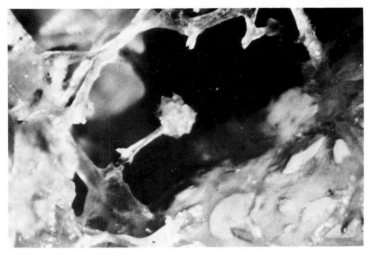

Fig. 6.12 Photograph of an individual trabecula of the subchondral cancellous bone, on which is seen a "cotton ball" swelling. This swelling is the result of callus formation around a fracture of the trabecula.

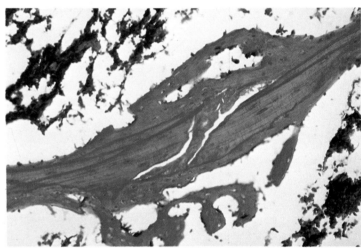

Fig. 6.13 Microscopic photograph of the fractured trabecula illustrated in Figure 6.12. Note the oblique fracture through the trabecula, as well as the surrounding new bone formation (callus).

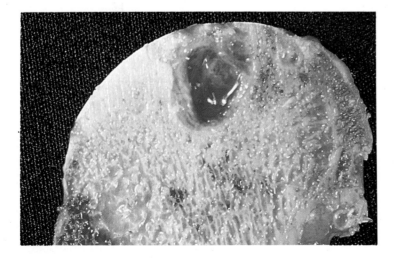

Fig. 6.14 An area of cystic degeneration is seen in the subchondral bone of the superior surface of a femoral head. Such cysts are, in general, present only in the absence of the overlying articular cartilage. Note also the large flat osteophyte on the medial surface.

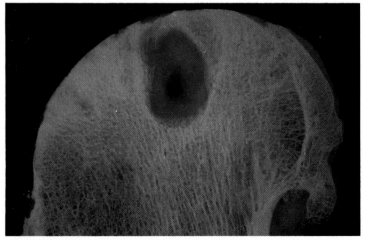

Fig. 6.15 A roentgenogram of the specimen shown in Fig. 6.14.

Reparative or reactive changes in the bone are seen as marked increases in osteoblastic activity, with new bone formation and thickened trabeculae (Fig. 6.18). The thickened trabeculae increase the strength of the bone.

The contour of the bone is altered by endochondral ossification. This process occurs through a proliferation of new cartilage at the periphery of the joint and over the less loaded areas of the joint, and the new cartilage is in turn

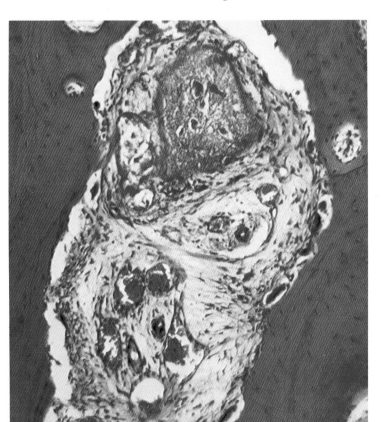

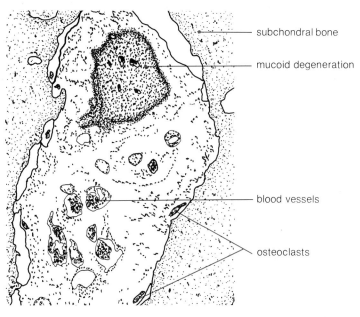

Fig. 6.16 Photomicrograph of early cyst formation in the subchondral bone underlying an area in which the cartilage has been eroded. One may note a proliferation of vascularized fibrous tissue with osteoclastic resorption of the surrounding bone and early mucoid degeneration in the fibrous tissue.

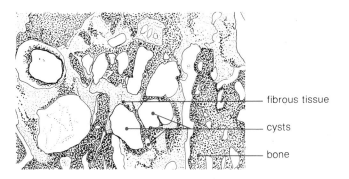

Fig. 6.17 Low power photomicrograph of a developed subchondral cyst, consisting of a fibrous cyst wall filled with a viscous fluid.

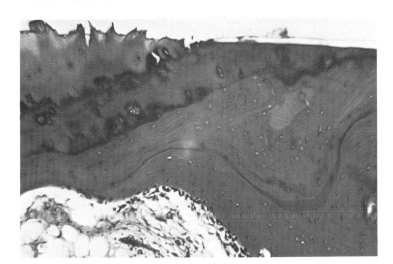

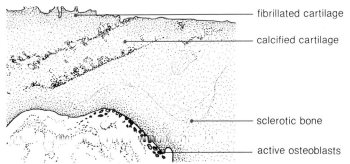

Fig. 6.18 Photomicrograph shows increased osteoblastic activity and trabecular thickening underlying an area of cartilage erosion. (Section taken from the edge of an eburnated area.)

replaced by bone. The resulting bony excrescences are called osteophytes (Figs. 6.19 and 6.20). The change in contour may be regarded as a mechanism that restabilizes the joint or equalizes the stress in the joint.

Synovium. Most arthritis is characterized by the breakdown of the articular surfaces of the joint, resulting in an increase in cellular debris. Consequently, in almost all forms of arthritis, hypertrophy and hyperplasia of the synovial cells occur, and the synovial lining of the joint is usually thrown into papillary folds (Figs. 6.21 and 6.22). Occasionally, giant cells may be seen in the synovial lining, and these cells are particularly prominent in certain

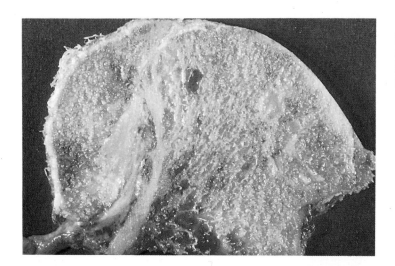

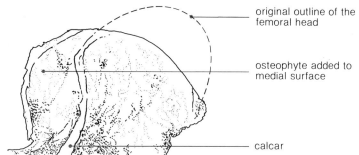

Fig. 6.19 Photograph of a slice through an arthritic femoral head in which, despite the loss of bone from the superior surface, the contour has been restored to something approaching sphericity by a large medial osteophyte, which is seen to extend well down the medial femoral neck.

original outline of the femoral head

osteophyte added to medial surface

calcar

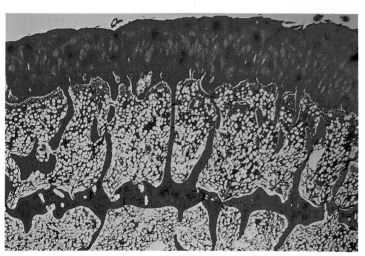

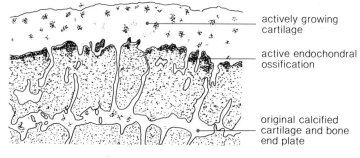

Fig. 6.20 Photomicrograph of a flat osteophyte on the medial surface of an osteoarthritic femoral head. Actively proliferating cartilage can be seen on the surface, which is being replaced by endochondral ossification. The original cartilage-bone interface is seen as a layer of calcified cartilage and a plate of underlying bone parallel to the new articular surface.

actively growing cartilage

active endochondral ossification

original calcified cartilage and bone end plate

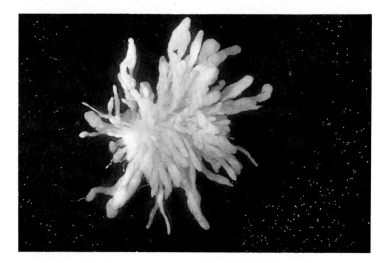

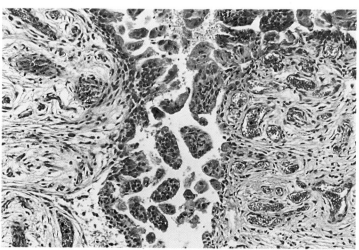

Fig. 6.21 The synovium from a patient with osteoarthritis reveals a marked villous pattern. Note that the villi are fine and delicate, an appearance that grossly reflects the lack of any significant cellular infiltrate in the subsynovium.

Fig. 6.22 Photomicrograph of the specimen shown in Fig. 6.21 demonstrates the overgrowth of the synovial lining cells without significant cellular infiltration of the subsynovial tissue.

diseases (e.g., rheumatoid arthritis) (Fig. 6.23). In patients in whom chronic hemorrhage in the joint has been a problem, deposits of hemosiderin are common. However, it should be pointed out that hypertrophied synovium is likely to be traumatized during articulation, and some degree of hemosiderin staining in the synovium is not unusual, whatever the etiology of the arthritic condition (Fig. 6.24). In those diseases in which a rapid breakdown of the bone and cartilage takes place (e.g., Charcot's joints or the arthritis associated with cortisone therapy), it is common to see large sequestered fragments of cartilage and bone within the synovium (Fig. 6.25).

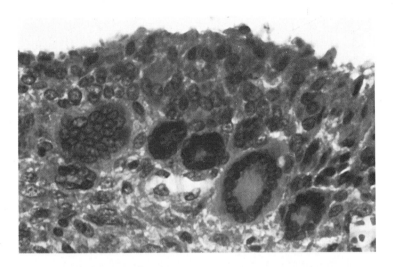

Fig. 6.23 Photomicrograph of the synovium from a patient with rheumatoid arthritis demonstrates marked hypertrophy and hyperplasia of the synovial lining, together with numerous giant cells. Giant cells may also be seen in specimens from individuals with osteoarthritis and other forms of synovitis in which hyperplasia is prominent, but this finding is not as common in patients with these conditions as it is in patients with rheumatoid arthritis.

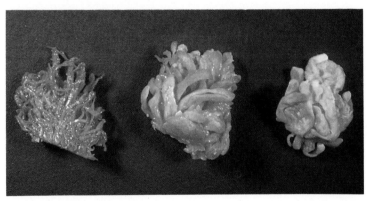

Fig. 6.24 Hemophilia *(left)*, pigmented villonodular synovitis *(center)*, rheumatoid arthritis *(right)*. In this photograph the synovial membrane from individuals with three different conditions is compared. In patients with hemophilia, the hemosiderin staining of the synovium results from excessive bleeding into the joint, but in individuals affected by the other two conditions, the hemosiderin staining is probably secondary to trauma to the hypertrophic synovium. The plump papillary appearance of the synovium in pigmented villonodular synovitis (PVNS) and rheumatoid arthritis, as opposed to the villous appearance of the synovium in hemophilia, reflects the considerable cellular infiltration of the subsynovium in patients with either of the first two conditions. (PVNS is discussed fully in Chapter 13.)

Fig. 6.25 Photomicrograph of the synovium from a patient with a rapidly destructive joint disease. Fragments of bone and cartilage, as well as foci of histiocytes and phagocytic giant cells, are present.

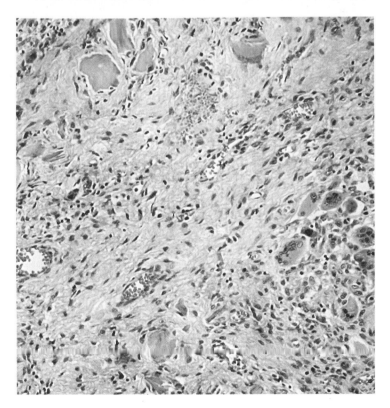

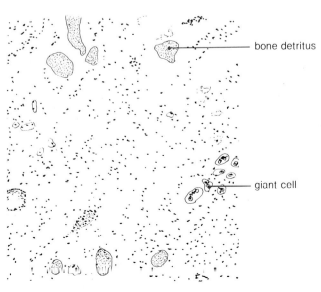

Synovial Fluid. Whatever the cause of arthritis, the synovial fluid will be affected (Fig. 6.26). Normal synovial fluid is a viscous, pale yellow, clear fluid, the volume of which, even in large joints, is normally very small. Normal synovial fluid is a dialysate of plasma to which hyaluronic acid produced by the synovial lining cells has been added (Table 6.1). In the inflammatory diseases the amount of hyaluronic acid is markedly diminished in the synovial fluid, which leads to the decrease in viscosity that is observed in connection with these conditions. In the degenerative forms of arthritis the amount of hyaluronic acid is increased, thereby producing an extremely viscous fluid. Table 6.2 shows the changes that occur in the synovial fluid in association with various conditions.

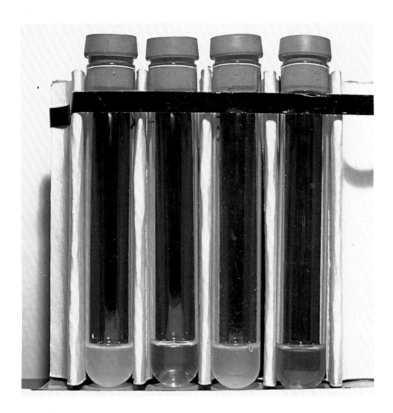

Fig. 6.26 Samples of synovial fluid from four patients.
Chondrocalcinosis: cloudy white fluid
Normal: clear white/amber fluid
Rheumatoid arthritis: cloudy yellow fluid
Traumatic arthritis: clear blood-stained fluid
The examination of synovial fluid can provide valuable information concerning the etiology of a patient's condition.

Table 6.1 Normal Synovial Fluid

	Range	Average
Physical Data		
Amount in knee (ml)	1.1	0.13–3.5
Specific gravity (20°C)		1.0081–1.015
Viscosity (37°C) relative to water	235	5.7–1160
Cell count per mm³	63	13–180
Differential %		
Lymphocytes	24.6	0–78
Monocytes	47.9	0–71
Polymorphonuclear leukocytes	6.5	0–25
Macrophages	10.1	0–26
Synovial lining cells	4.3	0–12
pH	7.434	7.31–7.74
Inorganic Substances		
Electrolytes (Na, K, Cl, CO_2)		Approximately the same as plasma
Calcium, phosphate, sulfate		Approximately the same as plasma
Organic Substances		
Hyaluronic acid (mg/ml)	4.0	
Nonprotein nitrogen		Approximately the same as plasma
Glucose		Approximately the same as plasma
Total lipid (mg/ml)	0.2	
Mucin nitrogen (mg/ml)	1.04	0.68–1.35
Mucin glucosamine (mg/ml)	0.74	0.12–1.32
Uric acid		Approximately the same as plasma

Source: Paget S, Bullough PG: Synovium and synovial fluid. In Owen R et al. (eds.) Scientific Foundations of Orthopaedics and Traumatology. Saunders, Philadelphia, 1980.

Table 6.2 Examination of Synovial Fluid

			Condition	
	Normal	**Noninflammatory**	**Chronic Inflammatory**	**Septic**
Clinical example		Osteoarthrosis	Rheumatoid arthritis	Bacterial infection
Cartilage debris	0	+	0	0
Volume (ml) (knee)	<3.5	>3.5	>3.5	>3.5
Color	Clear	Clear yellow	Opalescent yellow	Turbid yellow to green
Viscosity	High	High	Low	Low
WBCs per mm³	200	200–2000	2000–100,000	>100,000
Polymorphonuclear leukocytes (%)	<25	<25	50% or more	75% or more
Culture	Negative	Negative	Negative	Positive
Mucin clot	Firm	Firm	Friable	Friable
Fibrin clot	None	Small	Large	Large
Glucose (% of blood glucose)	~100	~100	75, may be less than 50	<50
Total protein		Equal to normal joint	Elevated	Elevated

Source: Paget S, Bullough PG: Synovium and synovial fluid. In Owen R et al. (eds.) Scientific Foundations of Orthopaedics and Traumatology. Saunders, Philadelphia, 1980.

Loose Bodies. Separated pieces of bone and cartilage may form loose bodies within the joint cavity (Fig. 6.27). (The cells on the surfaces of the loose bodies derive their nutrition from the synovial fluid.) These loose bodies tend to grow by the proliferation of immature cartilage cells on their surface (Fig. 6.28), and, as the loose body grows, its center becomes necrotic and calcified. In histologic sections it is possible to see the extension of the central calcification in the form of concentric rings that increase as the loose body grows larger (Fig. 6.29).

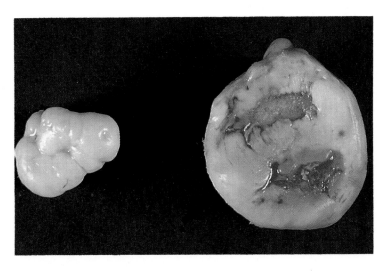

Fig. 6.27 In a patient with traumatic arthritis of the elbow, one sees a loose body *(left)* that has arisen from the portion of the articular surface seen to be missing from the radial head *(right)*.

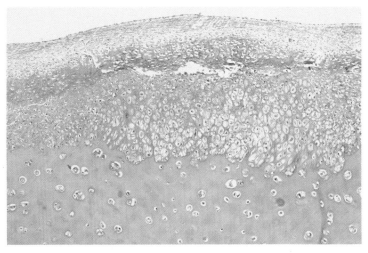

Fig. 6.28 Photomicrograph shows the proliferation of immature cellular cartilage on the surface of a loose body; the original cartilage is seen in the lower part of the picture. Through this process of cartilage cell proliferation, loose bodies may grow to an enormous size.

Fig. 6.29 Photomicrograph of a section through a loose body. One can discern the concentric rings of growth. The tissue toward the center of the loose body *(right)* is calcified.

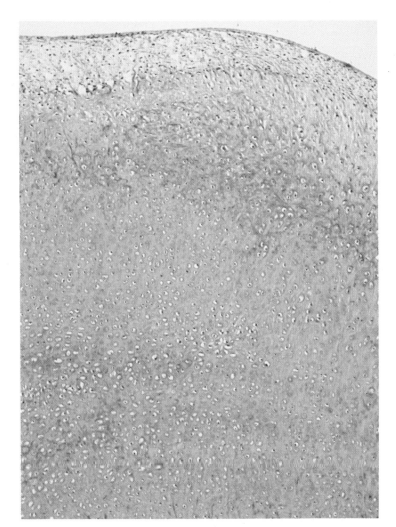

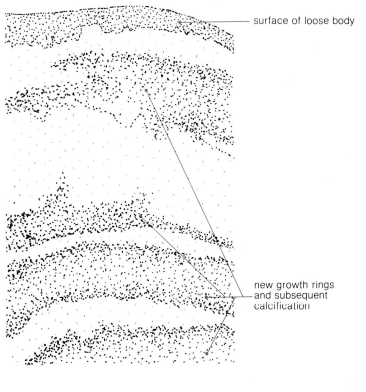

surface of loose body

new growth rings and subsequent calcification

Sometimes the loose body becomes reattached to the synovial membrane and invaded by blood vessels. If this process occurs, the calcified center becomes replaced by viable bone through endochondral ossification (Figs. 6.30 and 6.31).

In addition to cartilaginous and osseous loose bodies, loose bodies may result from excessive fibrinous exudation into the joint, as happens, for example, in patients with rheumatoid arthritis. In these circumstances numerous "rice body" configurations are produced (Fig. 6.32). Very occasionally a loose body is formed from a pedunculated synovial lesion.

(Loose bodies may also result from a primary disease of the synovial membrane called synovial chondromatosis, and this condition will be discussed later in Chapter 13.)

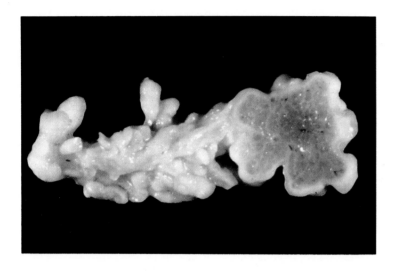

Fig. 6.30 The photograph shows a loose body *(right)* that has become attached to the synovium *(left)*. The specimen has been bisected and shows a viable osseous center that has resulted from the vascular invasion and endochondral ossification of the cartilaginous loose body.

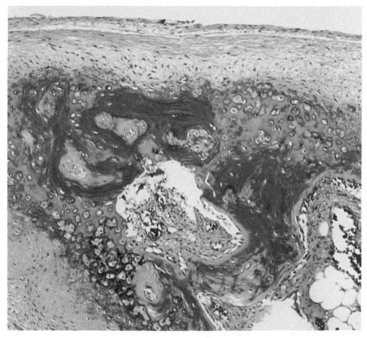

Fig. 6.31 Photomicrograph of the loose body shown in Fig. 6.30 demonstrates the formation of the osseous core by the process of endochondral ossification.

TRAUMATIC ARTHRITIS

Physical trauma to a joint may cause arthritis, and the underlying damage to the joint may occur in any of its several components: in the supportive tissues around the joint (for example, in ligamentous injuries), in the intra-articular structures (for example, the menisci or cruciate ligaments of the knee), in the articular cartilage alone, or in the articular cartilage and bone (Fig. 6.33). In all these instances the joint is rendered either unstable or irregular in contour, and in any case, signs of injury and repair will be found on morphologic examination of specimens from within the affected joint.

The breakdown of the extracellular matrix of bone and cartilage and the foci of cellular necrosis may be observed. Frequently, hemorrhage is present in the joint space; in injuries that have been present for some time, the synovium may be heavily stained with hemosiderin pigment. In more chronic cases of traumatic arthritis, the synovium will be observed to be proliferative, and the joint surface will show evidence of destruction and repair (apparent as osteophytosis around the periphery of the joint and proliferation of immature cartilage over some of the articulating surfaces).

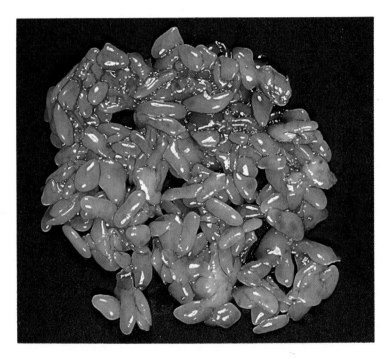

Fig. 6.32 Fibrinous loose bodies removed from a knee joint in a patient with rheumatoid arthritis.

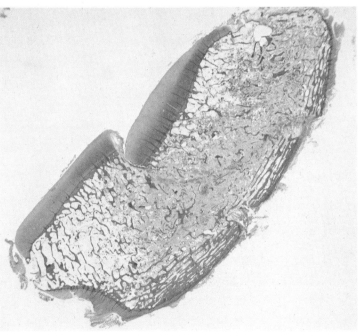

Fig. 6.33 A section through a patella that has sustained a transarticular fracture. Such a change in the contour of an articular surface will lead rapidly to degenerative arthritic changes.

INFLAMMATORY ARTHRITIS

Bacterial infections of the joint may result in the severe and rapid breakdown of the joint tissues, a development that leads to severe arthritis (see Chapter 9 under "Joint Infection").

The acute inflammatory infiltrate produces proteolytic enzymes that rapidly break down the articular cartilage and intra-articular structures (Fig. 6.34). Aspiration of the joint in such a case reveals a predominance of polymorphonuclear leukocytes, with a count usually well over 100,000/mm³ (see Table 6.2).

RHEUMATOID ARTHRITIS

Rheumatoid arthritis is a chronic systemic disease that frequently involves the peripheral joints and results in joint deformities (Fig. 6.35). It is two to three times more common in women than in men, and it is characterized by spontaneous remission and exacerbation. Seventy to 80 per cent of all affected individuals have histocompatibility antigen DW4, a finding that implies a strong hereditary component.

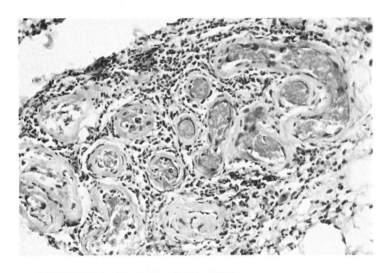

Fig. 6.34 Acute synovitis in early septic arthritis. Interspersed between the hypervascular stroma of this synovium are numerous polymorphonuclear leukocytes, the hallmark of acute bacterial infection.

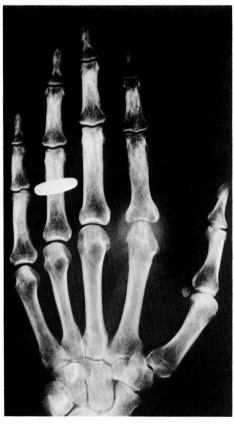

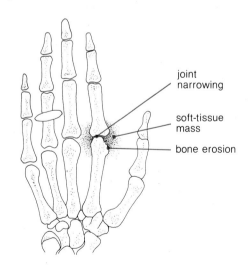

Fig. 6.35 Roentgenogram of the hand in a patient with early rheumatoid arthritis. Note the soft-tissue swelling, the reduction in the width of the joint space, and the erosion that has taken place at the margin of the metacarpophalangeal joint of the index finger.

joint narrowing

soft-tissue mass

bone erosion

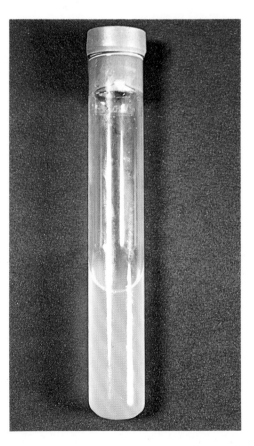

Fig. 6.36 Synovial fluid aspirate from a patient with rheumatoid arthritis. Note the turbidity of this specimen.

A clinical examination reveals the acutely affected joint to be hot, swollen, and tender. The synovial effusion is milky and turbid (Fig. 6.36). Compared with septic arthritis, in which the synovial fluid generally contains more than 100,000 white blood cells per cubic millimeter, at least 75 per cent of which are polymorphonuclear leukocytes, the rheumatoid joint effusion contains 20,000 to 50,000 inflammatory cells per cubic millimeter, about 50 per cent of which are polymorphonuclear leukocytes.

Cultures of the synovial fluid and synovial membrane for various organisms, including viruses, are generally negative.

The principal morphologic feature of rheumatoid disease is joint destruction (Fig. 6.37). Unlike the noninflammatory arthritides, there is little reparative activity, and osteophytes and new bone formation are not prominent (Figs. 6.38 and 6.39).

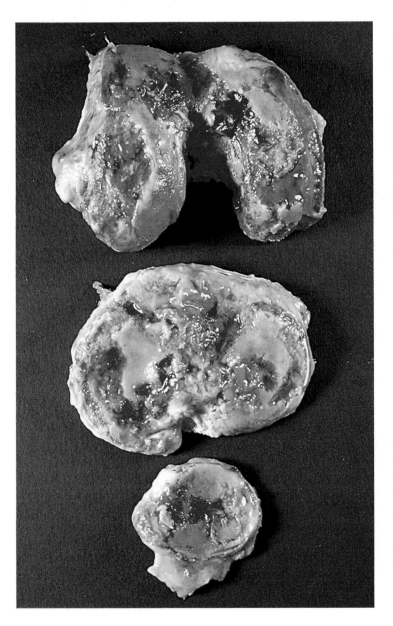

Fig. 6.37 Gross photograph of the articular surfaces of a knee joint from a patient with rheumatoid arthritis. The articular cartilage is destroyed more at the periphery of the joint, whereas the central areas are spared. This finding is characteristic of the inflammatory arthritides, and may be contrasted to the findings in patients with osteoarthritis, in whom the central cartilage is generally destroyed first and the periphery is spared.

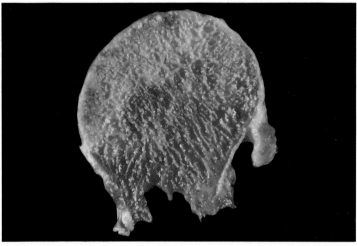

Fig. 6.38 Frontal section through a femoral head in a patient with rheumatoid arthritis. The joint surface is destroyed, but there is no evidence of osteophyte formation or bone sclerosis. The absence of these two features stands in marked contrast to the morphologic findings in patients with osteoarthritis.

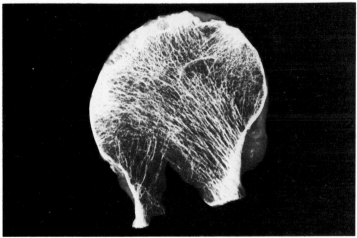

Fig. 6.39 Roentgenogram of the specimen shown in Figure 6.38.

The earliest histologic finding is a nonsuppurative chronic inflammation of the synovium characterized by (1) hypertrophy and hyperplasia of the synovial cells, resulting in a papillary pattern at the surface of the synovium (Figs. 6.40 and 6.41); (2) an infiltration of the synovial membrane with lymphocytes and plasma cells, the latter often containing eosinophilic inclusions of γ-globulin (Russell's bodies) (neutrophils, common in the synovial

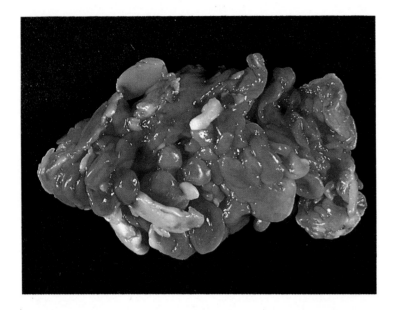

Fig. 6.40 Gross photograph of synovium from a patient with rheumatoid arthritis. The cinnamon color indicates the presence of posthemorrhagic hemosiderin deposits in the synovium. The plump papillae stem from the cellular overgrowth of the synovium, as well as from the lymphoid infiltration of the subintimal layer. The irregular white nodules on the surface are fibrin, the product of vascular exudation in the inflamed tissue.

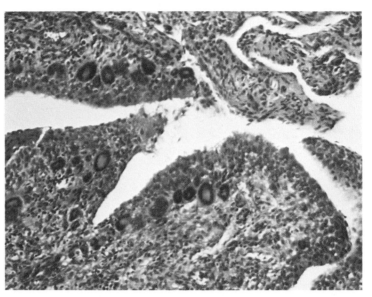

Fig. 6.41 Photomicrograph of a section of synovial membrane from a patient with rheumatoid arthritis. The increased number of lining cells (hyperplasia) and the increased size (hypertrophy) are evident. Many giant cells are also present just below the surface. In the subintimal tissue one may note a chronic inflammatory infiltrate.

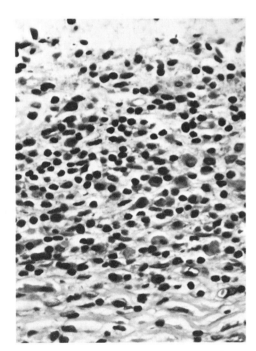

Fig. 6.42 Photomicrograph of the subintimal region of the synovial membrane in a patient with rheumatoid arthritis shows an infiltration of both lymphocytes and plasma cells.

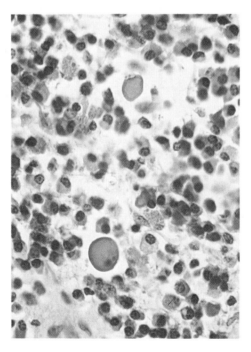

Fig. 6.43 Photomicrograph of inflammatory infiltrate in rheumatoid synovium reveals eosinophilic cytoplasmic inclusions (Russell's bodies) in the plasma cells.

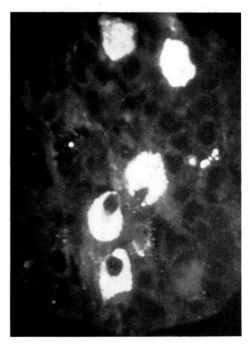

Fig. 6.44 The plasma cells and Russell's bodies contain rheumatoid factor (immunoglobulin including IgM) demonstrated here by staining with fluorescein-labeled antibody to rheumatoid factor. This specimen is viewed with ultraviolet light.

exudate, are much less common in the synovial membrane) (Figs. 6.42 to 6.44); (3) lymphoid follicles (Fig. 6.45); and (4) fibrinous exudation at the surface of the synovium and within the synovial tissue (Figs. 6.46 and 6.47).

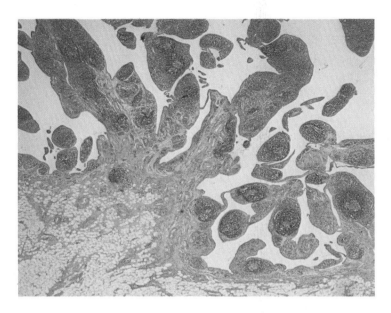

Fig. 6.45 Low power photomicrograph of synovium from a patient with rheumatoid arthritis demonstrates the distribution of lymphoid follicles (Allison-Ghormley bodies) in the subintimal tissue.

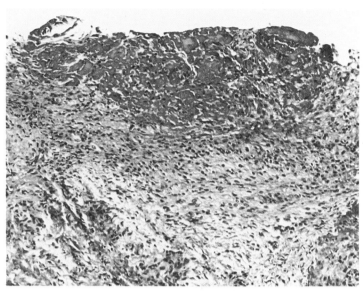

Fig. 6.46 Photomicrograph of the synovium shows the fibrinous exudate on the inflamed synovial surface.

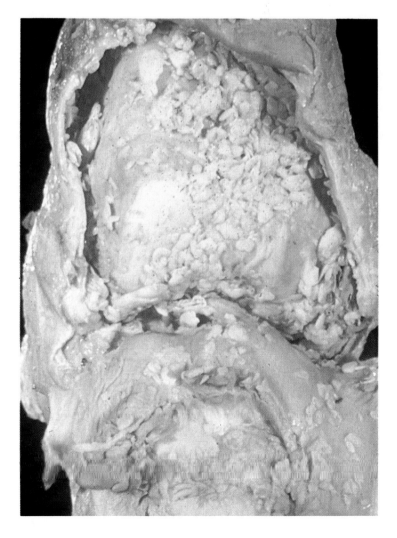

Fig. 6.47 Gross photograph of the suprapatellar pouch and synovium of a knee joint demonstrates copious fibrinous exudate on the surface of the synovium.

Later in the course of the disease, the hypertrophied, inflamed synovium extends over the articular surface (pannus) (Fig. 6.48), and destroys the underlying cartilage by interfering with chondrocyte nutrition and by the enzymatic degradation of the matrix (Figs. 6.49 and 6.50). The end result of this inflammatory destruction of the articular surfaces may be the fusion of the joint (ankylosis), either by fibrous granulation tissue or by bone (Fig. 6.51).

As well as destroying the cartilaginous surface of the joint, the rheumatoid synovium may invade and destroy the joint capsule and other periarticular supportive tissues. This process results in marked instability of the joint

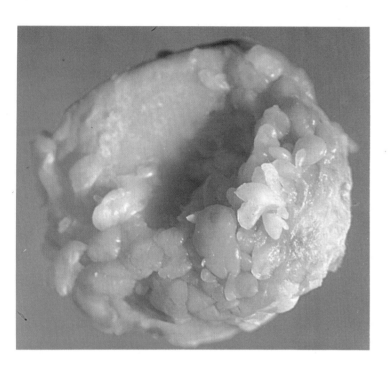

Fig. 6.48 Gross photograph of the radial head from an elbow in a patient with rheumatoid arthritis. The hyperplastic papillary synovium can be seen extending onto and over the articular surface.

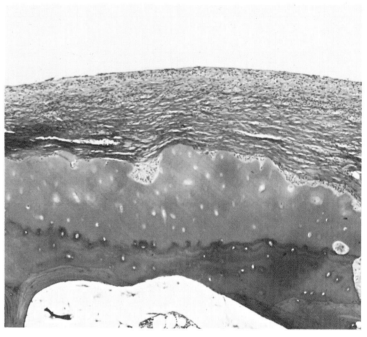

Fig. 6.49 Low power photomicrograph of a section of the synovium and underlying cartilage and bone from the specimen shown in Fig. 6.48. The inflamed synovium forms a covering or pannus over the cartilage, which in turn is being eroded.

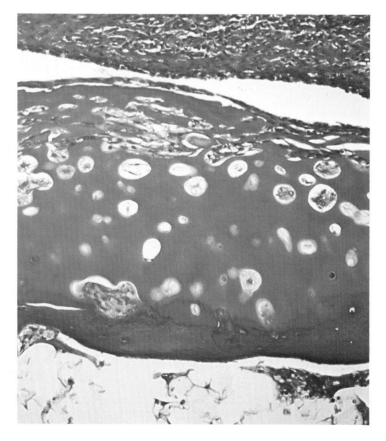

Fig. 6.50 Close-up of the section shown in Fig. 6.49. Not only is the cartilage being eroded from the surface, but the chondrocytes are seen to be mostly necrotic, and lysis of the matrix around the chondrocytes has occurred.

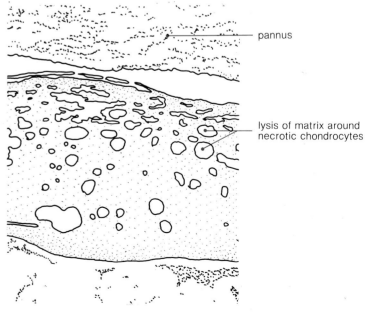

pannus

lysis of matrix around necrotic chondrocytes

and, frequently, subluxation or complete dislocation. The inflamed synovium also invades the bone at the articular margins, a change that appears on roentgenograms as a focal lysis.

Extra-articular synovitis may lead to carpal tunnel syndrome or "trigger finger," and these clinical syndromes may in some cases be heralds of rheumatoid arthritis.

In the subchondral bone not in contact with the articular margins, there may be considerable chronic inflammation and formation of lymphoid follicles (Fig. 6.52). This inflammation is confined to the subchondral bone and does not extend far into the underlying cancellous bone. In some cases, the inflammatory tissue may destroy the articular cartilage from below (Fig. 6.53).

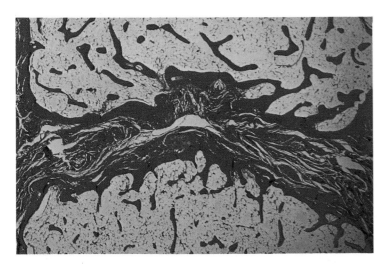

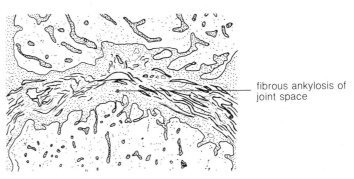

Fig. 6.51 Low power photomicrograph of a metacarpophalangeal joint with a fibrous ankylosis.

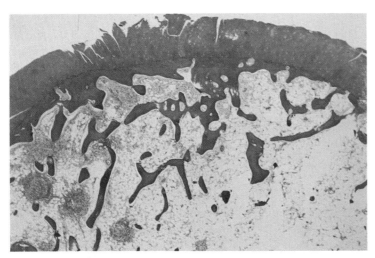

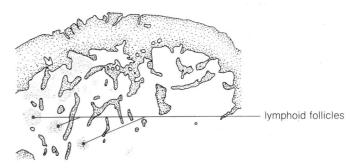

Fig. 6.52 Low power photomicrograph of a section through a joint in a patient with rheumatoid arthritis. Note the considerable chronic inflammatory infiltrate in the subchondral bone, as well as occasional lymphoid follicles.

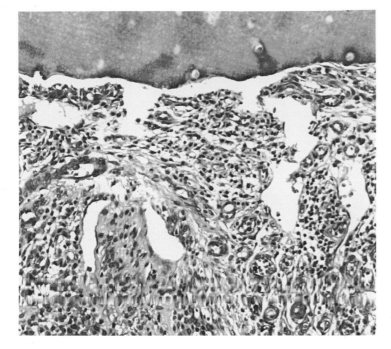

Fig. 6.53 Photomicrograph demonstrates the erosion of the articular cartilage by subchondral inflammatory tissue.

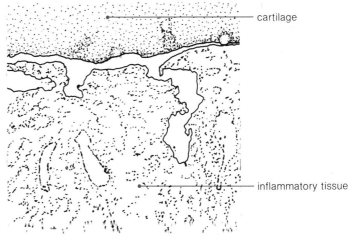

6.19

Roentgenograms of affected joints usually show osteopenia of the juxta-articular bone ends (Fig. 6.54). This finding may result from either the inflammation of the subchondral bone or hyperemia secondary to the inflammation of the synovium.

About 25 per cent of the patients with rheumatoid arthritis have subcutaneous nodules, most commonly over the extensor surfaces of the elbow and forearm (Fig. 6.55). The nodules may occur in other subcutaneous sites, as well as in the gastrointestinal tract, lungs, heart, and in

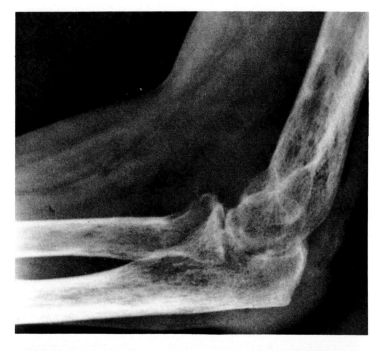

Fig. 6.54 Roentgenogram of the elbow in a patient with polyarticular rheumatoid arthritis. Note the loss of joint space resulting from destructive inflammatory synovitis. Considerable osteoporosis has occurred around the joint, a finding in marked contrast to the bony sclerosis associated with noninflammatory osteoarthritis.

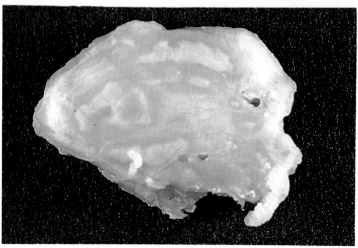

Fig. 6.55 Photograph of the cut surface of a subcutaneous nodule removed from a patient with rheumatoid arthritis. Note the multiple well-defined areas of necrosis with their irregular "geographic" outlines.

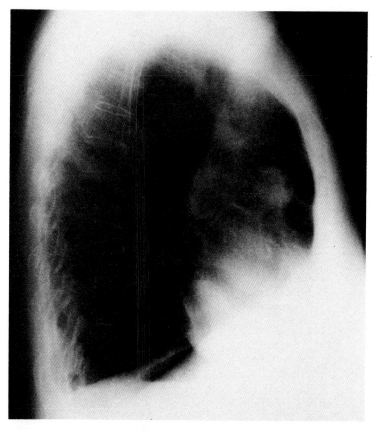

Fig. 6.56 Roentgenogram of a lateral projection of the chest shows a well-defined nodule in the anterior lung field.

the synovial membrane (Fig. 6.56). The nodules may be present before any other sign of rheumatoid disease.

The rheumatoid nodule is characterized histologically by an irregular shape and a central zone of necrotic fibrinoid material surrounded by histiocytes and some chronic inflammatory cells (Figs. 6.57 and 6.58). The long axes of these histiocytes are frequently radially disposed or palisaded. The fact that generalized vasculitis is much more common in patients with rheumatoid nodules is consistent with the belief that the nodules result from vascular damage.

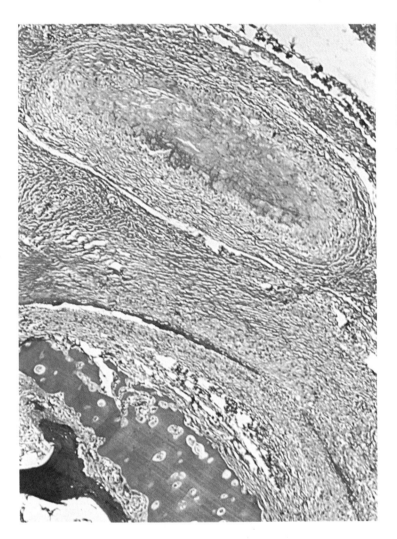

Fig. 6.57 Low power view of a rheumatoid nodule in the synovial membrane. At the bottom of the picture can be seen a portion of eroded and necrotic articular cartilage with overlying inflamed pannus, and at the top within the synovial membrane is a well-defined rheumatoid nodule with central fibrinous necrosis surrounded by a rim of cellular tissue.

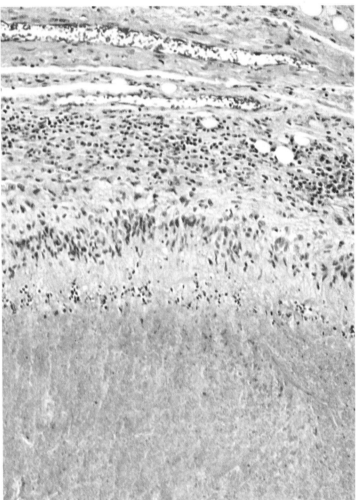

Fig. 6.58 Photomicrograph of a portion of a rheumatoid nodule demonstrates the well-defined zones of central fibrinoid necrosis surrounded by a layer of palisaded histiocytes, which in turn is surrounded by a layer of lymphocytes and dense fibrous connective tissue.

Although the ultimate cause of rheumatoid disease is unknown, there are two important contributory factors: an immunologic reaction and an increased number of degradative enzymes. Most patients with rheumatoid arthritis have a number of immunoglobulins in their serum and synovial fluid, the most common of which is IgM. These immunoglobulins are known as "rheumatoid factors"; they are produced by plasma cells in the synovium and lymphoid system, and they can be seen on microscopic examinations both within plasma cells and in the vicinity of plasma cells, as dense, homogeneous, eosinophilic globules (or Russell's bodies).

Rheumatoid factor complexes with IgG in a manner not unlike an antigen-antibody reaction.

In rheumatoid joints the level of the components of complement in the synovial fluid is reduced, in contrast to most other inflammatory joint diseases in which the complement levels are elevated in proportion to the increased serum proteins in the synovial fluid. Leukocytes are attracted to the immune complexes which, along with fibrin, form on the surface of the inflamed synovium. These cells, filled with particles of ingested fibrin and immune complex, may be found in the synovial fluid and are called "RA cells".

The lysosomal enzymes are released into the extracellular space following the destruction of the polymorphonuclear leukocytes, and they provoke an acute inflammatory response and tissue necrosis. These enzymes exist in large concentrations in both the synovial fluid and tissue of rheumatoid joints, and they play an important role in the tissue destruction that characterizes the disease.

In the late stages of rheumatoid arthritis the affected joint may show very little in the way of inflammation, and the disease may be anatomically indistinguishable from osteoarthritis.

A nonspecific, chronic inflammatory arthritis is sometimes seen in association with various systemic diseases, such as psoriasis, lupus erythematosus, and ulcerative colitis. Although the clinical presentation varies in these different inflammatory conditions, an examination of the joints generally shows a chronically inflamed and hyperplastic synovium, frequently with effusion and fibrinous exudation into the joint cavity, and a breakdown of the articular cartilage by enzymatic degradation.

7 Arthritis II

AVASCULAR NECROSIS

Segmental infarction, osteonecrosis

It is only recently that avascular necrosis of the bone has been appreciated as a significant cause of arthritis, not only of the hip, but of the knee and other major joints.

Areas of osteonecrosis that are immediately adjacent to an articular joint may result in arthritis owing to a fracture of the necrotic bone and subsequent collapse of the overlying articular surface (Figs. 7.1 to 7.5).

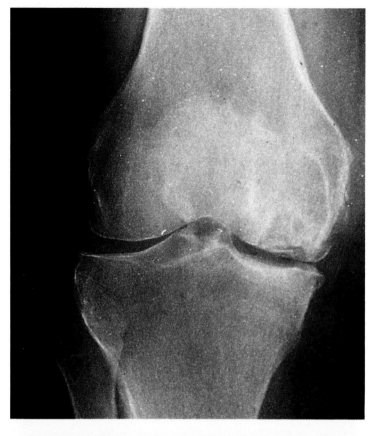

Fig. 7.1 Anteroposterior roentgenogram of the knee in a 58-year-old woman who complained of the sudden onset of pain in the knee. Inequality of the articular surface of the medial femoral cartilage is evident.

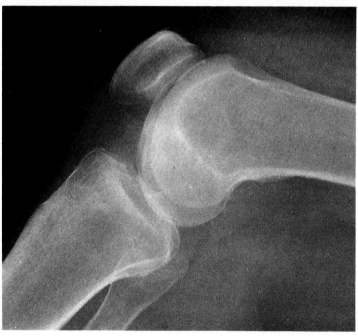

Fig. 7.2 Lateral view of the same knee shown in Fig. 7.1 reveals a subchondral fracture of a portion of the articular surface of the femoral cartilage.

The clinical onset of avascular necrosis is usually sudden. Furthermore, the duration of symptoms is shorter than that in either rheumatoid arthritis or osteoarthritis. The hip seems to be the joint most commonly affected by an infarct, which generally occurs in the femoral head rather than the acetabulum. In this regard, it is generally true that the convex surface of any joint is the one most often affected by osteonecrosis.

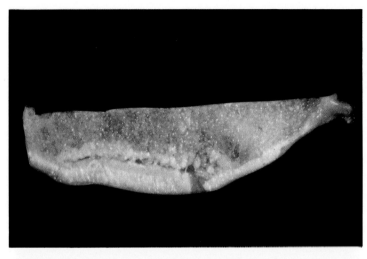

Fig. 7.3 A frontal slice taken through the medial condyle of a patient with osteonecrosis of the knee. The zone of bone necrosis is seen immediately under the articular surface, and is characterized by an opaque-yellow appearance. Immediately beyond the necrotic zone is a band of hyperemia. Separating the necrotic bone from the overlying cartilage is a gap created by the collapse of the bone trabeculae in the necrotic segment.

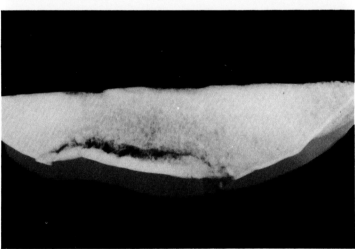

Fig. 7.4 A roentgenogram of the specimen illustrated in Fig. 7.3. Note that the subchondral bone end plate remains attached to the articular cartilage, and around the margin of the infarct the fracture can be seen to extend through the bone end plate, producing deformity of the articular surface.

Fig. 7.5 Histologic section through the specimen illustrated in Figs. 7.3 and 7.4.

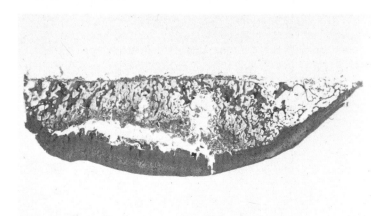

An infarction of the femoral head is a common complication of a subcapital fracture of the femoral neck. Following surgical reduction and internal fixation of these fractures, nearly 20 per cent of the patients develop clinical signs and symptoms of avascular necrosis. The overall frequency of femoral head infarction can be appreciated from the fact that, even when a fracture is excluded as an etiologic consideration, a segmental infarction is responsible for about 20 per cent of all hip disease requiring prosthetic replacement (in our experience).

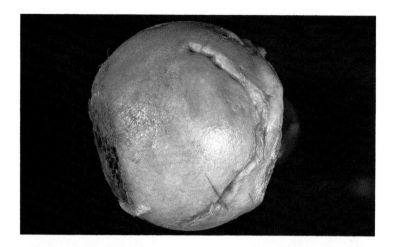

Fig. 7.6 Gross photograph of a femoral head removed surgically after clinical signs and symptoms of avascular necrosis were detected. (Three years previously, the femoral neck had been pinned following a fracture.) On the articular surface of the femoral head the fracture site is marked by a linear dimpling of the articular cartilage.

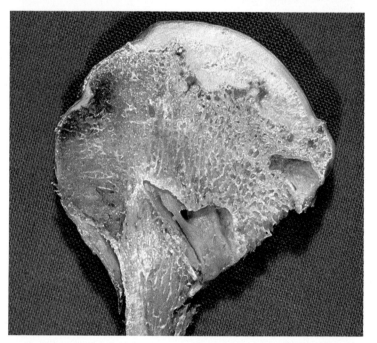

Fig. 7.7 Photograph of a slice through the femoral head shown in Fig. 7.6. The area of infarction is seen as a triangular, opaque-yellow area lying immediately beneath the articular surface. Also seen in this photograph is the track of the nail that was used for fixation of the fracture that preceded the necrosis.

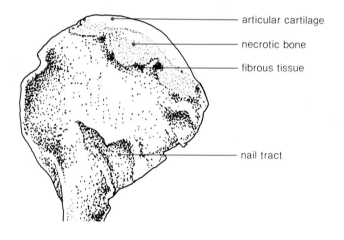

articular cartilage

necrotic bone

fibrous tissue

nail tract

Fig. 7.8 Roentgenogram of the specimen shown in Fig. 7.7. Note the unaltered trabecular pattern of the infarcted bone. The lucent area seen at the base of the infarction results from fibrous granulation tissue eroding the necrotic bone. The collapse of the necrotic segment is well demonstrated by the fracture through the subchondral plate, which is seen at both edges of the infarct. In contrast to the appearance of the infarct, the viable bone is seen to be dense, and this finding results from the formation of new bone in this area by the process of creeping substitution (see text).

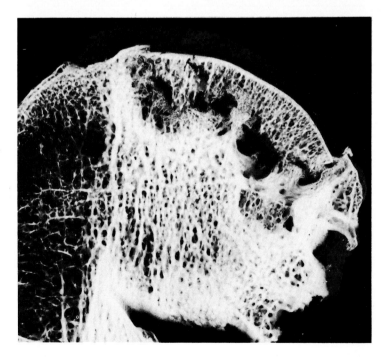

The radiologic features of avascular necrosis include a changed contour and increased density. The increased density results mainly from reparative new bone, with subsequent trabecular thickening surrounding the infarct (Figs. 7.6 to 7.8). The changes in the contour of the joint result from the failure of the reparative tissues to support the articular surface, with subsequent collapse of the infarcted area (Figs. 7.9 to 7.12).

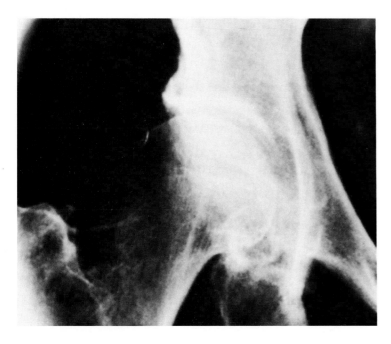

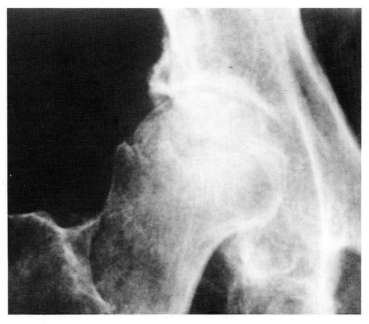

Fig. 7.9 Sequential roentgenograms in a patient who had osteonecrosis of the femoral head. In the film on the left, there are no visible radiologic changes. However, in the film on the right, taken only three months later, there is obviously increased density in the femoral head, which has also collapsed along its superior articular surface.

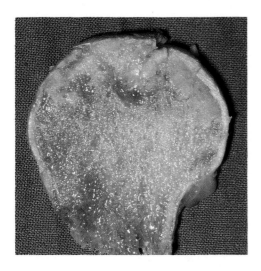

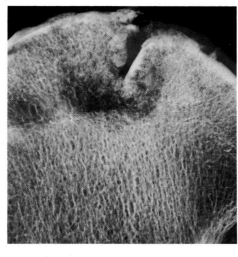

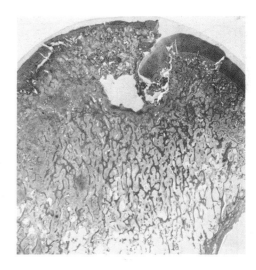

Fig. 7.10 Gross photograph of the femoral head removed from the patient in Fig. 7.9. In addition to flattening of the femoral head, a hyperemic granulation tissue is seen at the margin of the infarcted area. At the margin of the infarct an infolding of the articular cartilage can be appreciated.

Fig. 7.11 Roentgenogram of the specimen slice shown in Fig. 7.10. The osteolysis in the area of the hyperemic granulation tissue can be easily appreciated in this preparation.

Fig. 7.12 A histologic preparation of the specimen shown in Figs. 7.10 and 7.11.

It should be emphasized that the necrosis involves only bone and bone marrow, and not, except in rare cases, the articular cartilage, which receives its nutrition from the synovial fluid. Therefore, the joint space on roentgenograms remains intact, at least in the initial stages of the disease (Fig. 7.13). This radiologic feature clearly distinguishes early avascular necrosis from other forms of joint disease, in which the first radiologically evident change is a loss of articular cartilage and joint space narrowing.

A gross examination of a joint surface resected in a patient with early-stage clinical osteonecrosis is likely to reveal fairly intact articular cartilage, although some wrinkling of the surface that marks the edge of the necrotic area will probably be evident. On vertical sectioning, the infarcted zone exhibits a characteristic bright yellow, opaque appearance. If the infarct is recent, a hyperemic zone is present at its margin, to be replaced later by a zone of fibrous scarring (Figs. 7.14 to 7.16).

An infarct heals from the periphery by invading the necrotic marrow with granulation tissue and ensheathing the necrotic trabeculae by a layer of new bone (so-called

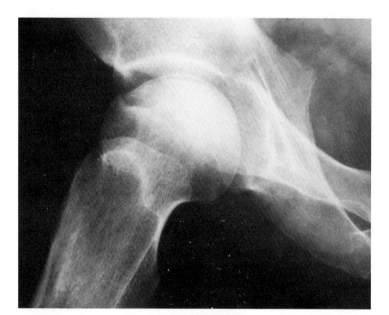

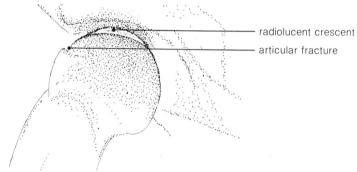

Fig. 7.13 Roentgenogram of a young black patient who complained of the sudden onset of pain in the hip. Note that the joint space is normal. However, in this frog-lateral view, a crescentic lucent zone outlining the articular surface can be appreciated on the superior aspect of the femoral head. This crescent sign is often an early radiologic manifestation of avascular necrosis and is best appreciated in the frog-lateral view.

radiolucent crescent
articular fracture

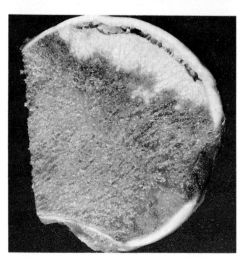

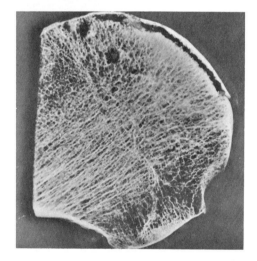

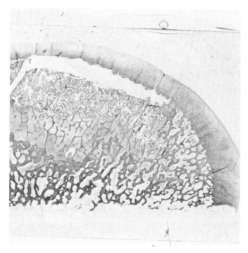

Fig. 7.14 Gross photograph of a slice taken through the femoral head removed from the patient shown in Fig. 7.13. The subchondral infarct is demarcated from the viable bone by a zone of hyperemia. The lucent crescent seen on the roentgenogram is appreciated as a space between the articular cartilage and the underlying infarcted bone.

Fig. 7.15 Roentgenogram of the specimen slice shown in Fig. 7.14. Again the crescent sign is clearly seen. The dense lucent line evident on the superior surface of the femoral head is an image of the subchondral bone end plate and the calcified cartilage, which remain adherent to the articular cartilage after the collapse of the infarcted area. After such a collapse the articular surface probably springs back like a ping-pong ball, giving rise to this radiologic phenomenon.

Fig. 7.16 A histologic preparation of the femoral head shown in the previous three figures. The thickened trabeculae of the viable bone can be clearly appreciated.

creeping substitution) (Figs. 7.17 to 7.20). Some infarcts heal without complication, and such instances are unlikely to be detected clinically since the process is generally asymptomatic. However, some cases are complicated by collapse, perhaps resulting from accumulated "fatigue" microfractures of the necrotic bone trabeculae.

With the progression of avascular necrosis, the collapse of the necrotic segment and flattening of the joint surface ensue. The articular cartilage detaches from the underlying bone, which in turn gradually fragments and erodes. These changes result in the gross destruction of the joint, which finally shows the signs of secondary osteoarthritis.

When a fracture is excluded from the etiologic considerations, the most frequently associated conditions in patients with avascular necrosis of the hip are systemic steroid therapy (usually for rheumatoid arthritis) and alcoholism. The other conditions associated with avascular necrosis, e.g., caisson disease, Gaucher's disease, and sickle cell disease, are much less common.

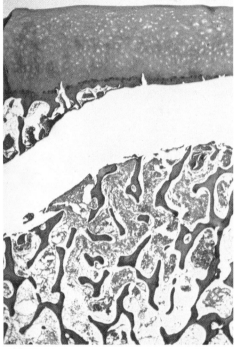

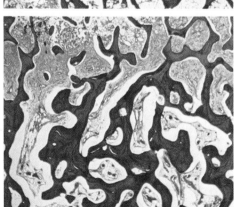

Fig. 7.17 High power photomicrograph of the specimen shown in Fig. 7.16. At the top one may note the necrotic bone and bone marrow of the infarcted area, together with the subchondral crescent; on the lower portion of the frame, one sees the junction between the necrotic and viable bone. At the bottom the thickened trabeculae of viable bone can be well appreciated. This thickening is the result of new bone deposition on the trabecular surfaces, which occurs as part of the healing of the infarct.

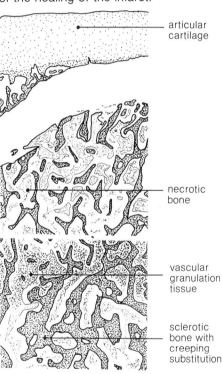

articular cartilage

necrotic bone

vascular granulation tissue

sclerotic bone with creeping substitution

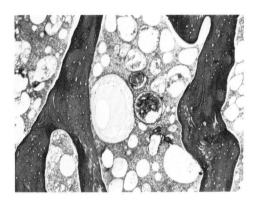

Fig. 7.18 High power view of infarcted bone and bone marrow reveals the acellular nature of the tissue, and large flat cysts characteristic of infarcted bone marrow.

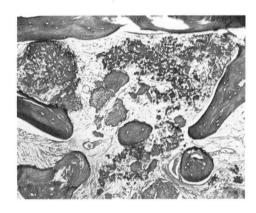

Fig. 7.19 Calcification is sometimes a prominent feature in infarcted bone marrow, and may on occasion give rise to increased density on roentgenograms.

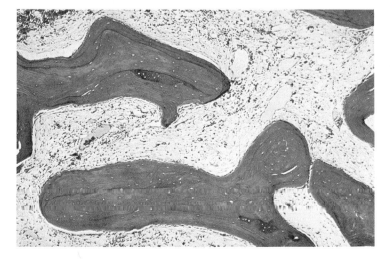

Fig. 7.20 In the process of healing an infarcted area of bone, a layer of living bone is deposited on the surface of the necrotic bone. This process, referred to as creeping substitution, gives rise to increased radiodensity at the healing margin of the infarct.

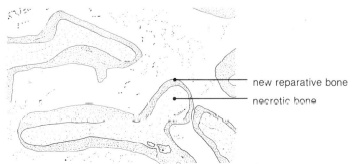

new reparative bone

necrotic bone

In cases of avascular necrosis associated with steroid therapy, and in those associated with alcoholism, fatty microemboli have been implicated as causative agents. Both steroid therapy and alcoholism lead to changes in the fat content in the liver, and in both conditions microemboli of fat have been found in many parenchymal organs at autopsy. Other theories suggest that the increased fat deposits in turn increase marrow pressure, which results in venous stasis, and that the alteration in fat metabolism affects cell function, with subsequent osteopenia and cumulative microfractures. That avascular necrosis is a systemic phenomenon is borne out by the observation that multiple joint involvement by infarcts is evident in about 50 per cent of the patients (Figs. 7.21 and 7.22).

LEGG-CALVÉ-PERTHES DISEASE

Osteonecrosis of the femoral head occurs in children who are usually between the ages of five and nine years. The disease is more likely to be found in boys, and in about 13 per cent of the patients the condition is bilateral.

Since the growth plate of the femoral head is above the insertion of the capsule of the hip joint in children, and since the epiphyseal plate acts as a firm barrier between the metaphysis and the epiphysis with regard to blood flow, it can be seen that the femoral head is dependent upon vessels that track along the surface of the neck of the femur to enter the epiphysis above the growth plate. Injection studies have demonstrated that the most important vessels supplying the epiphysis are the lateral

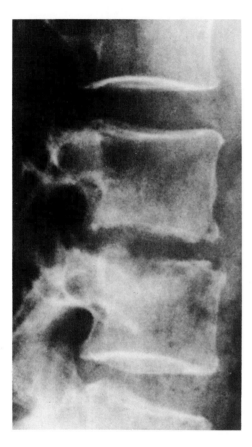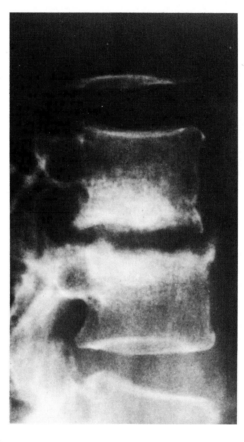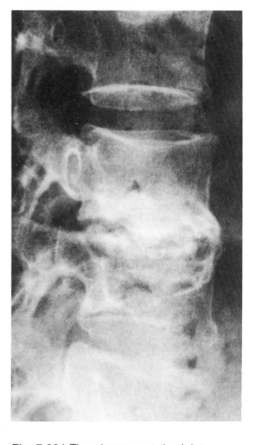

Fig. 7.21 Sequential radiographs of a 50 + -year-old man receiving cortisone therapy for a chronic skin condition. The time interval between the first and second films is 8 months, and the time between the second and third films is 2 years. At the time of the second examination the patient began to complain of pain in the shoulder. (Radiograph of the shoulder is shown in Fig. 7.22.) The changes at the joint surfaces resulted from osteonecrosis secondary to cortisone therapy, though at first the radiologic changes were considered results of tuberculosis.

Fig. 7.22 Roentgenogram of the shoulder from the patient in Fig. 7.21.

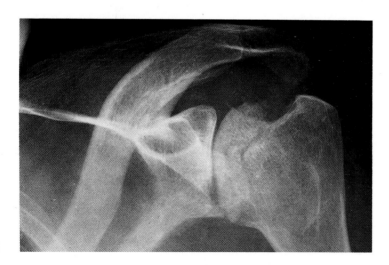

epiphyseal vessels, and it can be appreciated that these vessels are vulnerable to interruption of blood flow from trauma or increases in intra-articular pressure (Fig. 7.23).

One of the earliest radiologic signs of Legg-Calvé-Perthes disease is widening of the joint space. This appearance probably results from the cessation of endochondral ossification, which means that no cartilage is converted to bone. Therefore, the continuous growth of cartilage will be appreciated as an increase in the width of the joint space on the radiologic film (Fig. 7.24). The bony epiphysis may undergo collapse and subsequent deformation, but deformity may also result from the irregular growth of new bone on the surface of the necrotic secondary center of ossification (Fig. 7.25). Characteristic

radiologic changes in patients with Legg-Calvé-Perthes disease include some widening of the epiphysis of the femoral neck and, often, lytic lesions in the metaphysis. Since the growth plate is dependent upon its epiphyseal supply for growth and nutrition, it is to be expected that following necrosis of the epiphysis secondary changes will occur in the growth plate.

Arthritis secondary to osteonecrosis is rarely detected in joints other than the hip, the knee, and the shoulder. However, there are three other sites in which osteonecrosis may occasionally be the cause of disease: the carpal lunate bone (Kienböck's disease), the head of a metatarsal bone—usually the second (Freiberg's disease), and the tarsal navicular bone (Köhler's disease).

Fig. 7.23 Blood supply to the femoral head in a child.

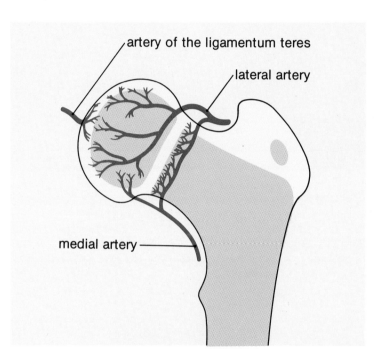

artery of the ligamentum teres

lateral artery

medial artery

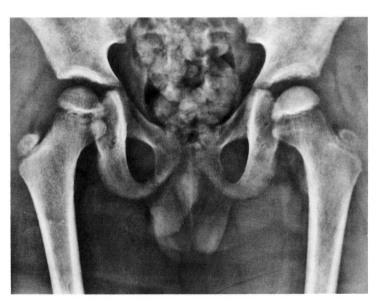

Fig. 7.24 In the early stages of Legg-Calvé-Perthes disease, before any obvious deformity of the secondary center of ossification occurs in the epiphysis, one may observe a widening of the joint space and an apparent increase in the density of the secondary center of ossification. However, this "increase in density" is only the result of osteopenia in the surrounding bone. The secondary center retains its density, probably because it is nonviable.

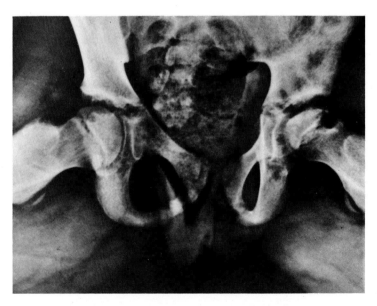

Fig. 7.25 In the late stages of Legg-Calvé-Perthes disease, the secondary center of ossification appears smaller and has an irregular outline resulting from collapse of the epiphysis and lack of growth. However, new bone formation does take place between the cartilage and the underlying necrotic, distorted secondary center of ossification, and eventually this process results in a "head within a head" appearance. Note also the large cyst in the region of the growth plate that extends into the metaphysis.

OSTEOARTHRITIS

Degenerative joint disease, osteoarthrosis

Osteoarthritis is generally regarded as a noninflammatory condition that begins as a disruption of the weight-bearing surfaces of the articular cartilage, and ends with the disintegration of the mechanical joint. In about one-fifth of the patients, it is evident to the clinician that there was an antecedent condition causally related to the osteoarthritis, which can be considered secondary osteoarthritis (Table 7.1, Fig. 7.26). Individuals affected by secondary osteoarthritis are likely to be about 10 years younger than those with primary (idiopathic) osteoarthritis, who are generally over 60 years of age.

A patient with clinical osteoarthritis complains of pain and disability. Movement of the affected joint may be limited, and the patient often lacks the capability for full flexion or extension. The most characteristic radiologic

Table 7.1	Conditions that May Precede Osteoarthritis (Secondary Osteoarthritis)
	Hip dysplasia
	Congenital dislocation or subluxation of the hip
	Perthes' disease
	Slipped capital femoral epiphysis
	Intra-articular fracture: traumatic dislocation
	Radiation damage
	Infection
	Metabolic diseases (e.g., gout, CPPD, ochronosis)
	Unrecognized avascular necrosis
	"Burnt-out" rheumatoid arthritis

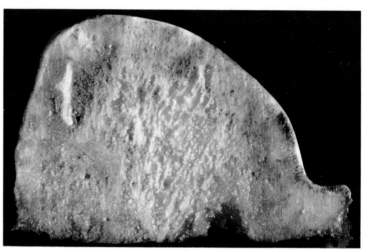

Fig. 7.26 A slice through a severely deformed femoral head with extensive osteophyte formation and flattening of the superior surface. In this patient the osteoarthritis was secondary to Paget's disease of the bone, a diagnosis that can be appreciated in the altered texture and trabecular architecture seen in this specimen.

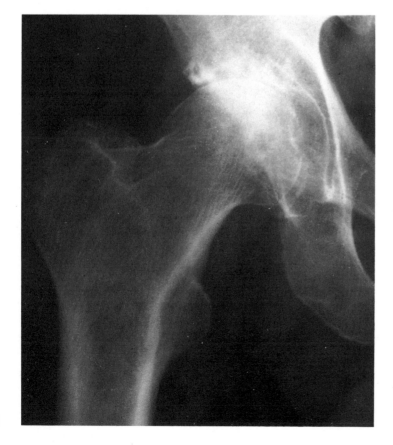

Fig. 7.27 Roentgenogram of the hip joint in a patient complaining of pain and limitation of motion in that joint. Note the diminished joint space in the superior aspect of the joint, together with sclerosis evident on both the acetabular and femoral sides of the joint. In this patient there has been no significant migration of the joint, either medially or laterally, and this finding may be considered characteristic of the early stage of osteoarthritis of the hip joint.

finding in patients with osteoarthritis is the loss of the joint space, usually in the superior part of the joint, but occasionally medially or concentrically. In the majority of patients, bony osteophytes will also be seen around the periphery of the joint, particularly on the acetabular margin and on the medial surface of the femoral head. Both on the acetabular side of the joint and on the femoral head in the superior quadrant, the bone will be observed to have increased density, and, frequently, cystic lesions can be noted in the subchondral bone region, either in the acetabulum or in the femoral head or in both.

The examination of a joint removed at surgery or autopsy shows that the most significant features of an osteoarthritic joint are alterations in the shape of the articular surfaces and damaged cartilage. In the weight-bearing areas of the joint, the cartilage may be entirely absent, and the exposed subchondral bone has a dense, polished appearance like marble (eburnation) (Figs. 7.27 to 7.31).

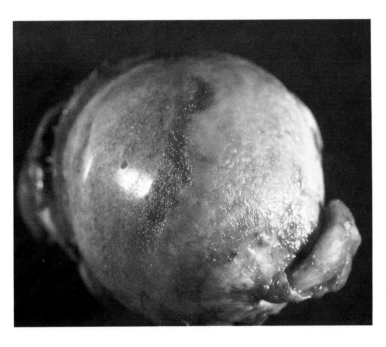

Fig. 7.28 Gross photograph of the femoral head removed from the patient shown in Fig. 7.27. Note the absence of the articular cartilage on the superior and lateral aspect of the femoral head, and the polished appearance of the exposed bone (eburnation). The remaining surrounding cartilage has a somewhat yellow color, and its surface is roughened.

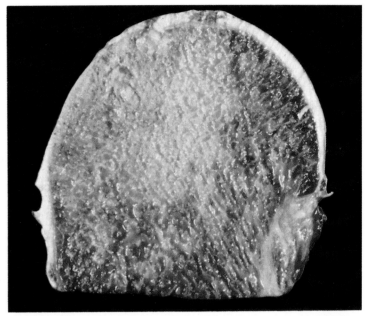

Fig. 7.29 A slice through the femoral head shown in Fig. 7.28 reveals the absence of the articular cartilage over the superior-lateral surface. However, the sphericity of the joint is fairly well maintained, and there is no significant osteophyte formation. This finding is in keeping with the lack of significant migration seen in the radiograph. (In later stages of the disease when migration has occurred, osteophyte formation is prominent.)

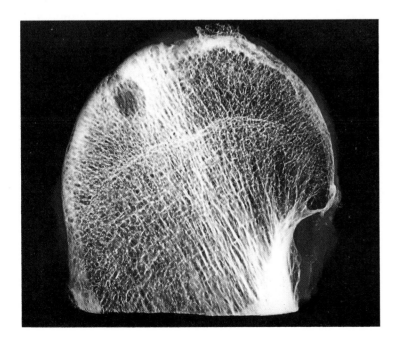

Fig. 7.30 Roentgenogram of the specimen shown in Fig. 7.29. Note the sclerosis of the bone underlying the superior-lateral surface of the femoral head. Within this sclerotic bone, a cyst can be seen. (The specimen roentgenogram will often reveal gross anatomic features more clearly than the specimen itself.)

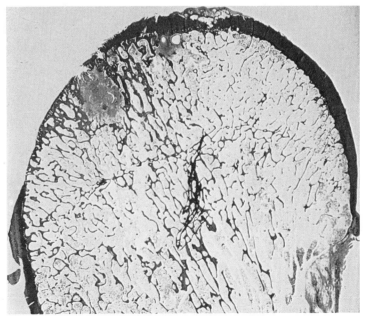

Fig. 7.31 A histologic preparation of the specimen shown in the previous three figures. The sclerosis of the bone in the eburnated portion of the femoral head and the fibrous filled area of bone lysis are evident.

In these areas of absent cartilage, the bone is usually markedly thickened (sclerotic); adjacent to the surface, cystic defects filled by loose fibromyxoid tissue (or sometimes, a thick fluid) may be found (Figs. 7.32 to 7.35). In the eburnated areas, the superficial bone may be seen to be necrotic when it is examined microscopically. In the areas of the joint that do not bear weight, and around its margins, bony and cartilaginous overgrowths (osteophytes or exostoses) develop, which on the medial and inferior aspect of the femoral head may occur in the form of very large, flat plaques of bone and cartilage (Figs. 7.36 and 7.37).

The remaining cartilage, when viewed under a microscope, will be found to have many clefts in its substance, most but by no means all of which are vertically disposed. The cartilage cells far from the areas of eburnation may

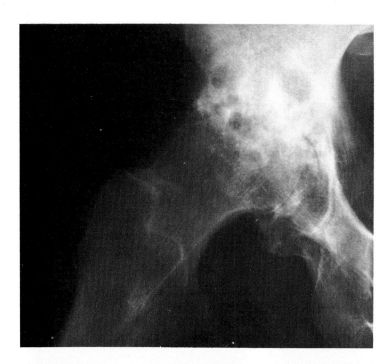

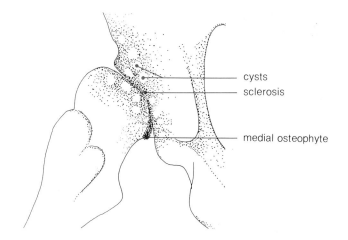

Fig. 7.32 Roentgenogram of a patient with more advanced osteoarthritis of the hip joint. Note the increased deformity of the femoral head, with marked sclerosis on both sides of the joint, and radiologic evidence of cyst formation. Some lateral subluxation has taken place, and a medial osteophyte is apparent.

cysts
sclerosis
medial osteophyte

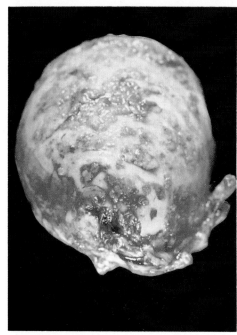

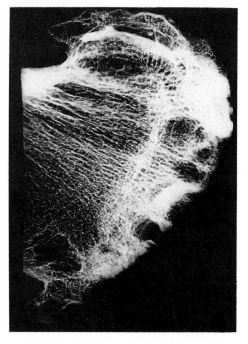

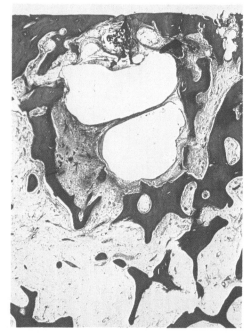

Fig. 7.33 Gross photograph of the femoral head removed from the patient shown in Fig. 7.32. One may observe marked irregularity and flattening of the superior-lateral surface of the femoral head. As shown in this photograph, small plaques of fibrous tissue are often present on the eburnated surface.

Fig. 7.34 Roentgenogram of a slice taken through the femoral head shown in Fig. 7.33. The considerable flattening of the superior surface of the femoral head can be appreciated, together with marked subchondral sclerosis and cyst formation. On the medial side of the joint one may note osteophyte formation.

Fig. 7.35 Photomicrograph of one of the subchondral bone cysts seen in the specimen radiograph shown in Fig. 7.34.

show considerable replication, with the formation of prominent cell nests (Fig. 7.38). However, adjacent to the eburnated areas, cell replication does not usually occur (Fig. 7.39). Generally, the proteoglycan staining ability of the matrix will be found to be diminished, though there is evidence from radioactive SO_4 uptake studies that the amount of proteoglycan produced by the chondrocytes in osteoarthritis may be increased. Presumably, the proteoglycan is either enzymatically degraded or it leaks into the joint space through the damaged articular surface. The synovial membrane shows some villous proliferation and slight hyperplasia of the intima. A mild chronic inflammation may be noted (Fig. 7.40). Small osteochondral loose bodies are commonly found in the synovium and in the joint.

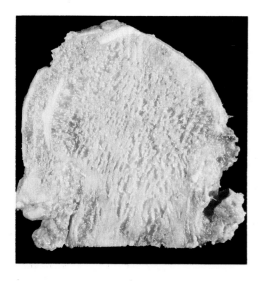

Fig. 7.36 Associated with subluxation of the femoral head in a patient with osteoarthritis of the hip is the formation of a large, flat, medial osteophyte. The osteophyte can be seen to extend from the joint margin to the region of the fovea. The residual cartilage of the medial surface of the femoral head can still be seen.

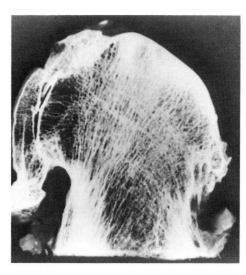

Fig. 7.37 Roentgenogram of the tissue slice shown in Fig. 7.36 again illustrates the large medial osteophyte. Notice that the loss of bone on the superior and lateral surfaces seems to equate with the gain of bone on the medial surface, so the sphericity of the femoral head remains.

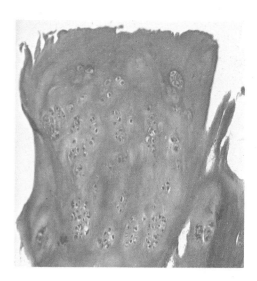

Fig. 7.38 Photomicrograph of fibrillated cartilage away from the eburnated area shows a considerable proliferation of chondrocytes within the cartilage matrix. Many of the chondrocytes can be seen to form cellular nests or clones.

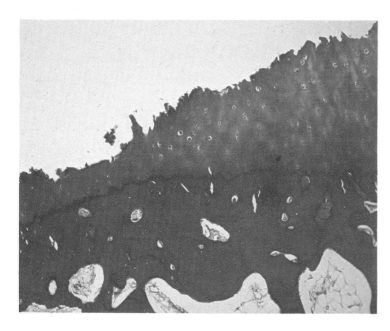

Fig. 7.39 A section through the articular cartilage at the margin of the eburnated area shows thinning and irregularity of the surface of the cartilage without obvious chondrocyte proliferation.

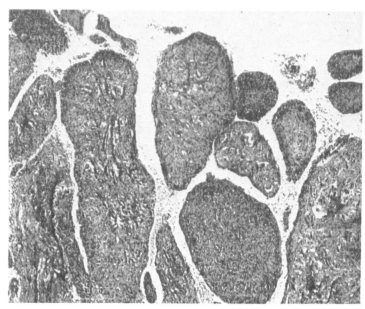

Fig. 7.40 Photomicrograph of the synovial membrane in a patient with osteoarthritis. The villous pattern of the synovium and hyperplasia of the synovial lining cells can be appreciated. In this patient, as in many patients with osteoarthritis, one may also note a mild chronic inflammatory infiltrate in the synovial tissue. (This inflammation can be quite severe in some individuals.)

7.13

It has been found that a significant number of patients who appear by all histologic criteria to have an inflammatory arthritis have been diagnosed on the basis of their clinical picture as having osteoarthritis. It is important, when considering the etiology and pathogenesis of osteoarthritis, to take into account these cases of so-called inflammatory osteoarthritis (or rapidly progressive osteoarthritis).

Some patients with osteoarthritis have a tendency to improve spontaneously by both clinical and radiologic criteria. We have observed that in advanced stages of the disease, eburnated areas tend to resurface with fibrocarti-

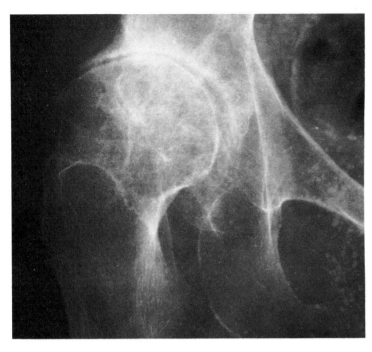

Fig. 7.41 Advanced osteoarthritis of the hip joint. Note narrowing of the joint space, subchondral sclerosis, and cyst formation.

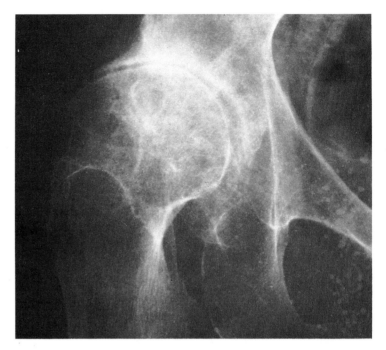

Fig. 7.42 Roentgenogram of the hip joint shown in Fig. 7.41, taken three and one-half years after the first film. The patient had received no treatment, but it can be appreciated that there has been a reduction in the subchondral sclerosis, and the subchondral cysts are no longer obvious.

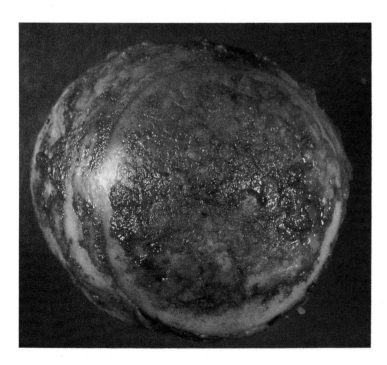

Fig. 7.43 Gross photograph of the femoral head removed from the patient shown in Figs. 7.41 and 7.42. Most of the superior-lateral surface of the femoral head can be seen to be covered by an irregular layer of tissue, which seems to be growing in the form of small tufts from many focal areas in the bone.

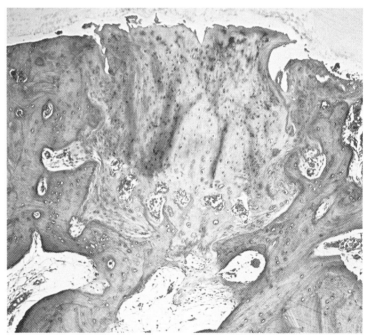

Fig. 7.44 Photomicrograph of one of the tufts shown in Fig. 7.43. The tuft is formed of fibrocartilaginous tissue extending from the marrow onto the joint surface. On either side is eburnated bone.

lage, which explains the radiologic improvement seen in some late cases (Figs. 7.41 to 7.46). This finding also suggests that osteoarthritis is not necessarily a progressive and continually degenerative process. Rather, it should be said that there are two opposing processes occurring in a joint: the degenerative process of mechanical breakdown and repair. In the arthritic joint, when breakdown occurs faster than repair, the joint deteriorates. Sometimes the processes come into balance, and the disease stabilizes. In some patients, the reparative process gains ascendency, and there is morphologic and perhaps even clinical improvement (Fig. 7.47).

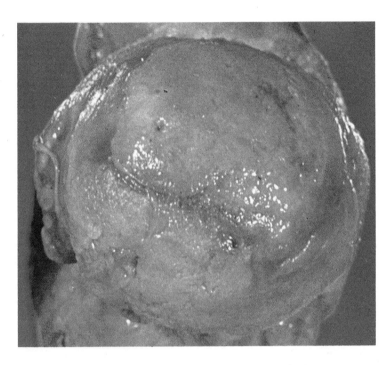

Fig. 7.45 In some occurrences of osteoarthritis, and even in untreated patients, the superior surface of the femoral head may be entirely covered by a layer of fibrocartilaginous tissue, as seen in this example.

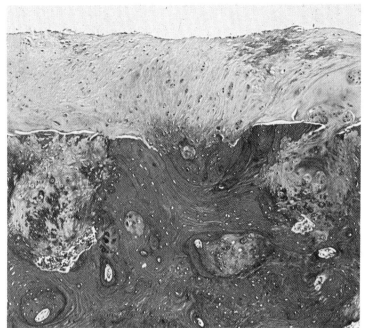

Fig. 7.46 Photomicrograph of the fibrocartilage seen in Fig. 7.45 reveals the extension over the previously eburnated bone of cartilaginous tissue, presumably derived from the underlying subchondral bone.

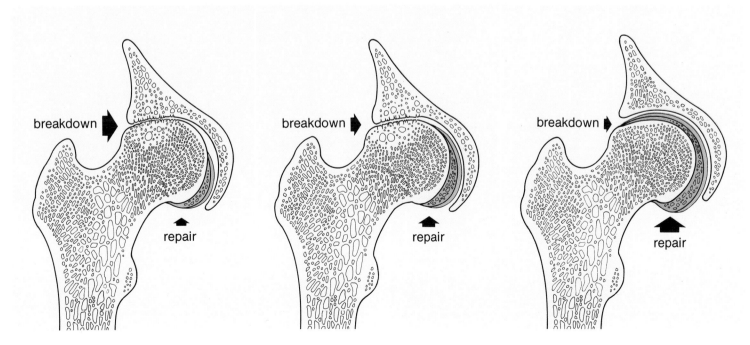

Fig. 7.47 The roentgenographic and clinical signs of arthritis depend, to some extent, on the balance between injury to the joint and repair of the joint. (Left) Deterioration is taking place because breakdown (i.e., loss of cartilage, bone, and bone shape, as well as bone necrosis) is proceeding more rapidly than repair (i.e., regeneration of cartilage and formation of new bone). (Center) Both injury and repair are proceeding at about the same pace, and the joint is stabilized. (Right) Repair is proceeding more rapidly than injury, leading to morphologic and perhaps clinical improvement.

7.15

CHARCOT'S JOINTS

Extreme cases of osteoarthritis seen in association with a neurologic deficit are known as Charcot's joints. The underlying neurologic disorder may be one of several conditions: peripheral neuropathy and spinal cord degeneration (seen in association with pernicious anemia and diabetes mellitus), or syringomyelia. In patients with these neurologic problems, one may observe a rapidly destructive osteoarthritis, complicated by the production of multiple loose bodies, severe subluxation, and even dislocation of the joint (Figs. 7.48 to 7.50).

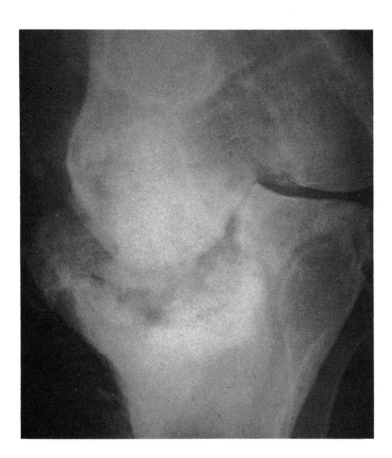

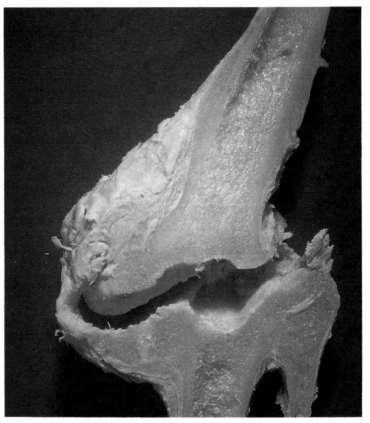

Fig. 7.48 Roentgenogram of the knee in a patient with both diabetes and a history of pernicious anemia. The patient presented with grossly deformed and unstable knees; however, the condition was painless. Note the severe destruction of the medial compartment of the knee and the multiple loose bodies.

Fig. 7.49 Coronal section through a grossly discombobulated knee joint (Charcot's joint). Both subluxation and severe destruction of the joint surfaces are evident. The synovium is hypertrophic; and in such a joint, loose bodies are often numerous.

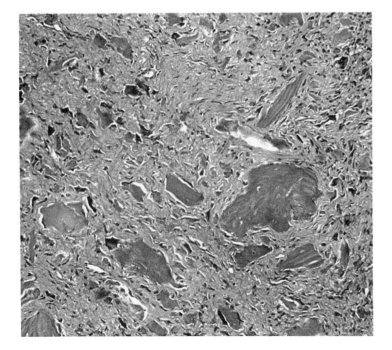

Fig. 7.50 Photomicrograph of a portion of the synovium in a Charcot's joint. The scarred and chronically inflamed synovium is filled by multiple irregular fragments of bone and cartilage. The finding of bone and cartilage detritus in the synovial membrane usually denotes a rapid breakdown of the joint. Sometimes this breakdown is seen in patients with rheumatoid arthritis. In instances of rapid breakdown of the joint, as seen in patients with a Charcot's joint, the detritus is copious. In patients with osteoarthritis it is rare to find any significant degree of detritus.

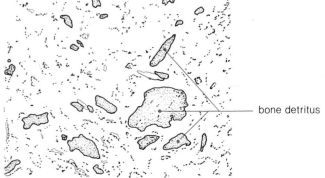

bone detritus

8 Arthritis III

TISSUE RESPONSE TO ARTIFICIAL JOINT IMPLANTS

Perhaps one of the most important therapeutic advances in the past 20 years has been the development of artificial joints, and in most orthopaedic services, endoprosthetic replacements probably account for up to one-third of all surgical procedures. For the pathologist this therapeutic progress means a considerable increase in the amount of orthopaedically related tissue specimens to be studied and documented (Fig. 8.1). The prostheses are manufactured from relatively noncorrosive metals, high density polyethylene, and silicone, either alone or in various combinations.

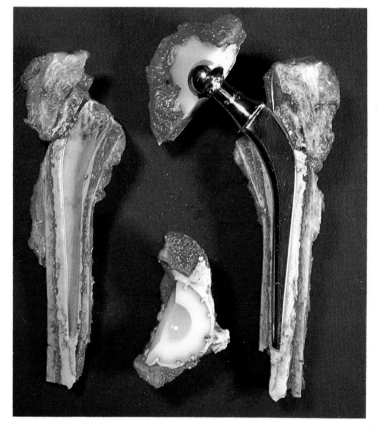

Fig. 8.1 In this photograph the components of a total hip replacement are seen attached to the bone. Between the plastic acetabular component and the metal stem of the femoral component, a layer of cement is interposed between the prosthesis and the bone in order to obtain a close (optimally immobile) fit of the prosthesis. Looseness of the prosthetic parts is a significant cause of failure in such operations.

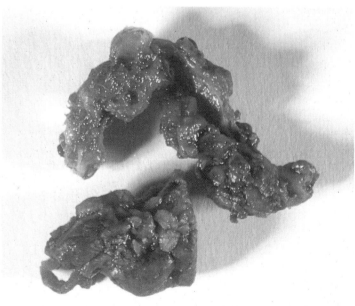

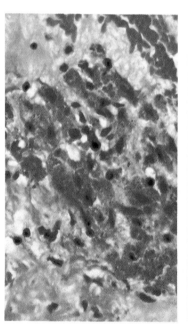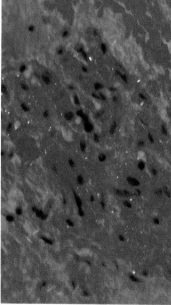

Fig. 8.2 Specimen of synovium removed from the hip joint of a patient with a prosthetic hip comprised of a metallic acetabular component articulating against a metallic femoral head. One may note black staining of the synovial lining surface resulting from wear products generated by the metallic articulating surfaces and then taken up into the synovial membrane.

Fig. 8.3 Photomicrograph of a histologic preparation obtained from the gross specimen shown in Fig. 8.2. A large number of darkly stained histiocytes are seen, and, within the cytoplasm of these cells, small black specks can be appreciated. When this tissue is examined under polarized light (*right*), the small black particles appear as refractile specks.

In patients who have had a prosthesis in which metal articulates on metal, it is not uncommon to see a distinct gray-black discoloration at the synovial surface (Fig. 8.2). A microscopic examination of tissue removed from the area shows irregular metal fragments that measure between 1 and 3μm, mostly within histiocytes (Fig. 8.3).

The synovial fluid may be cloudy, and a microscopic examination reveals the presence of metal particles (Fig. 8.4). By transmission electron microscopy, metal granules smaller than the limits of the resolution of the optical microscope can be seen within phagolysosomes (Fig. 8.5).

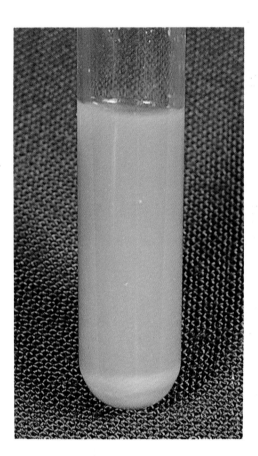 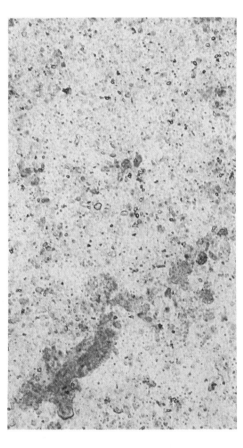 

Fig. 8.4 A synovial effusion removed from a patient with a metal-on-metal prosthesis may be quite turbid, giving the mistaken impression that one is dealing with an infection (*left*). However, a microscopic examination of the fluid fails to reveal polymorphonuclear leukocytes, but does reveal numerous fragments of fine amorphous debris (*center*). When these fragments are viewed under polarized light, they are seen to be refractile. This appearance results from refraction at the edge of the opaque metal particles (*right*).

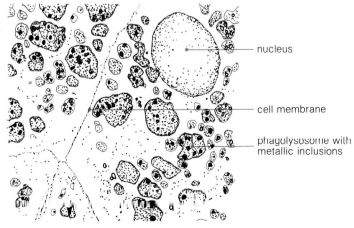

Fig. 8.5 Electron photomicrograph of synovial cells from a patient with a total hip replacement shows an accumulation of electron-dense material in phagolysosomes in the cytoplasm. These dense particles are metallic.

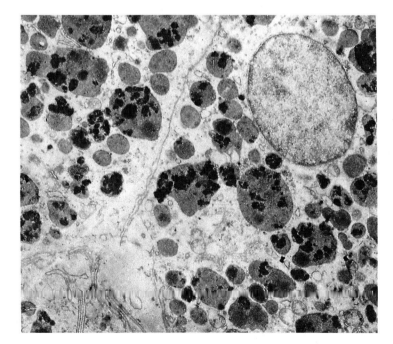

nucleus

cell membrane

phagolysosome with metallic inclusions

Wear particles of the components manufactured from high density polyethylene are visible only when the tissue is examined under polarized light (Fig. 8.6). These particles are mostly intracellular, threadlike, and measure about 1μm in width and 4 to 10μm in length. A severe histiocytic response in the synovium is frequently observed, and foreign body giant cells are common (Figs.

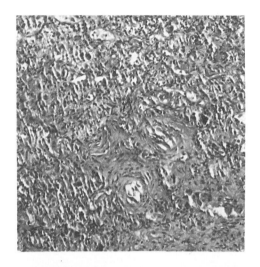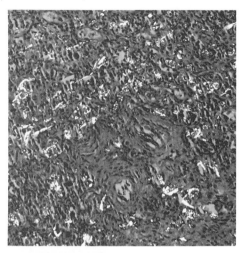

Fig. 8.6 Photomicrograph of a histologic section taken from the synovium of a patient with a hip prosthesis in which the acetabular component was made of polyethylene (*left*). In the transmission light photograph shown here, the subsynovium is seen to be infiltrated by large numbers of histiocytes and some chronic inflammatory cells. On polarized light microscopy the cells are seen to be filled with threadlike particles of refractile material, which are derived from wear of the polyethylene surface (*right*).

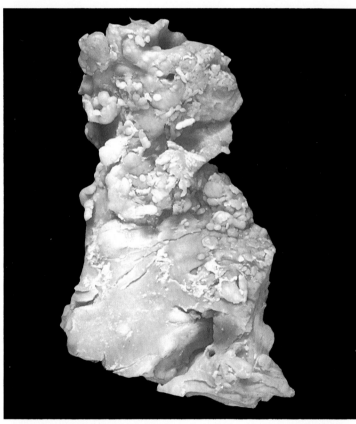

Fig. 8.7 Specimen of synovium removed from the knee of a patient with a total knee prosthesis in which the tibial component was polyethylene. The synovium is markedly hyperplastic and papillary, and on the surface one may observe a fibrinous exudate, grossly resembling the appearance of synovium in a patient with rheumatoid arthritis. However, all these changes can be attributed to a histiocytic and foreign body giant-cell reaction in the synovium resulting from polyethylene debris.

Fig. 8.8 Photomicrograph of a giant cell in the patient shown in Fig. 8.7 reveals fine threadlike particles of polyethylene within the cytoplasm.

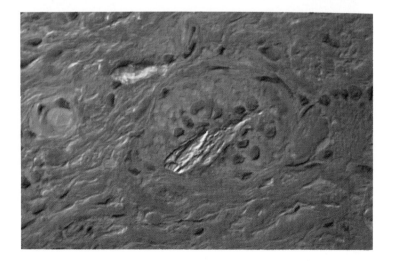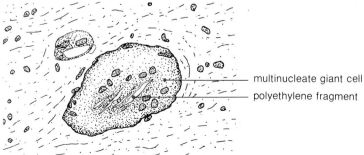

multinucleate giant cell
polyethylene fragment

8.7 and 8.8). Occasionally, the tissue reaction to polyethylene has resulted in pseudotumors in the capsule and erosions of the periarticular bone (Figs. 8.9 and 8.10).

Both the plastic and metallic components of an artificial joint are usually keyed to the underlying bone by an interposed layer of methyl methacrylate cement (Fig. 8.11).

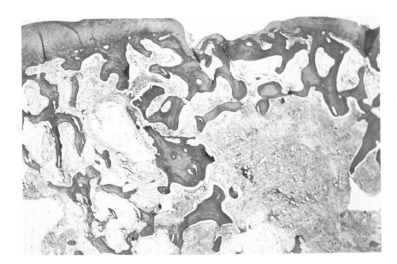

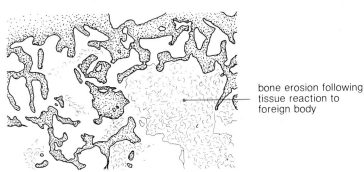

Fig. 8.9 Photomicrograph of a section taken through the articular surface of a patella in a patient with a total knee replacement. In the subchondral bone there is a tumorlike accumulation of cellular tissue.

bone erosion following tissue reaction to foreign body

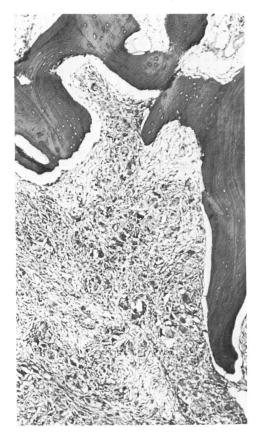
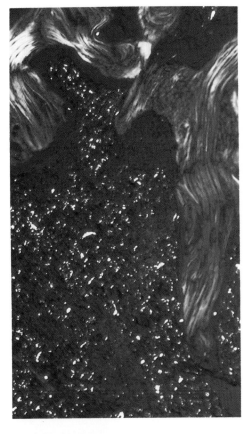

Fig. 8.10 High power view of the tissue seen in Fig. 8.9. Left: note histiocytic replacement of the bone and bone marrow. Right: polarized light microscopy reveals highly refractile particles of polyethylene debris within the histiocytes and giant cells of the tissue.

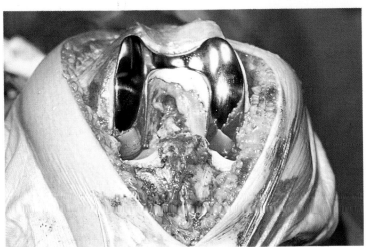

Fig. 8.11 Total knee replacement seen at necropsy. A large amount of cement can be seen extruded around the prosthetic parts. Such excess cement is likely to break up and be ground between the articular surfaces into a fine powder, which will eventually be incorporated into the synovium and will also cause wear between the articulating surfaces of the artificial joint. In joint replacement procedures, the use of cement should be kept to a minimum, and any extruded cement, particularly around the prosthesis, should be carefully cleared from the joint before closure.

Methyl methacrylate is prepared by mixing liquid mono-mer with a polymer powder (Fig. 8.12). In the routine preparation of histologic sections, any cement in the tissue will be dissolved out by the solvents used in the processing, and a microscopic examination will reveal only spaces where the cement had previously been (Fig. 8.13).

Fortunately, it usually leaves behind a marker in the form of insoluble barium sulfate, which is put into the cement to render it radiopaque (Fig. 8.14).

Fragmentation of the cement usually results when an excess of cement is left around the implant bed (Figs. 8.15 to 8.18). Often the fragments are fairly small (10 to

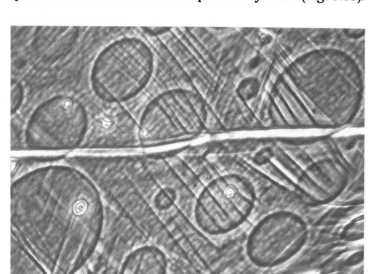

Fig. 8.12 Histologic section of a piece of cement reveals the "two-phase" characteristic of this material. The spherical objects are the microscopic equivalent of the beadlike polymer, and the material between is the polymerized monomer.

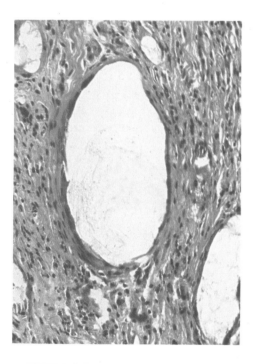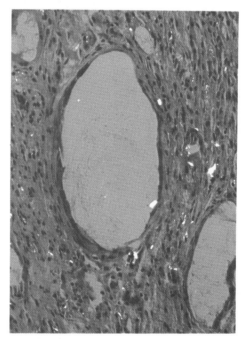

Fig. 8.13 In this photomicrograph large spaces surrounded by giant cells are seen within synovial tissue (*left*). These spaces were filled with methyl methacrylate cement; however, during the processing of the tissue for histologic examination, such material was dissolved away by the organic solvents used in the process. The same tissue viewed by polarized microscopy reveals that there is no refractile cement within these spaces (*right*). However, a few particles of refractile polyethylene are seen in the histiocytes of the intervening tissue.

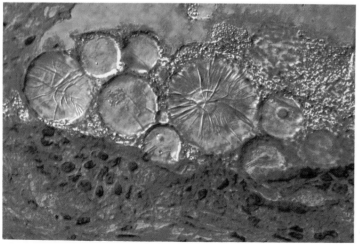

Fig. 8.14 Photomicrograph of a specimen of synovium cut by frozen section without the use of solvents demonstrates cement in situ. The polymer balls are evident, and between these spheres a finely granular yellow material may be seen. This appearance results from the barium sulfate that is mixed with the cement to render it radiopaque.

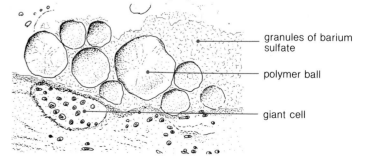

granules of barium sulfate

polymer ball

giant cell

30μm), in which case they are surrounded by recognizable giant cells. Sometimes the pieces are very large (100μm or more), and in these instances histologic sections reveal large irregular spaces surrounded by flattened giant cells.

Silicone elastomer has been used for the manufacture of implants in the fields of plastic surgery, neurosurgery, cardiac surgery, and orthopaedic surgery. In orthopaedic surgery this material is used particularly in the manufacture of prostheses to replace the small joints of the hand.

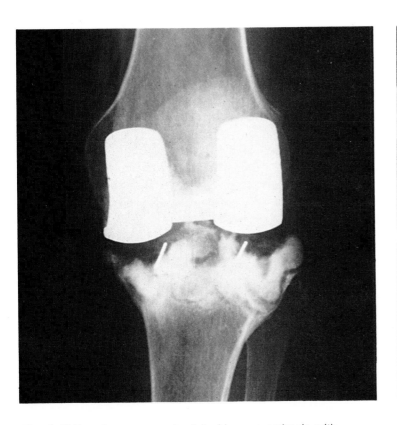

Fig. 8.15 Roentgenogram of a failed knee prosthesis with marked loosening of the tibial components. Note the lucent line around the cement and the displacement of the tibial components.

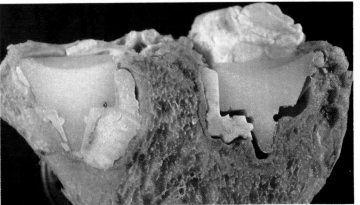

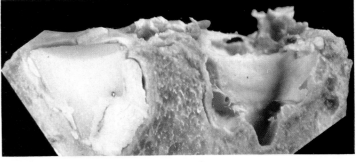

Fig. 8.16 Gross photograph of the tibial plateau in the patient shown in Fig. 8.15. The knee has been sagittally sectioned, and the tibial components are seen surrounded by a thick layer of cement. Adjacent to the cement, between the cement and the bone, a thick layer of fibrous tissue is apparent. In the lower photograph the polyethylene component has been removed to better demonstrate this fibrous membrane. In patients in whom a radiolucent line is seen surrounding the cement, the histologic equivalent of this line is generally a fibrous membrane. It is probable that the fibrous membrane develops in response to micromotion at the cement-bone interface, rather than as a result of a chemical reaction.

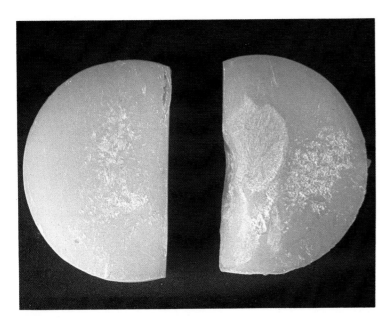

Fig. 8.17 The tibial components of a total knee prosthesis show extensive wear and scuffing of the articular surfaces by the polyethylene components. The material generated by this wear process is taken up by the synovium and results in a considerable synovial reaction. Significant wear results from fragments of cement that are caught between the articular surfaces and ground into the polyethylene.

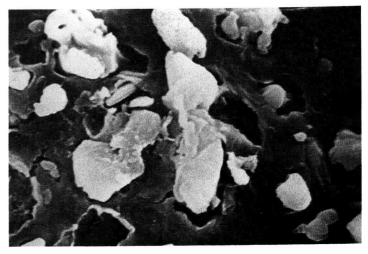

Fig. 8.18 Scanning electron photomicrograph shows cement particles buried in the polyethylene surface of a total joint replacement.

Fragmentation of the silicone material leads to a severe histiocytic and giant-cell reaction; the particles of silicone have a characteristic bosselated, faintly yellow appearance (Figs. 8.19 and 8.20). The material is not birefringent when examined by polarized light microscopy.

In all the removed prostheses we have examined, wear debris in the synovium, bone, or surrounding soft tissue was present on histologic examination. There was good correlation between the amount of wear debris and the patient's activity and age. The more active the patient (as determined by distance walked and other physical activities, e.g., dancing or sports), the more wear debris and tissue reaction were present. There is also a correlation with age; over 50 per cent of the patients in the fourth and fifth decades, and over 30 per cent of the patients in the sixth and seventh decades showed considerable wear debris with moderate to severe tissue reactions. Patients in the eighth and ninth decades showed only insignificant wear debris and tissue reaction. The patient's weight and the duration of the implant have failed to show a direct relationship to the presence of wear debris and tissue reaction.

DISEASES OF THE SPINE

Disease presenting primarily in the vertebral column may result from any of a vast number of conditions: tuberculosis and pyogenic infections of the bone; metabolic disturbances such as rickets, osteomalacia, hyperparathyroidism, ochronosis, or chondrocalcinosis (all of which have been previously referred to in the text); a tumor, either primary or secondary; trauma to the spine; disease of the intervertebral disc; or various connective tissue diseases or degenerations. In this section we will discuss those diseases of the spine that result from abnormalities of the intervertebral disc, degenerative arthritis, diffuse idiopathic skeletal hyperostosis (Forrestiere's disease), and ankylosing spondylitis.

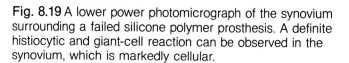

Fig. 8.19 A lower power photomicrograph of the synovium surrounding a failed silicone polymer prosthesis. A definite histiocytic and giant-cell reaction can be observed in the synovium, which is markedly cellular.

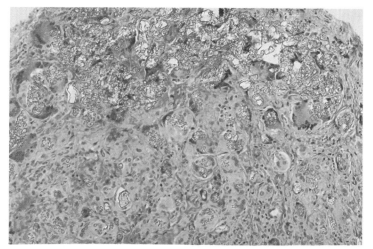

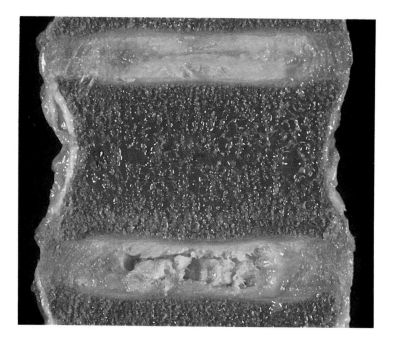

Fig. 8.20 A high power view of the giant cells from the tissue shown in Fig. 8.19. Within the cytoplasm of the giant cells can be seen bosselated inclusions of a yellowish-gray material. This microscopic appearance is typical of silicone breakdown, and similar inclusions may be found around silicone injections used in plastic surgery procedures.

Fig. 8.21 Vertebral body and adjacent intervertebral discs obtained at autopsy from a 65-year-old man. Note the yellowish color of the discs and the degenerative changes in the nucleus pulposus. These findings are characteristic in elderly people.

Intervertebral Disc Disease. The normal intervertebral disc is formed of a central nucleus pulposus, which is composed of a large amount of proteoglycan, little collagen, and diffuse rounded chondrocytes; the nucleus pulposus is bounded by the anulus fibrosus, a dense fibrous tissue in which alternating layers of collagen are seen to lie circumferentially and longitudinally. When the spine is sectioned in young people, the intervertebral disc is seen to bulge away from the vertebrae on either side, and the nucleus pulposus has a bluish white, translucent appearance. However, in older individuals the intervertebral disc is seen to be diminished in height, to have a yellowish color, and, on cut section, rather than bulging away from the surface, it tends to sink into the surface (Fig. 8.21).

One of the most common abnormalities seen in the disc at autopsy is the herniation of the disc tissue into the adjacent vertebral body. Such herniations are known as Schmorl's nodules (Fig. 8.22). (If these herniations are large, they may mimic tumors on radiologic films. So before diagnosing a lesion of the vertebra as a chondrosarcoma, it is important to be sure that the lesion is not a Schmorl's nodule.)

Posterolateral herniation of the nucleus pulposus through the anulus fibrosus (Fig. 8.23) may result in pressure on the nerve roots (a so-called "slipped" disc). In the acute phase such a herniation may well result in significant local inflammatory response, causing pressure on the nerve. In late stages of the disease, the prolapsed intervertebral disc tissue often shows signs of cellular proliferation (Fig. 8.24). This finding suggests that the size of the prolapse may increase, not because of continuing herniation, but because of the growth of the prolapsed tissue in a way similar to that of the growth of loose bodies within joints.

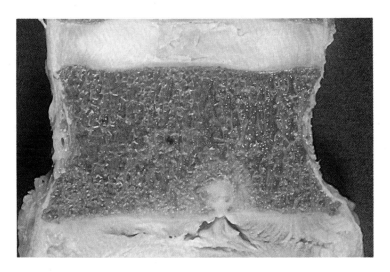

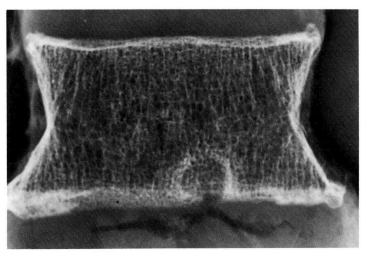

Fig. 8.22 Photograph and roentgenogram of a segment of spine removed at autopsy demonstrate herniation of the intervertebral disc into the adjacent vertebral body. Such herniations are commonly found at autopsy and are known as Schmorl's nodules.

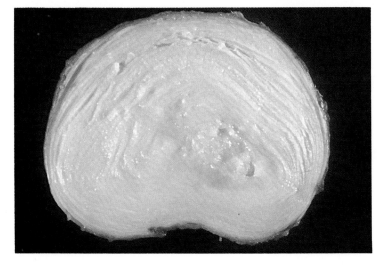

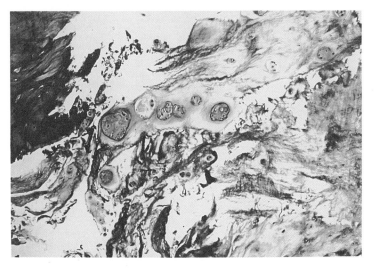

Fig. 8.23 Photograph of a slice taken through the center of an intervertebral disc shows the surrounding anulus fibrosus and central nucleus pulposus in an elderly person. Note the yellowish color and granular appearance of the nucleus pulposus. Extension of the nucleus pulposus posteriorly and laterally into the anulus fibrosus is occurring. Complete herniation of the nucleus pulposus may result in pressure on the nerve roots.

Fig. 8.24 Photomicrograph of tissue removed at surgery from a herniated intervertebral disc. Note the irregular fibrillated matrix of the nucleus pulposus, which appears largely necrotic but has foci of proliferating cartilage cells.

Degenerative Disease of the Spine. Degenerative disease of the spine includes a number of distinct but often overlapping conditions. In association with the degeneration of the intervertebral disc (which occurs with aging as has been described), reactive sclerosis of the end plate of the adjacent vertebral body is frequently seen. In addition, peripheral osteophytosis around the vertebral body is a common finding at autopsy in elderly people (Figs. 8.25 and 8.26). The vertebral column also includes synovial joints, both the apophyseal joints and the costovertebral joints. These joints may be involved with osteoarthritis, in which case changes are observed that are similar to those already described and commonly associated with disease of the hip, knee, and small joints of the hand. Disease of the diarthrodial joints of the spine may well be a significant cause of chronic backache.

Diffuse Idiopathic Skeletal Hyperostosis (DISH). This condition is a disease of older individuals, predominantly men. It is characterized by the presence of calcification and ossification along the anterolateral aspect and/or along the posterior longitudinal ligament of several contiguous vertebral bodies. These changes occur in the

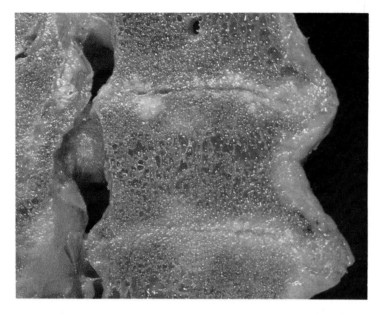

Fig. 8.25 A segment of the vertebral column removed from an elderly person at autopsy. Narrowing and degeneration of the intervertebral discs are frequently associated with bony proliferation at the margins of vertebral bodies.

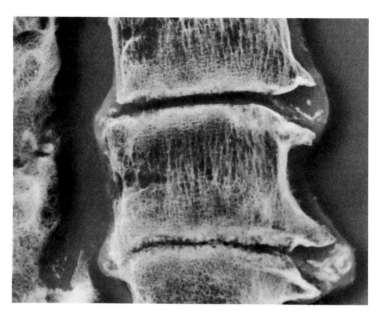

Fig. 8.26 Roentgenogram of a portion of the specimen shown in Fig. 8.25 shows the bony osteophytes developed at the margin of a degenerated disc. Such beaking is a common radiologic finding in the vertebral bodies of older people, particularly in the cervical and lumbar regions.

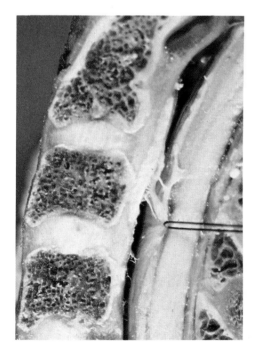

Fig. 8.27 Gross photograph of the upper cervical spine in a 43-year-old woman shows ossification of the posterior longitudinal ligament in a patient with diffuse idiopathic skeletal hyperostosis (DISH).

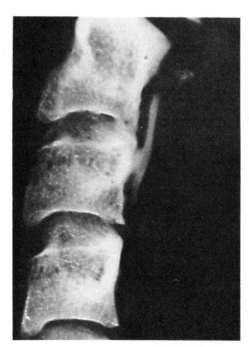

Fig. 8.28 Roentgenogram of the specimen shown in Fig. 8.27. (Figures 8.27 to 8.29 courtesy of Prof. K. Terterayama.)

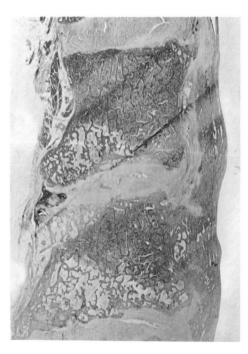

Fig. 8.29 Photomicrograph of the specimen shown in Fig. 8.27 reveals extensive ossification of the ligament, resulting in the immobilization of this section of the spine.

presence of relative preservation of the intervertebral disc. One also commonly sees calcification and ossification at ligamentous and tendinous insertions, particularly around the major joints (Figs. 8.27 to 8.29).

The bony excrescences around the vertebrae (referred to as syndesmophytes) are seen to be vertically disposed, in contrast to the horizontal osteophytes of degenerative joint disease. The principal complaint of patients with this condition is spinal stiffness.

Ankylosing Spondylitis. Ankylosing spondylitis is generally a disorder of young men, although women may be affected much more commonly than has been thought. The disease often manifests as a low backache and early morning stiffness, and usually progresses to involve more and more of the spine, which eventually becomes ankylosed (Figs. 8.30 to 8.33). With ankylosis of the spine, there is frequently a further complication of restriction of chest movement, and in the late stages of the disease, peripheral joint involvement may add to the problems. (Occasionally, patients may first present with peripheral joint involvement.)

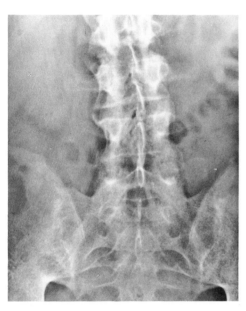

Fig. 8.30 Roentgenogram of the sacroiliac joints and lumbar vertebrae of a patient with ankylosing spondylitis. Note the bony fusion of the sacroiliac joints as well as the intervertebral disc spaces.

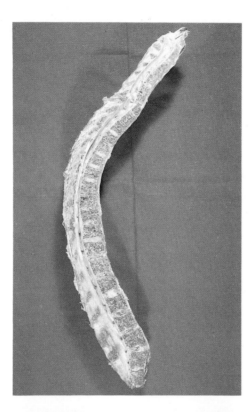

Fig. 8.31 A sagittal section through the vertebral column removed from a patient with ankylosing spondylitis. The vertebral column is fused into complete immobility. The exaggerated kyphosis seen in this specimen is characteristic of patients with ankylosing spondylitis. In the upper thoracic spine there is some angular deformity, the result of a previous fracture through this area.

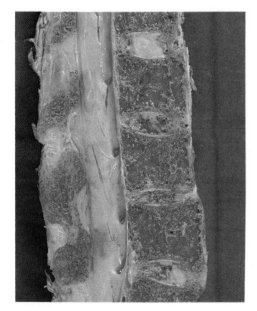

Fig. 8.32 Close-up of the lumbar region in the spine shown in Fig. 8.31. It can be appreciated that osseous fusion has taken place across the intervertebral discs. Some remnants of intervertebral disc remain, but, for the most part, the discs have been obliterated by osseous tissue.

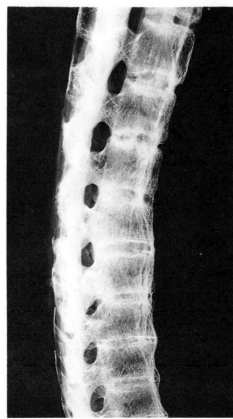

Fig. 8.33 Specimen radiograph of a spine removed from a patient with ankylosing spondylitis reveals osseous fusion across the discs and marked thickening of the anterior cortex of the vertebral bodies. The fusion of the discs changes the mechanics of the spine, so that the spine comes to resemble (in function) a long tubular bone. In reflection of this change in functional activity, the cortices become markedly thickened, particularly on the side of compression.

Over 90 per cent of the patients with ankylosing spondylitis carry the HLA B27 antigen. The disease is often seen in association with other disorders, including psoriatic arthritis, Reiter's syndrome, ulcerative colitis, Crohn's disease, Whipple's disease, Behcet's syndrome, and acute anterior uveitis.

The striking morphologic feature is the ankylosis, which occurs first in the sacroiliac joint and later in the intervertebral discs, and which may also involve the diarthrodial joints (Fig. 8.34). A histologic examination of the affected joints demonstrates active endochondral ossification taking place across the articular cartilage or intervertebral discs (Fig. 8.35). Inflammatory changes may be seen in the synovium and also in the subchondral bone, although the changes are generally less severe than those that are present in patients with rheumatoid arthritis. (In patients with rheumatoid arthritis, ankylosis is actually uncommon.)

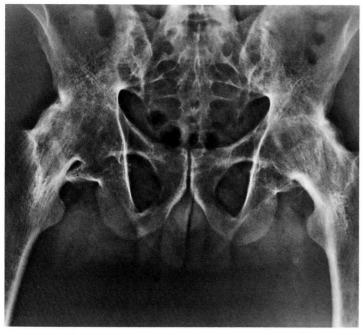

Fig. 8.34 Roentgenogram of the pelvis in a 50-year-old man with advanced ankylosing spondylitis. Note the fusion of the sacroiliac joints (usually the first joints to be affected in this condition) together with the fusion of the lumbar vertebrae. In this patient with advanced disease both hip joints are also ankylosed.

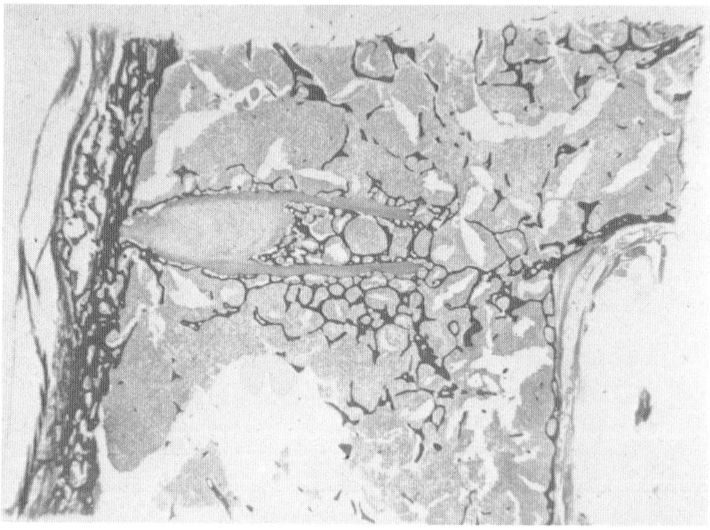

Fig. 8.35 A histologic section of two adjacent vertebrae with the intervening disc largely replaced by osseous tissue.

9 Bone and Joint Infections

Experiments conducted in the late nineteenth century demonstrated that bone infection (osteomyelitis) results from microbes, and that the disease tends to involve the extremities and the juxtaepiphyseal area of the bone. Before the era of antibiotics, bone and joint infections commonly occurred, and they presented serious clinical problems leading to high rates of morbidity and mortality. Nowadays, the incidence of osteomyelitis and the mortality resulting from it have decreased dramatically; however, even with the use of antibiotics, the morbidity connected with the disease remains high.

The proper diagnosis and management of osteomyelitis depends on careful correlation of clinical, radiologic, and histopathologic findings. Occasionally, problems in differential diagnosis may occur, especially with respect to differentiating osteomyelitis from round-cell tumors and eosinophilic granuloma.

The majority of bone and joint infections result either from organisms which are pus-producing (pyogenic infections) or from organisms which produce multiple nodules or granules in the tissue (granulomatous infections). In general, pyogenic infections more commonly result in bone disease, whereas granulomatous infections result in joint disease.

PYOGENIC INFECTIONS OF BONES AND JOINTS

CLINICAL CONSIDERATIONS

Infection of the skeletal tissues results from microbial organisms that are either blood-borne (hematogenous infection) or implanted directly into the bone. The latter occurs most often as a complication either of a compound fracture or of surgery.

Hematogenous Osteomyelitis. The majority of patients with acute hematogenous osteomyelitis are children, and they usually present with high fever and local pain. The organism responsible for the infection in patients over age 3 is, in most cases, *Staphylococcus aureus* (coagulase-positive). The most frequent sites of infection in children are the lower end of the femur and the upper end of the tibia, areas of both rapid growth and, especially in children, increased risk of trauma. It has been suggested that the large caliber of the metaphyseal veins in children results in marked slowing of blood flow, and consequently predisposes to posttraumatic thrombosis and colonization by blood-borne bacteria (Fig. 9.1).

Hematogenous osteomyelitis is uncommon in otherwise healthy adults. However, cases of acute hematogenous osteomyelitis are sometimes seen in debilitated

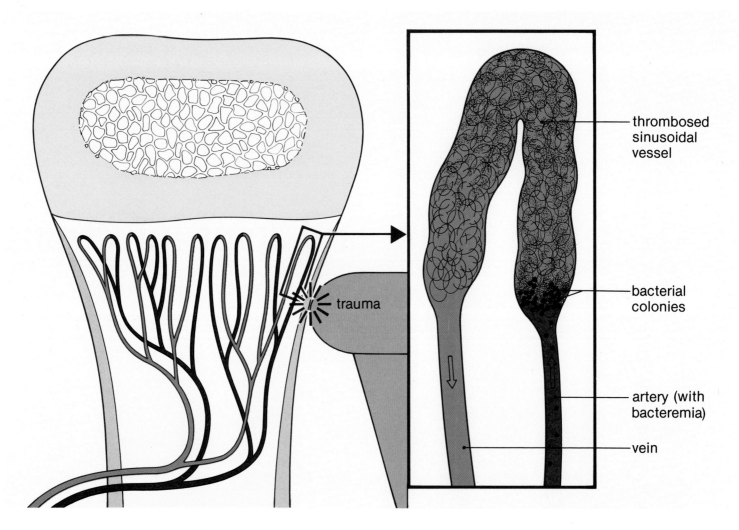

trauma

thrombosed sinusoidal vessel

bacterial colonies

artery (with bacteremia)

vein

Fig. 9.1 In children, following mechanical trauma to the bone, the large venous channels in the metaphysis are liable to thrombose (see vein on right). In the presence of bacteria from infection elsewhere in the body, such a site of thrombosis can act as a nidus for bacterial growth and the subsequent development of osteomyelitis.

adults, for example, those with chronic disease or drug addiction (Fig. 9.2).

In debilitated elderly adults with genitourinary infections, spinal osteomyelitis is not uncommon. In such patients, the responsible organisms (usually gram-negative) probably gain access to the spine via Batson's venous plexus (Fig. 9.3).

Another group of elderly patients in whom osteomyelitis may be a problem are those with peripheral vascular insufficiency, which in many cases is associated with diabetes. In these patients, the bone infection frequently results from polymicrobial infiltration, probably of anaerobic organisms.

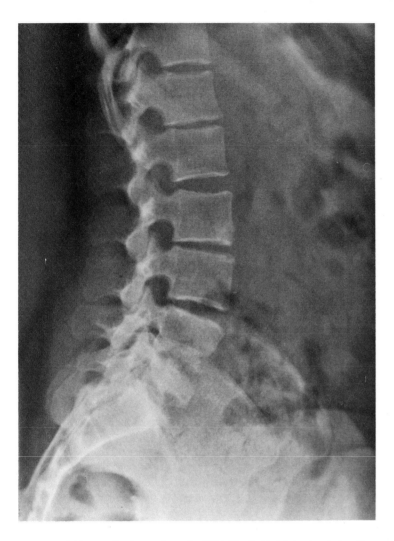

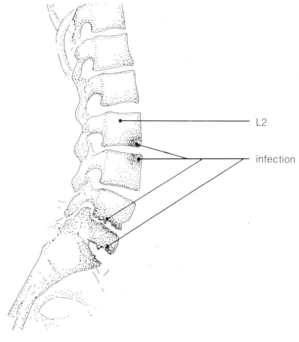

Fig. 9.2 Roentgenogram of a lateral projection of the spine in a young drug addict shows bone destruction anteriorly on both sides of the disc between L2 and L3, and extensive destruction at L4–L5 and L5–S1, with collapse of L5. Bacteriologic culture showed that the offending organism in this case was *Staphylococcus aureus*.

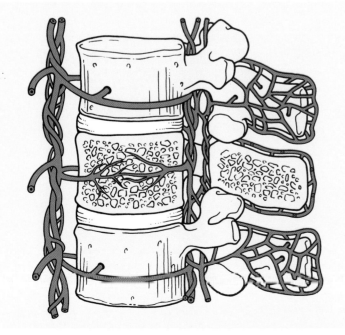

Fig. 9.3 The veins of the vertebral column form intricate plexuses around the column, along the spinal canal, and through the bone substance. These venous plexuses, also known as Batson's plexus, freely communicate with the segmental systemic veins and with the portal system. Because of these anastomoses and lack of valves in these veins, retrograde flow may frequently occur and result in metastatic infection, as well as metastatic tumors to the vertebral bodies, spinal cord, brain, and skull.

Recent studies of osteomyelitis in drug addicts have shown pseudomonas to be the responsible organism in the majority of affected individuals. In most of these patients, fever and chills were conspicuously absent, and local pain was often the sole clinical finding suggesting osteomyelitis. In drug addicts, the focus of osteomyelitis is usually the spine or the pelvis, although the disease may occur anywhere in the skeletal system (sometimes in unusual sites, such as the clavicle). Organisms are carried from the skin and from unclean hypodermic needles. In addition, the intravenous injection of drugs—often cut with other particulate matter—may produce microvascular occlusion, thereby providing a site for bacterial colonization.

It is important to realize that adult patients with bone infections frequently present only with pain; therefore, the diagnosis of osteomyelitis is often not made immediately. In these patients, roentgenographic changes in the bone may be misinterpreted by the radiologist as resulting from a malignant tumor (Fig. 9.4).

Joint Infection. Joint infection (septic arthritis) may result from hematogenous infection of the synovium, from decompression of contiguous osteomyelitis (Fig. 9.5), or as a consequence of direct inoculation of a joint following trauma. This disease often occurs in neonates and infants, most frequently affecting the hip, knee, and ankle. (In patients with neonatal septic arthritis, severe residual growth disturbances frequently result from damage to the growth cartilage. For this reason, the importance of early diagnosis and treatment cannot be overemphasized.) Another group of patients who are particularly susceptible to developing septic arthritis are older adults with rheumatoid arthritis or other chronic joint diseases.

The diagnosis is established by joint aspiration, preferably assisted by radiologic image intensification and performed under strict antiseptic conditions. The aspirate should be sent immediately to the laboratory for direct smear, aerobic and anaerobic cultures, and antibiotic sensitivity analysis. To increase the chance of bacterial growth, the aspirate should be inoculated into the medium as soon as possible. (The phenomenon of an apparently sterile infection may well result from difficulties in recovering and growing the bacteria.) The hip joint, situated deep in the body, is difficult to examine, and thus the diagnosis of septic arthritis in this joint tends to be delayed, particularly in newborns and infants.

Since cartilage is susceptible to the action of enzymes released by bacteria and disintegrating inflammatory cells, and consequently is rapidly destroyed in patients with septic arthritis, the treatment of the disease consists of immediate surgical incision and drainage, followed by

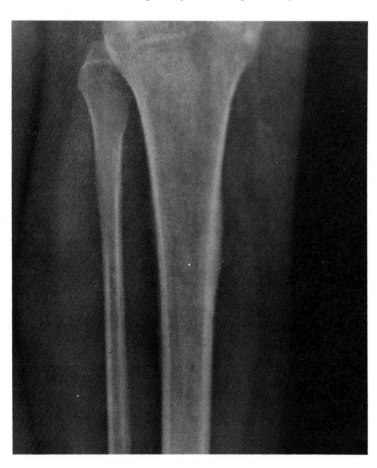

Fig. 9.4 Roentgenogram of a young woman who complained of pain in the upper end of the tibia shows extensive periosteal reaction along the tibia. Clinical examination of the area showed a degree of tenderness and swelling, though the patient's general health appeared good. The differential diagnosis was between a round-cell tumor (e.g., non-Hodgkin's lymphoma) or infection. Biopsy proved the lesion to be infective in nature.

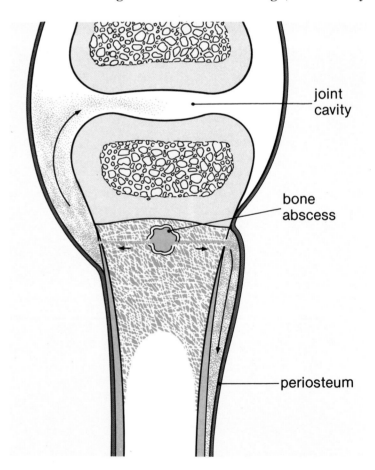

joint cavity

bone abscess

periosteum

Fig. 9.5 In patients with osteomyelitis, infected fluid material tracks through the bone to the bone surface, initially elevating the periosteum, and finally breaking through the periosteum into the soft tissues to drain onto the skin surface. In those instances where the capsule of the joint is attached below the growth plate (as in the hip), the infection may extend directly into the joint cavity, giving rise to secondary septic arthritis.

immobilization of the affected bone. Antibiotic therapy alone is usually insufficient.

Neonatal Osteomyelitis. Neonatal osteomyelitis, which also generally involves the joint adjacent to the involved bone (see Fig. 9.5), is usually the result of hematogenous infection by one of three organisms: *Staphylococcus aureus,* group B streptococcus, or *Escherichia coli.* Group B streptococcus is commonly found in the vagina, and presumably the unborn child is infected during delivery. *E. coli,* a common contaminant at the time of delivery, is pathogenic in the neonatal period because of the child's lack of immunity, a condition that persists for the first 30 days or so of neonatal life.

In the case of *S. aureus* and *E. coli* infections, about 40 per cent of the patients show polyostotic involvement (Fig. 9.6). (Polyostotic involvement with osteomyelitis is extremely rare in all but neonatal patients.) When streptococcus is the causative organism, usually only a single bone is involved. Heel punctures in young children may result in iatrogenic infection of the os calcis (Fig. 9.7).

In some cases of neonatal osteomyelitis, the absence of systemic symptoms may delay the clinical diagnosis.

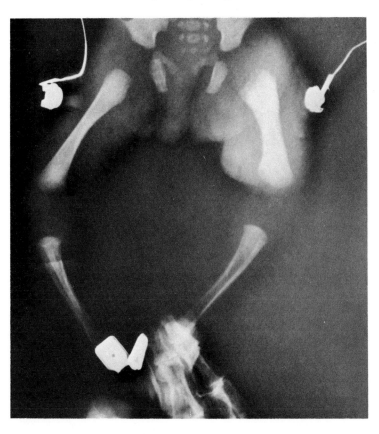

Fig. 9.6 Polyostotic involvement in neonatal osteomyelitis. Roentgenogram of the lower limbs of a newborn child (*left*) shows marked periosteal reaction all along the left femur.

Roentgenogram of the chest (*right*) shows involvement of some ribs as well as the right clavicle.

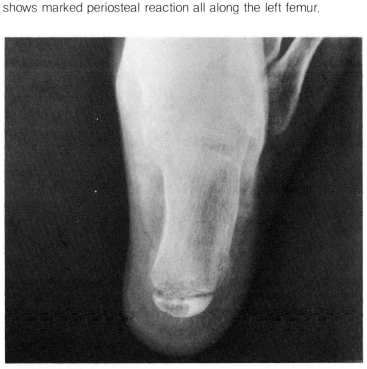

Fig. 9.7 Roentgenogram of the heel in a 7-year-old child shows a lytic lesion in the apophysis of the os calcis, which proved on biopsy to be due to infection.

Joint Infection following Venereal Disease. Suppurative arthritis, which had been a frequent complication of gonorrhea, is now decidedly rare, presumably as a result of early and efficient chemotherapy. However, it is an important diagnostic alternative to bear in mind, since the true nature of the disease is likely to be missed unless a careful history is taken. As with other forms of bacterial arthritis, the knee joints are usually the first to be affected, but multiple joint involvement is much more common in patients with gonorrhea than in those with other types of infection. (In the acute stage of gonorrhea, transient arthritis may be a complication, and arthritis may also complicate nonspecific urethritis. However, in neither of these cases does the arthritis result from bacterial infection of the joint.)

Patients with syphilis may also develop arthritis, either as a result of the extension of gummatous osteitis into a joint, or as a complication of congenital syphilis. (Charcot's joint, a rapidly destructive noninfectious arthritis that frequently complicates tabes dorsalis, was discussed in Chapter 7.)

Osteomyelitis Resulting from Direct Inoculation of Bacteria. Acute hematogenous osteomyelitis of childhood, which used to be regularly encountered in orthopaedic practice, is now much less common, at least in the developed Western countries. However, posttraumatic osteomyelitis has become much more of a clinical problem, usually resulting from infections following traffic accidents and iatrogenic infections.

Most traffic accidents involve high-impact collisions that result in compound and comminuted fractures. Usually a significant amount of foreign material, including pieces of automobile, pieces of clothing, soil, etc., can be found in these wounds.

It is important to recognize the polymicrobial nature of the infection in accident cases: Both staphylococcus and streptococcus may be expected, and in addition, gram-negative organisms (including pseudomonas) are often present. The most important procedure in the treatment of such infections is the removal of all foreign and dead matter, for without this step, the elimination of the infection is difficult, if not impossible. It should be emphasized

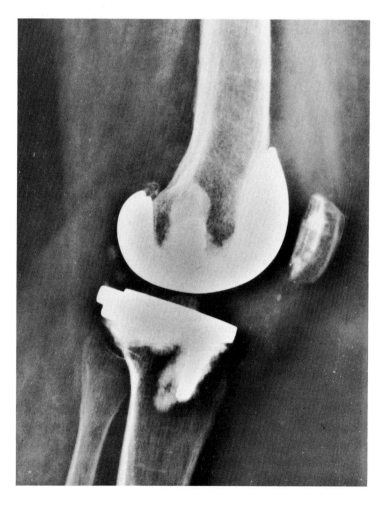 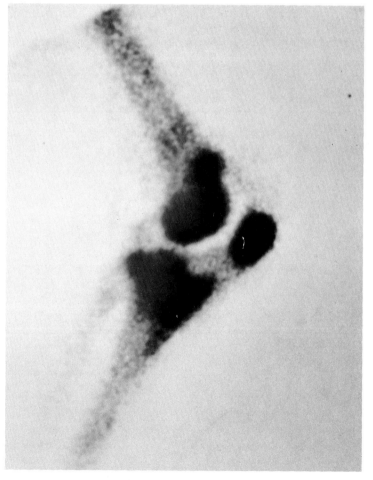

Fig. 9.8 Roentgenogram of a patient with a total knee prosthesis inserted 18 months previously *(left)*. The patient had recently experienced increasing pain in the knee; on the roentgenogram, evidence of osteolysis can be seen around the prosthesis, particularly in the area of the tibial component. Such osteolysis may result from either infection or mechanical loosening. An isotope scan shows intense uptake around *all* the components of the knee joint, typical of infection *(right)*. In the case of prosthetic loosening, increased isotope uptake would·also occur; however, one would expect it to be limited to the component that had been loosened (usually, in the case of the knee, the tibial component), and to be focal at the sites of maximal movement of the prosthesis.

that antibiotic therapy should not be continued for longer than is necessary to eliminate the signs of sepsis; otherwise, secondary contamination of the wound by resistant organisms may be expected. (Although it is important not to continue the administration of antibiotics too long in treating open wounds, antibiotic therapy should be continued for at least six weeks in treating closed wounds before a more definitive course is determined.)

In patients who have osteomyelitis as a complication of a fracture, it is important to achieve complete immobilization of the fracture fragments. Without immobilization, any reestablishment of the vascular supply necessary to deal adequately with the inflamed and infected tissues cannot be expected.

Iatrogenic infections result from surgical intervention: either the internal fixation of a simple or compound fracture, or, more recently, around a prosthetic joint replacement. (More than 150,000 prosthetic joint replacements are completed every year in the United States alone.) Following a total joint replacement procedure, infection may occur as an acute complication of the operation, or it may present insidiously many months (or even years) later (Fig. 9.8). The organisms commonly found in such cases are staphylococcus (both coagulase-negative and coagulase-positive), pseudomonas, and a variety of anaerobic organisms.

Chronic Osteomyelitis. Although the mortality of acute hematogenous osteomyelitis has been reduced to almost zero, between 15 and 30 per cent of patients with this disorder still develop chronic disease. Frequently, chronic osteomyelitis results from inadequate treatment with antibiotics, and the failure to adequately surgically debride necrotic bone contributes to its development. (The sequestrum provides a harbor for the bacteria in which they are inaccessible, even to high levels of antibiotics.) In patients with chronic relapsing osteomyelitis due to staphylococcus, the organisms that are isolated in the microbiology laboratory, even after many years, are of the same phage type as the original infecting organisms.

Squamous cell carcinoma has been reported as a late sequela of chronic osteomyelitis in about 1 per cent of patients, occurring up to 30 to 40 years after the original infection (Figs. 9.9 to 9.11). Systemic amyloidosis may also be a complication of chronic osteomyelitis.

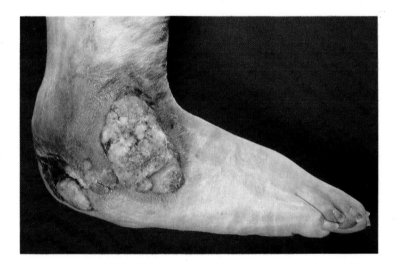

Fig. 9.9 Gross photograph of the foot and ankle in a patient with long-standing osteomyelitis. An overgrowth of partially ulcerated hyperkeratotic skin is seen in the area of the ankle joint.

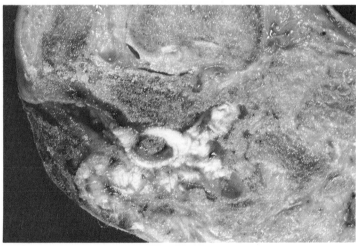

Fig. 9.10 Sagittal section of the foot shown in Fig. 9.9. A draining sinus from the infected bone opens onto the ulcerated skin. There is invasion of firm white tissue from the skin surface into the underlying soft tissue and bone.

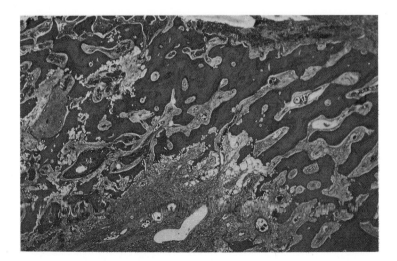

Fig. 9.11 Photomicrograph of the bone from the patient in Figs. 9.9 and 9.10 shows that the bone is being invaded by a well-differentiated epidermoid carcinoma.

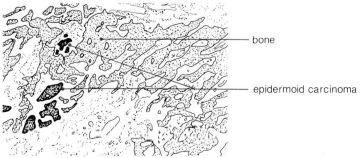

ROENTGENOGRAPHIC CHANGES

In the early stages of osteomyelitis, no radiologic changes are visible on roentgenograms or tomograms. The morphologic changes in individuals with this disease cannot be demonstrated on roentgenograms until the disease is well established, significant bone destruction has occurred, and there is reactive new bone formation. These difficulties in radiologic diagnosis have been partly solved by the considerable progress achieved in radionuclide imaging, which permits earlier detection of osteomyelitic foci. Of the many radioactive substances used, technetium polyphosphates seem to produce the best results. In clinical studies, radionuclide uptake has been shown to occur in a sizable percentage of cases 10 to 14 days before changes are evident on roentgenograms (Fig. 9.12).

Despite its usefulness, radionuclide imaging has important limitations. First, in some patients, multiple "hot spots" are detected radiologically at an early stage of *Staphylococcus aureus* septicemia, but these "spots" do not progress toward clinical osteomyelitis. (It is not known whether these areas represent false-positive results or aborted bone infection.) Second, experimental and clinical studies have documented rare cases of osteomyelitis that have been confirmed by bacteriologic and histologic studies, even though bone scans were initially negative. (This phenomenon may be explained by impaired blood supply to, or infarction of, the infected area.) Third, technetium polyphosphate bone scanning performed after fracture or bone surgery does not differentiate bone repair from bone infection.

In joint infections, the early stage of disease is usually seen roentgenographically as a bulging of the joint cavity (Fig. 9.13). Later in the disease process, destruction of the articular cartilage and involvement of the subchondral bone result in severe destructive joint disease (Fig. 9.14).

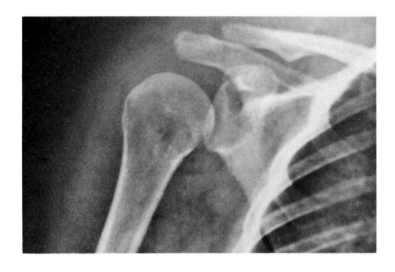

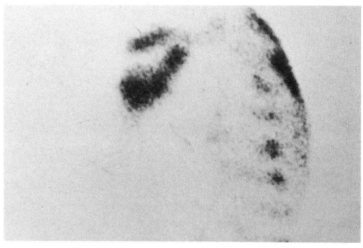

Fig. 9.12 Roentgenogram of the shoulder in a patient with fever, and pain and tenderness at the upper end of the humerus (*left*). Although some osteolysis may be present, it is difficult to define a lesion. No obvious periosteal reaction has occurred. However, in the isotope scan, an intense uptake of radioactive isotope is evident at the upper end of the humerus (*right*). (A scan frequently demonstrates the presence of osteomyelitis before any changes are evident on roentgenograms.)

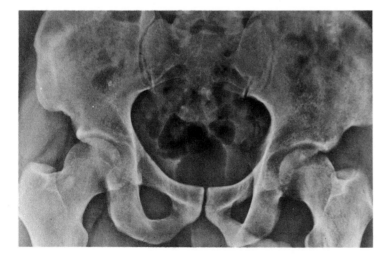

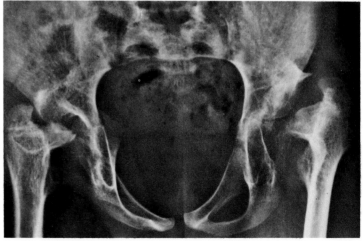

Fig. 9.13 Roentgenogram of the pelvis shows localized osteoporosis on both sides of the hip joint. The joint space is still intact.

Fig. 9.14 Roentgenogram of a 7-year-old boy with a history of multiple joint infections shows total disappearance of both femoral heads and disintegration of the hip joints, characteristic of late septic arthritis.

BACTERIOLOGIC DIAGNOSIS

The conclusive bacteriologic diagnosis of septic arthritis or of osteomyelitis depends on the isolation of the pathogen from the lesion or from blood cultures (Fig. 9.15). The blood culture is positive in only about 50 per cent of the patients with acute, untreated hematogenous osteomyelitis. In patients in whom osteomyelitis is a likely diagnosis based on clinical data, direct bone aspiration or a surgical biopsy should be carried out when blood culture testing is negative. The importance of immediate inoculation of the material suspected of being infected cannot be overemphasized. Delays in plating out and inoculating medium from swabs and the tissue obtained from the diseased area may result in a reduction in viable organisms, and, consequently, a reduction in positive cultures.

THE MORBID ANATOMY OF OSTEOMYELITIS

As is the case with most sites of infection, the clinical course of bone infection depends upon the interplay between the injurious agent and the host tissue. In other words, in a patient with osteomyelitis, the severity of the signs and symptoms depends on the virulence of the invading organism, the site of infection, and the patient's age and general health. The presence of bacteria in a bone does not necessarily result in osteomyelitis, and it is generally believed that trauma is an important associated condition, perhaps because it produces venostasis or thrombosis.

The initial local response to infection with pyogenic bacteria is acute inflammation, which results in the production of an exudate containing polymorphonuclear leukocytes (neutrophils) and fibrin (Fig. 9.16). The bacterial products, the vascular ischemia, and the enzymes released from the disintegrating tissue and neutrophils singly and in combination result in local bone and bone marrow necrosis.

If the infection is localized, an abscess (Brodie's abscess) will form. The roentgenographic differential diagnosis of Brodie's abscess includes osteoid osteoma, eosinophilic granuloma, and malignant small-cell tumors (Fig. 9.17).

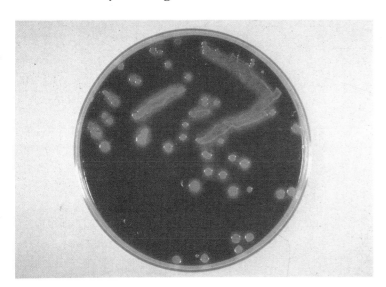

Fig. 9.15 A blood-agar plate shows growth of beta-hemolytic staphylococci.

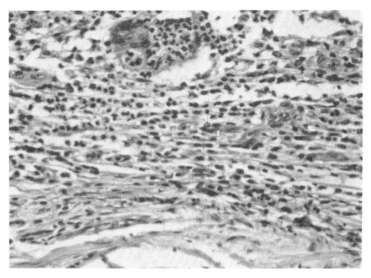

Fig. 9.16 Photomicrograph of a bone biopsy from a patient with acute osteomyelitis shows a polymorphonuclear leukocyte exudate in the marrow space.

Fig. 9.17 Roentgenogram of the ankle in a patient complaining of a dull aching pain in the lower leg reveals a lytic lesion with a well-defined sclerotic margin. Biopsy proved this lesion to have resulted from infection.

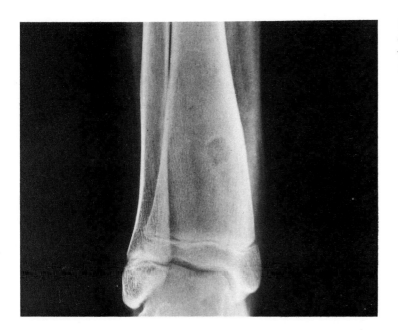

In most cases, however, infection of the bone does not result in a localized abscess. Continuing exudation raises the tissue pressure and, because of the inexpandable form of the bone, this pressure cannot be relieved by swelling, as it is in most tissues. Instead, the only potential space—the vascular space—is compromised, resulting in widespread bone death (Fig. 9.18). Indeed, the major problem in treating patients with osteomyelitis is the extent of the resulting osteonecrosis that interferes with the access of antibiotics.

Eventually, the exudate will be forced through the medullary canal and the haversian systems of the cortical bone to the bone surface. In children, the cortex is thin, and the periosteum is only loosely attached, so it is easily elevated (Fig. 9.19). New bone from the cambium layer of the periosteum produces a sleeve of reactive bone (the involucrum) around the affected area. In very young children, the involucrum may be quite massive (Fig. 9.20). Alternatively, in adults (in whom the periosteum is firmly attached to the cortical bone), the periosteal elevation and new bone formation may be minimal. In children, the necrotic medullary bone becomes isolated within a large cavity and is referred to as the sequestrum (Fig.

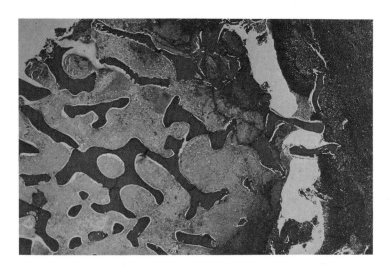

Fig. 9.18 Photomicrograph demonstrates an area of necrotic bone surrounded by an acute inflammatory exudate (pus). A focus of necrotic bone such as this allows the sequestration of bacteria, and unless it is surgically removed from the bone, antibiotic therapy may not prevent the development of chronic relapsing osteomyelitis.

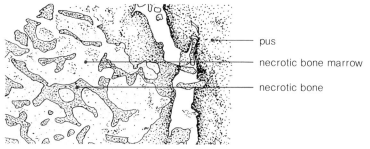

pus

necrotic bone marrow

necrotic bone

Fig. 9.19 As illustrated in this diagram, increased pressure in the medullary cavity eventually results in extension of the inflammatory exudate through the haversian systems of the cortex and beneath the periosteum. The elevated periosteum will lay down a sleeve of new bone (involucrum) around the infected segment. In children, this reaction is likely to be prominent; in adults, much less so.

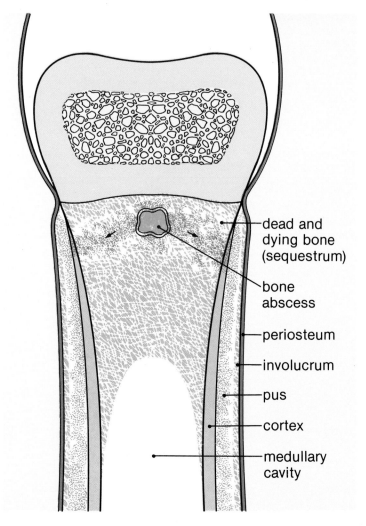

dead and dying bone (sequestrum)

bone abscess

periosteum

involucrum

pus

cortex

medullary cavity

9.21). In adults, a large involucrum and the associated sequestrum formation are much less common.

Osteomyelitis is often seen as a complication in other bone diseases that tend to result in vascular insufficiency. In the United States, perhaps the most common of these diseases is sickle cell anemia (Fig. 9.22). Patients with sickle cell anemia often experience repeated attacks of bone infection; among the organisms that may be isolated from these cases of osteomyelitis, the salmonella are important to consider. It has been postulated that salmonella organisms gain access to the blood through microinfarcts of the bowel. However, it should be pointed out that salmonella is not the most common organism in patients with sickle cell disease; staphylococci are still the most common bacteria cultured from patients with osteomyelitis complicating sickle cell disease.

Two other bone diseases which may be complicated by infection are Gaucher's disease and osteopetrosis. In patients with Gaucher's disease, osteomyelitis sometimes follows a biopsy procedure. Therefore, if a biopsy is being considered for such a patient, the strictest asepsis is necessary (and perhaps even antibiotic coverage should be considered). In patients with osteopetrosis, it is the jaw that is often affected, probably via tooth infections.

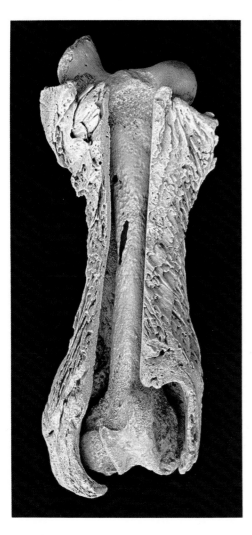

Fig. 9.20 Gross photograph of a femur from a calf with osteomyelitis. The periosteal reaction has resulted in an extensive sleeve of new bone (the involucrum) which surrounds the necrotic, partially destroyed diaphysis of the femur (the sequestrum).

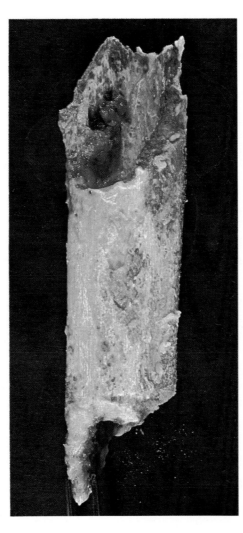

Fig. 9.21 Gross photograph of a sequestrum removed from a patient with chronic osteomyelitis of the femur. It is important to remove such a focus of dead bone from an individual with osteomyelitis if persistent, chronic infection is to be avoided.

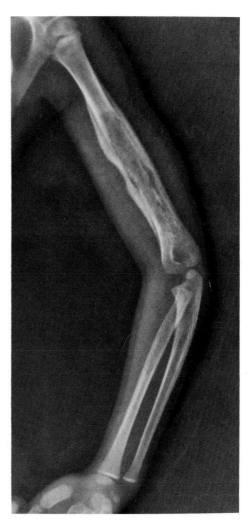

Fig. 9.22 Roentgenogram of the arm in a patient with sickle cell disease shows permeative bone destruction of the humerus, with involucrum formation and extensive sequestration. At surgery, these complications were shown to be due to infection.

GRANULOMATOUS INFLAMMATION OF BONES AND JOINTS

CLINICAL CONSIDERATIONS

Tuberculosis. Before the advent of modern chemotherapy for tuberculosis, and before the elimination of bovine tuberculosis in milking herds, bone and joint tuberculosis was one of the most common indications for admission to an orthopaedic service, and in less developed countries this is still the case.

Nowadays, in developed countries, tuberculosis has become unusual enough that there is a real risk that cases may go clinically undetected. Therefore, not until the

pathologist has examined the tissue does the true nature of the disease become apparent. In individuals with chronic debilitating conditions (including narcotic addicts and patients receiving cortisone therapy, i.e., immunosuppressed patients), an increased incidence of tuberculous infection exists.

Osseous tuberculosis results from the metastatic spread of the disease from elsewhere in the body, usually from the lungs. In most patients, bony foci of infection coexist with arthritis, and multiple skeletal lesions are not uncommon. Skeletal manifestations of tuberculosis most often occur in the spine (Figs. 9.23 and 9.24); the next most commonly affected area is the hip (Figs. 9.25 and 9.26),

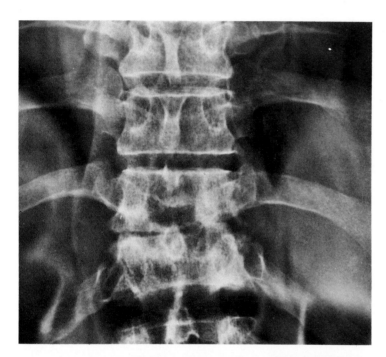

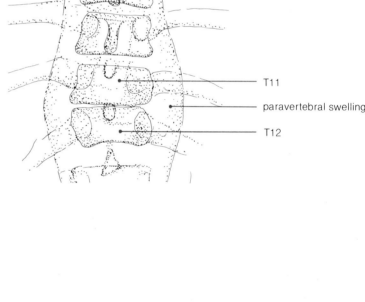

Fig. 9.23 Anteroposterior roentgenogram of the spine *(upper)* shows narrowing and destruction of the intervertebral disc at the level of T11–T12. Note also the paravertebral soft-tissue swelling. In the lateral roentgenogram *(lower)*, destructive bone disease is seen anteriorly in both the 11th and 12th thoracic vertebrae. This lesion was proved to be due to tuberculosis.

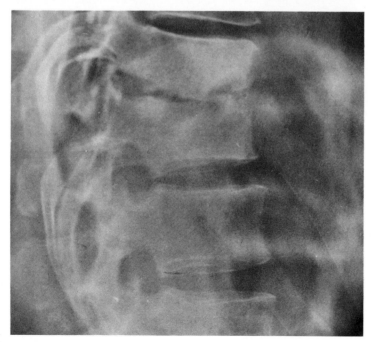

followed by the knee (Fig. 9.27). However, any joint may be involved, including those of the hand.

In general, tuberculosis is a disease of young people, and both sexes are equally affected. Most patients are under the age of 25 at diagnosis; however, the disease may occur at any age. Tuberculosis of the spine and hip is more common in children; tuberculosis of the knee is most common in adults.

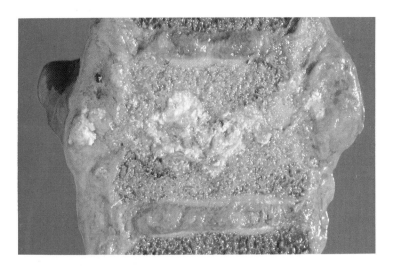

Fig. 9.24 Gross photograph of a portion of the spine removed at necropsy from a patient with tuberculosis reveals destruction of the intervertebral disc space and contiguous bone, and the presence of a cheesy necrotic tissue (caseation necrosis). The caseating tissue can be seen extending into the soft tissue on either side of the spinal column.

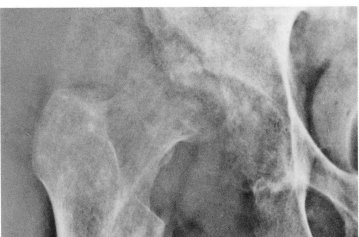

Fig. 9.25 Roentgenogram of a patient with long-standing pain and limitation of motion in the right hip. Destructive joint disease with involvement of the bone is evident in both the femoral head and the acetabulum. In addition, a dislocation of the femoral neck has occurred. These are common manifestations of tuberculosis.

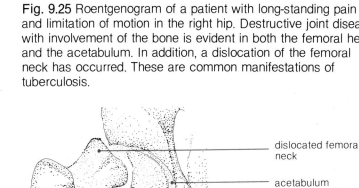

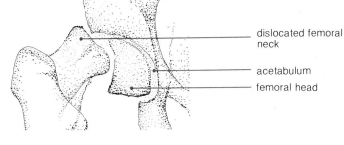

dislocated femoral neck

acetabulum
femoral head

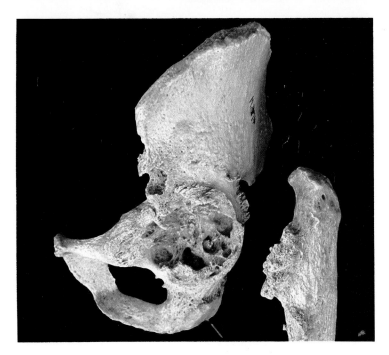

Fig. 9.26 A macerated bone specimen obtained at necropsy demonstrates destructive disease of the hip joint in a patient with tuberculosis. Total destruction of the femoral head has occurred, with only a stump of the femoral neck remaining attached to the shaft of the femur.

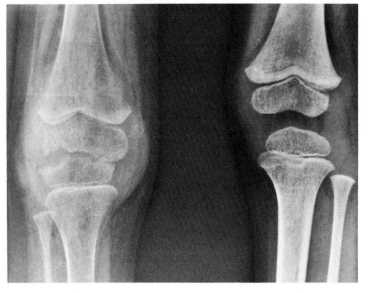

Fig. 9.27 Roentgenogram of the knees in a child complaining of pain, swelling, and limitation of motion in the right knee. Note the narrowing of the joint, resulting from the destruction of cartilage and bone, that is evident in the right knee. (The destruction is particularly obvious at the margins of the joint.) In addition to the destructive changes, the roentgenogram also shows marked soft-tissue swelling. These changes were proven to be due to tuberculosis.

Spinal tuberculosis usually involves the lower thoracic and upper lumbar spine. The disease often begins in one vertebral body, but spreads underneath the spinal ligaments to affect other vertebrae. In untreated patients, this course eventually leads to vertebral collapse and angulation of the vertebral column (Pott's disease) (Fig. 9.28). Compression of the spinal cord with consequent neurologic defects may occur, or the disease may spread to the meninges with subsequent tuberculous meningitis. Because the initial lesion is most often seen in the lower thoracic spine, the psoas muscle sheath is frequently affected. In cases where treatment is delayed, the infection may track down the psoas muscle and form a so-called "cold" abscess in the groin.

In tuberculous infections of the hip and knee, both the bone and the synovium are involved. Roentgenographic examination of the involved joint shows osteoporosis and soft-tissue swelling early in the disease. These changes are followed by the marginal erosion of the bone, and destruction of the subchondral bone with narrowing of the joint space. Gross examination of the areas affected by tuberculosis is likely to show a thickened edematous tissue, frequently studded with grayish small nodules, sometimes with white opaque centers (granulomas). These granulomas frequently become confluent and produce larger areas of white necrotic material, so-called caseation (or cheesy) necrosis. In the joint, the separation of the articular cartilage that is dissected from the under-

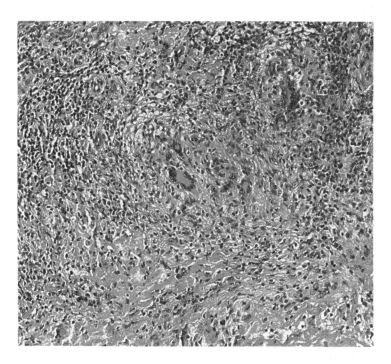

Fig. 9.29 Photomicrograph of granulomatous tissue obtained from the synovium of a knee joint in a patient with tuberculosis. Numerous Langerhans-type giant cells are seen, as are nodular collections of histiocytes and an infiltration of chronic inflammatory cells.

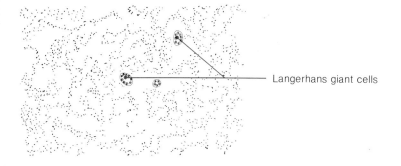

Langerhans giant cells

Fig. 9.28 A macerated specimen of spine removed at autopsy from a patient with chronic tuberculosis. Severe kyphosis and fusion of several vertebral bodies may be observed.

lying bone by granulomatous tissue is a characteristic feature. In the later stages of untreated disease, ankylosis is a frequent complication.

On microscopic examination, the typical tubercle (Fig. 9.29) is formed of a central necrotic area surrounded by pale histiocytes, sometimes referred to as epithelioid cells. Among the epithelioid cells are some scattered giant cells, the nuclei of which are typically arranged at the margin of the cell. At the periphery of the tubercle a rim of mixed chronic inflammatory cells is present. Often the tubercles are confluent, resulting in extensive central caseation. The acid-fast bacilli may be demonstrated with the Ziehl-Neelsen stain, and are characteristically seen in the giant cells and at the margin of the caseous area.

Occasional bone infections may result from atypical mycobacteria, and in this instance typical granulomas may not form. However, acid-fast staining will show large numbers of organisms, many more than can be seen in a patient with tuberculosis (Fig. 9.30). Atypical myco-bacteria may be difficult to culture from synovial fluid. For this reason, synovial biopsy may be necessary for diagnosis.

Fungal Infections. If granulomatous infection is found or suspected, it is important to make direct smears as well as prepare cultures not only for acid-fast organisms but also for fungi. The common fungal conditions that have been found to be responsible for granulomatous infections include blastomycosis (Fig. 9.31),

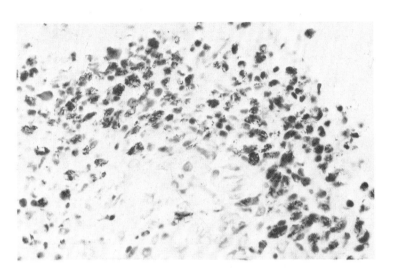

Fig. 9.30 Photomicrograph of a specimen obtained from a patient with an atypical mycobacterial infection of the ankle joint. Innumerable acid-fast bacilli are present, and most of them are within histiocytes (Ziehl-Neelsen stain).

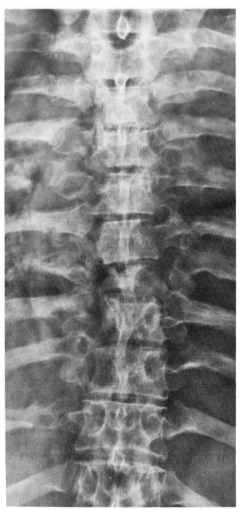
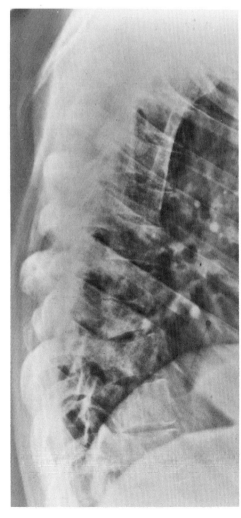

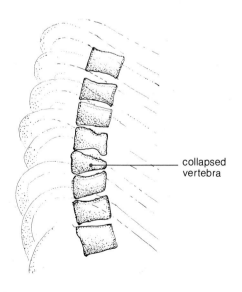

Fig. 9.31 Anteroposterior (*left*) and lateral (*right*) roentgenograms of the thoracic spine demonstrate multiple destructive lesions involving several vertebral bodies, some of which are partially collapsed. Biopsy proved this to be due to blastomycosis.

collapsed vertebra

coccidioidomycosis (Figs. 9.32 and 9.33), cryptococcosis, and rarely, actinomycosis. Sporotrichosis infection may result from the direct contamination of a joint by a puncture wound from the thorn of a contaminated plant (often a rose).

Patients with long-term indwelling intravenous catheters (e.g., for parenteral nutrition) occasionally develop bone and joint infections due to candida or aspergillus.

Since blood cultures are likely to be negative with fungal infections, biopsy may be necessary for diagnosis.

Sarcoidosis. About 10 per cent of the patients with sarcoidosis have joint involvement. In most cases, this condition is a migratory polyarticular disease, often symmetrical and of only a few weeks' duration. In a small number of patients one may see a chronic granulomatous arthritis. Most often this form of the disease is seen in the

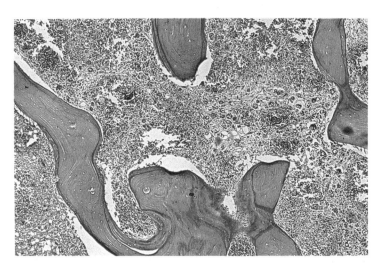

Fig. 9.32 Low power photomicrograph of tissue obtained from a patient with chronic spinal disease resulting from infection with *Coccidioides immitis.* The marrow space is infiltrated by chronic inflammatory tissue.

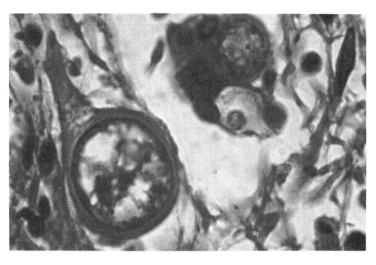

Fig. 9.33 High power view of the tissue shown in Fig. 9.32 reveals two rounded, thick-walled fungal organisms containing endospores.

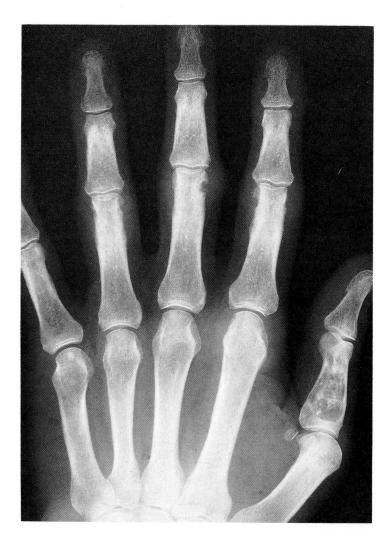

Fig. 9.34 Roentgenogram of the hand in a patient with sarcoidosis demonstrates the two types of lesions which may be seen in this condition. Punched-out cortical erosions, some with obvious overlying soft-tissue lesions, are evident at the distal end of the proximal phalanx in the index, middle, and ring fingers. In the thumb can be seen a central lytic lesion of the proximal phalanx, similar in appearance to the lesions of dactylitis tuberculosa seen in young adults.

patient's fingers, where it clinically resembles rheumatoid disease (Fig. 9.34). The involvement of the synovium of large joints is rare, and therefore may lead to the mistaken diagnosis of tuberculosis (Figs. 9.35 and 9.36). However, there are histologic features that help to distinguish sarcoidosis, e.g., the lack of caseation necrosis, the increased prominence of large, pale epithelioid cells with fewer chronic inflammatory cells, and the absence of acid-fast bacilli. (With regard to this last point, it should be noted that it is frequently difficult to demonstrate acid-fast bacilli in patients with bone and joint tuberculosis. In any individual suspected of having granulomatous tissue, smears should be taken for direct examination, and cultures for tuberculosis, brucellosis, fungus, and atypical mycobacteria should be prepared. Generally, a firm diagnosis can be made only when positive cultures have been obtained.)

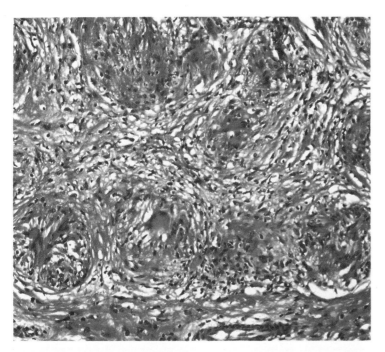

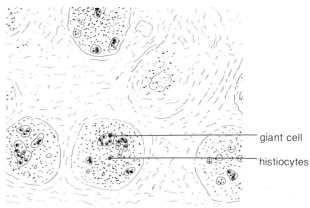

Fig. 9.35 Photomicrograph of the synovium from a patient with sarcoidosis of the knee joint. Multiple nodules composed of pale histiocytes and giant cells are evident.

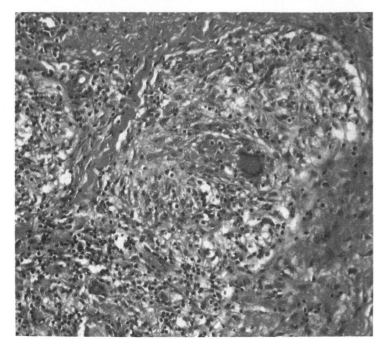

Fig. 9.36 The noncaseating character of the granulomas may be seen in this higher power photomicrograph of the specimen shown in Fig. 9.35. Note also the lack of lymphocytic cuffing of the granulomas. The rareness of sarcoidosis in large joints is likely to result in the misinterpretation of the lesion as some other form of granulomatous inflammation.

Echinococcal Cysts. Echinococcal cysts (hydatid cysts) are not uncommonly seen in the bones of patients from those countries in which the disease is endemic. The cyst is often seen initially at the epiphyseal end of the bone. It is usually a multiloculated lesion, with an irregular outline that may be easily confused with a tumor on roentgenograms (Figs. 9.37 to 9.39).

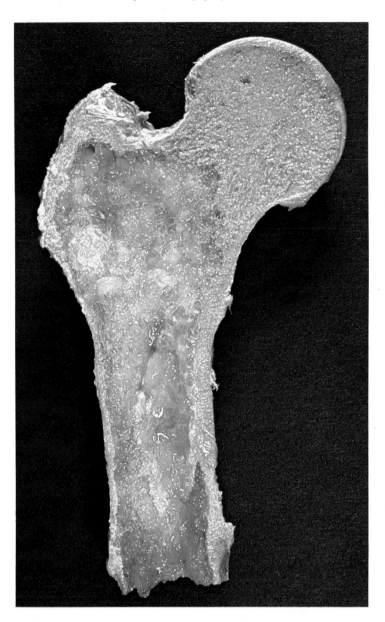

Fig. 9.37 Gross photograph of the upper end of a femur removed at necropsy from a patient with hydatid disease. The medullary cavity is filled by a glistening white nodular tissue, which on closer examination is found to be made up of fibrous, walled cysts.

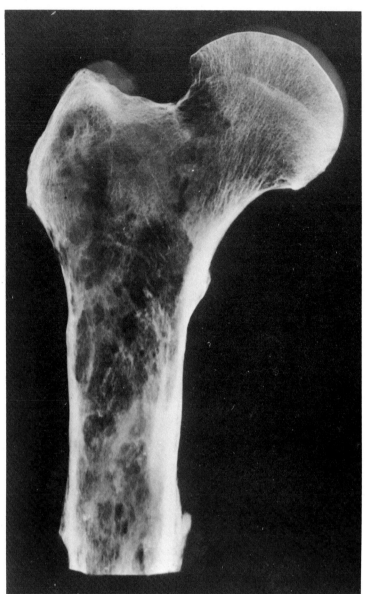

Fig. 9.38 Roentgenogram of the specimen shown in Fig. 9.37. Note the multiloculated lytic appearance and the irregular thinning of the cortices. In those parts of the world where the occurrence of hydatid disease is rare, such roentgenographic findings will probably be interpreted by the radiologist as a tumor.

Fig. 9.39 Photomicrograph of material removed from a hydatid cyst reveals a scolex with hooklets.

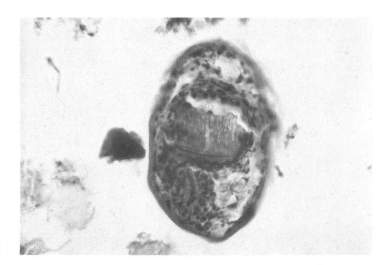

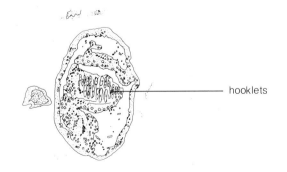

hooklets

10 Skeletal Hamartomas and Other Benign Tumorous Conditions I

When considering the diagnosis in a patient with a localized bone tumor, after ruling out metastatic disease, the most commonly occurring lesions are not neoplasms but developmental malformations (hamartomas) or other benign conditions. These conditions will be discussed in detail in the following two chapters.

EPIDERMOID INCLUSION CYST

Epidermoid inclusion cysts are bound by a wall of stratified squamous epithelium and filled with keratin debris (Fig. 10.1). Although these lesions are rarely seen in bone, when they are present they are usually evident radiologically as sharply outlined, intraosseous lytic areas found most commonly in the distal terminal phalanx (Fig. 10.2) or the calvarium.

The differential diagnosis of an epidermoid inclusion cyst in the finger includes enchondroma (seen in the proximal portion of the distal phalanx only), giant-cell reparative granuloma, and intraosseous extension of a glomus tumor (Figs. 10.3 and 10.4).

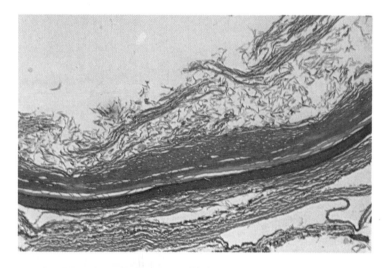

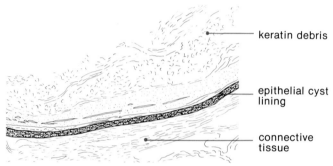

Fig. 10.1 Photomicrograph of an epidermoid inclusion cyst. The central space is lined by stratified squamous epithelium and filled with keratin debris.

keratin debris

epithelial cyst lining

connective tissue

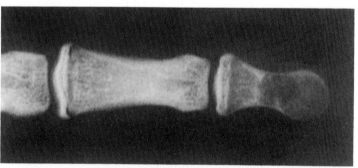

Fig. 10.2 Anteroposterior (*upper*) and lateral (*lower*) roentgenograms showing an epidermoid inclusion cyst. A well-circumscribed lucent defect with a thinned cortical rim is present in the distal portion of the terminal phalanx. No calcification is evident, and this fact, together with the location, help to differentiate this lesion from an enchondroma.

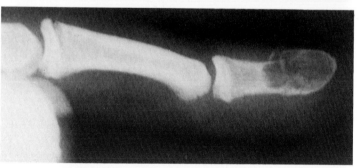

Fig. 10.3 Although glomus tumors may appear to be intraosseous, they are more typically seen subcutaneously, where they may cause pressure erosion of the terminal phalanx of a finger (as seen in this example). Note the slight irregularity in the cortical surface.

GANGLIONIC CYSTIC DEFECTS OF BONE

Intraosseous ganglionic cysts are uniloculated or multi-loculated, well-demarcated lytic defects with a rim of sclerotic bone. These lesions most frequently appear at the epiphyseal end of long bones, commonly in the medial malleolus of the ankle (Fig. 10.5). Despite its proximity to a joint, a ganglionic cyst rarely involves the joint. Occasionally, an overlying soft-tissue ganglion is present, and it may communicate with the intraosseous ganglion.

Patients with this disorder are middle-aged, and they usually present with mild localized pain that increases with weight bearing.

The lesion is a unilocular or multilocular cyst lined by a thick fibrous membrane and filled with a whitish or yellowish gelatinous material. Upon microscopic examination, the wall of a ganglionic cyst is found to be composed of a dense, fibrous connective tissue layer with focal mucoid degeneration, flattened membrane-lining cells, and occasional mononuclear inflammatory cells (Fig. 10.6).

Both the lack of communication between the cystic bone defect and the articular cavity and the absence of arthritic changes distinguish this disorder from marginal cysts and subchondral bone cysts associated with degenerative joint disease.

Treatment by curettage or excision has been curative. Recurrences are rare.

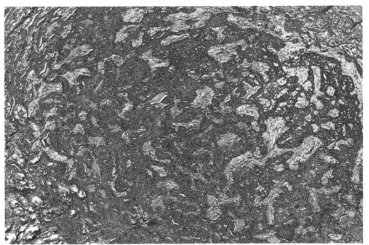

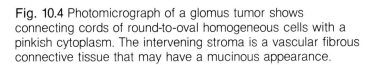

Fig. 10.4 Photomicrograph of a glomus tumor shows connecting cords of round-to-oval homogeneous cells with a pinkish cytoplasm. The intervening stroma is a vascular fibrous connective tissue that may have a mucinous appearance.

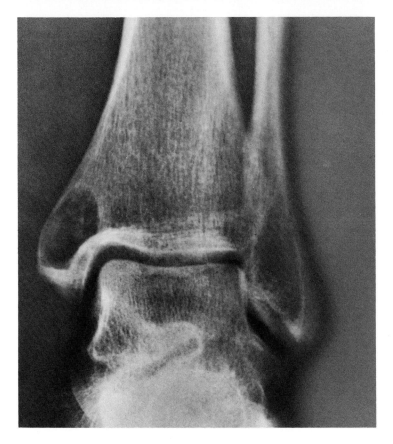

Fig. 10.5 Ganglionic cyst of bone. In this roentgenogram of the lower end of the tibia, a well-demarcated, roundish lucent area is evident. Note that although this lesion is close to the joint space, the joint space is not narrowed. This finding differentiates a ganglionic cyst from an osteoarthritic cyst.

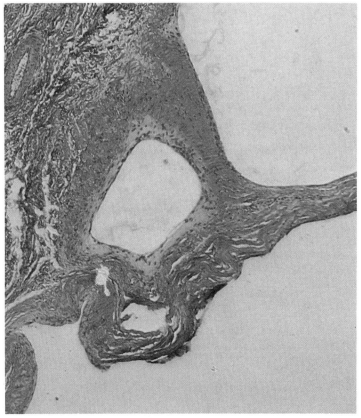

Fig. 10.6 Microscopic examination of a ganglionic cyst of bone reveals the walls of the lesion to consist of fibrous connective tissue with focal areas of mucoid degeneration and patchy dense collagen. The membrane may be lined with flattened lining cells.

UNICAMERAL BONE CYST
Solitary cyst, simple bone cyst

A simple bone cyst is a benign, solitary cystic defect in the metaphyseal region of long bones in children and adolescents (Fig. 10.7). The classic location for such a lesion is the proximal humerus (Figs. 10.8 and 10.9), and the most common reason for clinical presentation is a fracture through the area of weakened bone. On roentgenographic studies, the lesion presents as a well-defined lucent area with a thin sclerotic margin. A pseudoloculated appearance may result from the irregular thinning of the cortex by the expanding cyst.

Upon gross inspection, an unaltered lesion appears as a clear, fluid-filled cyst lined with a thin fibrous membrane (Figs. 10.10 and 10.11). However, since fractures are common complications, one may observe "secondary"

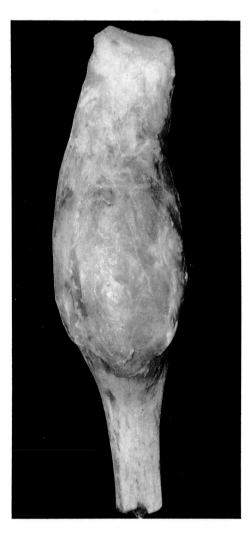

Fig. 10.7 Gross photograph of fibula with a central bulblike expansion due to a simple bone cyst. Note the pink color at the margin of the cyst due to periosteal bone formation.

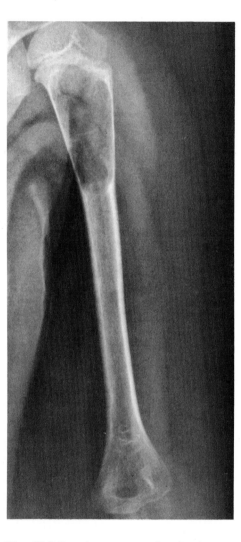

Fig. 10.8 Roentgenogram of a simple bone cyst in the proximal humerus of an 8-year-old boy reveals a well-circumscribed lucent area in the metaphysis extending to the diaphysis. Note that although the lesion extends up to the epiphysis, the epiphysis is not involved. Thinning of the cortex is evident. (Since these lesions present typically following a fracture, the radiologic appearance may be complicated by callus formation.)

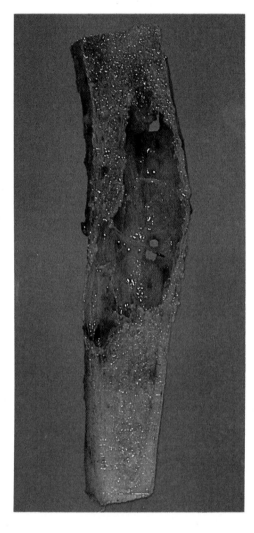

Fig. 10.9 Longitudinal section of a segment of resected humerus reveals a well-demarcated cystic cavitation in the medullary portion of the bone, with cortical thinning and periosteal elevation leading to a bulging cortex. Note also the glistening cystic lining. (These lesions usually contain a clear serous-like fluid.)

changes such as hemorrhage and hemosiderin deposits, granulation tissue, cholesterol clefts, fibrin, calcification, and reactive bone (Fig. 10.12). In such instances, the lesion may mimic the histologic features of an aneurysmal bone cyst or even a giant-cell tumor. A rarely observed histologic feature is an accumulation of calcified amorphous material that resembles the contents of a cementoma of the jaw (Fig. 10.13).

The lesion, when observed in serial roentgenograms, appears to migrate from the epiphyseal plate, although, in reality, the growth plate grows away from the cyst. Although the entity is benign, there is a high rate of recurrence following surgery, particularly in children under 10 years of age, in whom the lesion is characteristically juxtaepiphyseal.

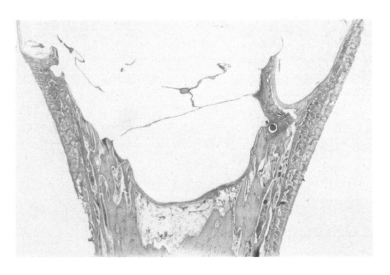

Fig. 10.10 Low power photomicrograph of a simple bone cyst reveals a fibrous membrane. The erosion of the cortex is evident, as is the periosteal bone formation.

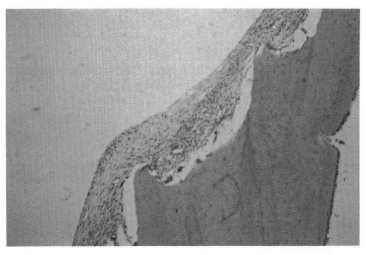

Fig. 10.11 High power view of the fibrous lining of a simple bone cyst.

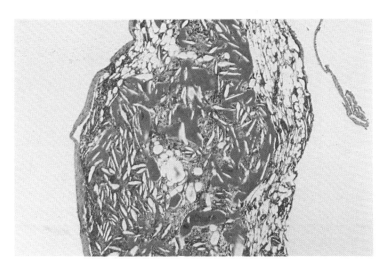

Fig. 10.12 Photomicrograph of tissue curetted from a simple bone cyst following fracture. Local hemosiderin deposits, chronic inflammation with many cholesterol clefts, and a rapidly forming callus are evident.

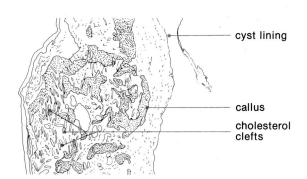

Fig. 10.13 The membranous wall of this simple bone cyst reveals a peculiar, irregularly arranged calcific matrix that morphologically resembles the tissue present in a cementoma of the jaw.

10.5

ANEURYSMAL BONE CYST

An aneurysmal bone cyst is a solitary, generally eccentric, expansile entity of unknown etiology. The lesion most commonly involves long bones or the spine, but any bone may be involved, including flat bones. On serial roentgenographic films, the lesion is seen as a rapidly expansile, eccentric, lucent lesion in the shaft of a long bone (Fig. 10.14). In the spine, the lesion may involve the body, arch, or transverse and spinous processes of the vertebrae. Aneurysmal bone cysts are most commonly seen in individuals in the second and third decades of life, and swelling, pain, or tenderness may be observed clinically in these patients.

A macroscopic examination of one of these lesions reveals a multiloculated bloody cavity (Fig. 10.15), which

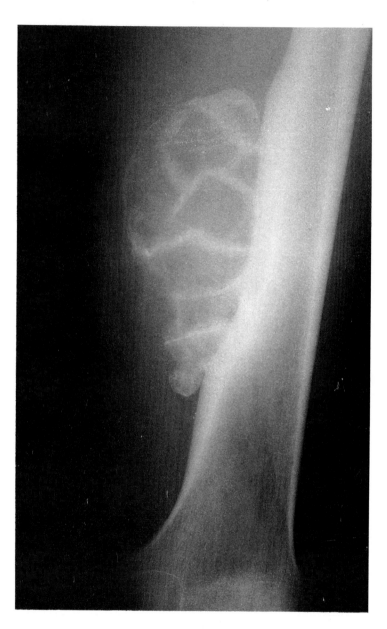

Fig. 10.14 Roentgenogram of an aneurysmal bone cyst shows a septated, subperiosteal blowout lesion. Note the irregular cortical margins at the lesion's interface with the shaft of the bone.

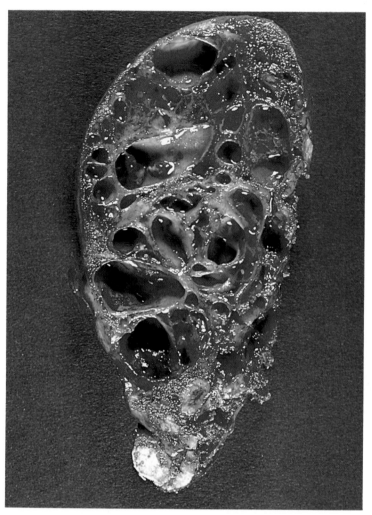

Fig. 10.15 Viewed grossly, the lesion resected from the patient shown in Fig. 10.14 is a spongy, honeycombed, blood-filled mass with cystic spaces of varying size, some containing osseous tissue within the septated walls.

on histologic examination is found to contain cystic spaces of different sizes that are filled with blood but are not lined by vascular endothelium. Between the blood-filled spaces are fibrous septa containing giant cells and foci of immature bone or osteoid (Figs. 10.16 and 10.17). Focal or diffuse collections of hemosiderin or reactive foam cells and chronic inflammatory cells may be seen in the septal zone. Characteristically, the cellular mor-

phology appears innocuous. In some instances it is clear from histologic examination that the lesion coexists with another benign tumor, such as an osteoblastoma or a chondroblastoma. In about 50 per cent of patients, the lesion may recur once or several times following curettage.

It is important to differentiate this lesion microscopically from a telangiectatic osteosarcoma, a differential diagnosis that may be difficult.

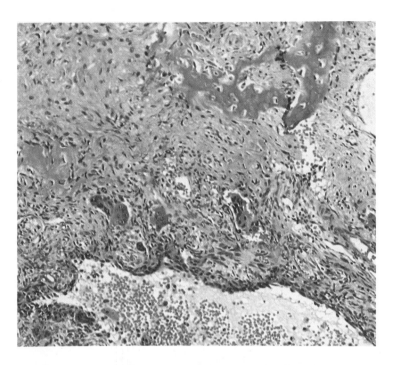

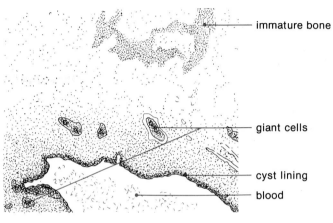

Fig. 10.16 Low power photomicrograph reveals that the lining tissue of an aneurysmal bone cyst contains a cellular stroma, often with numerous giant cells and new bone formation.

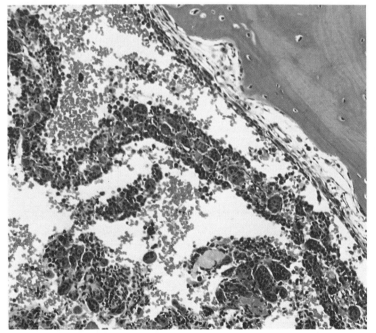

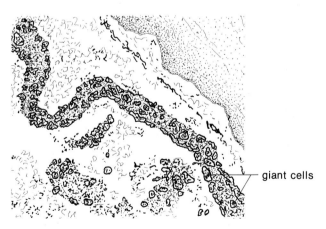

Fig. 10.17 Higher power photomicrograph demonstrates the numerous giant cells lining the septa. This feature distinguishes an aneurysmal bone cyst lining from the fibrous lining space of a simple bone cyst.

GIANT-CELL REPARATIVE GRANULOMA

A giant-cell reparative granuloma is a benign, nonneoplastic, intraosseous lesion most commonly seen in the mandible or maxilla, but also reported in the small bones of the hands and feet (Fig. 10.18). The clinical signs of this lesion are localized pain and swelling of variable duration. A roentgenographic examination reveals a lucent defect expanding the bone. The cortex is thinned, and there is little evidence of bone destruction and no surrounding sclerosis.

The gross appearance of tissue obtained from a giant-cell reparative granuloma is grayish-brown, and it is often friable. Upon microscopic observation of the tissue, one may find varying degrees of cellularity, with predominantly unremarkable fibroblast-like spindle cells (Figs. 10.19 and 10.20). Histiocytes are also present. Characteristically, giant cells are scattered throughout the tissue of the lesion, but they are usually clustered in areas of hemorrhage. Mitotic activity is rare. New bone formation and osteoid may be seen, usually at sites of hemorrhage.

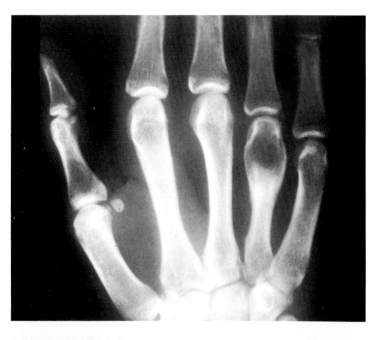

Fig. 10.18 Roentgenogram of a giant-cell reparative granuloma of the fourth metacarpal. A lucent lesion expands the bone, and there is thinning and expansion of the cortex. No calcification has occurred. The shaft of the bone is protruding into the expansile lesion, resembling a finger inside a balloon. This radiologic finding is also common in aneurysmal bone cysts when they affect small tubular bones, and it is evidence of rapid growth.

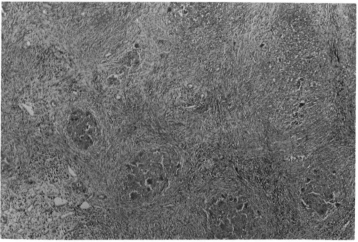

Fig. 10.19 Low power photomicrograph of a giant-cell reparative granuloma. Spindle-shaped fibroblasts constitute the bulk of the lesion. Foci of giant cells can be seen, particularly in areas of extravasated blood (often accompanied by iron deposits).

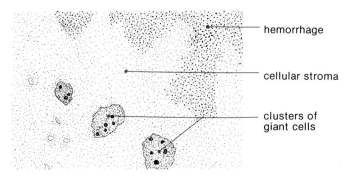

hemorrhage

cellular stroma

clusters of giant cells

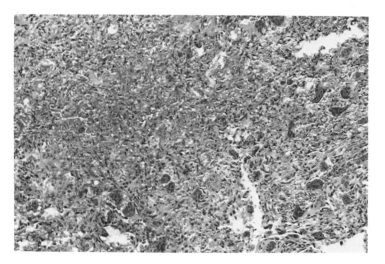

Fig. 10.20 High power photomicrograph of a giant-cell reparative granuloma. The cellularity varies, but hypervascularity is usually evident. Changes typical of reactive tissue include focal chronic inflammation. The histologic differential diagnosis includes giant-cell tumors and aneurysmal bone cysts.

Focal or scattered lymphocytic infiltration has been noted. The differential diagnosis of giant-cell reparative granuloma includes "brown" tumor of hyperparathyroidism, giant-cell tumor, and aneurysmal bone cyst.

The following considerations may prove helpful in sorting through the differential diagnosis of a suspected giant-cell reparative granuloma. The clinical presentation of a solitary lesion, as well as laboratory findings of normocalcemia and normophosphatemia, mitigate against a "brown" tumor of hyperparathyroidism. A giant-cell tumor has a more homogeneous morphology, with diffuse but uniform distribution of the giant cells; the stromal cells of a giant-cell tumor are more rounded and less spindle-shaped, and little or no inflammation is evident. A giant-cell reparative granuloma lacks the large blood-filled channels seen in aneurysmal bone cysts, and, in addition, the locations of the lesions are different.

Treatment consists of curettage or excision of the involved bone; however, recurrences are common in curetted lesions of the small bones of the hands and feet.

HEMANGIOMA OF BONE

Intraosseous hemangiomas are vascular hamartomas that are usually asymptomatic and solitary. These lesions typically affect the vertebral bodies or the skull, and if one presents clinically, it is usually in patients in the middle years of life. There is no familial tendency in these lesions.

The entity is characterized roentgenographically by a relatively lytic defect with a coarse, trabeculated bone pattern, often producing a honeycomb appearance (Fig. 10.21). Cortical expansion may be seen in flat bones such as the ribs and skull.

On gross examination of hemangioma, one notes a cystic, dark-red cavity (Fig. 10.22). The microscopic structure of this cavity consists of thin-walled cavernous blood vessels or proliferating capillaries lined by thin, flattened epithelium (Fig. 10.23).

Hemangiomas usually follow an indolent course, but they may be complicated by a fracture or extraosseous extension.

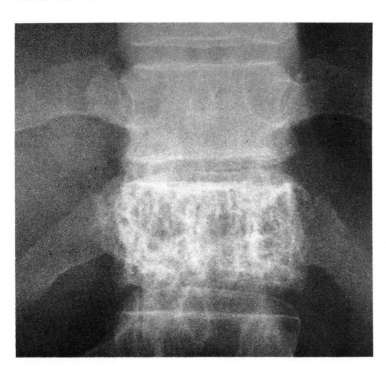

Fig. 10.21 Roentgenogram of a hemangioma of a vertebral body demonstrates the characteristic, accentuated, coarse trabecular pattern of the lesion.

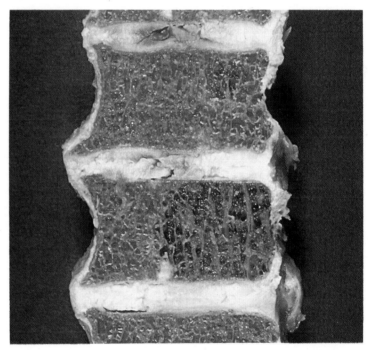

Fig. 10.22 Gross photograph of hemangiomas of the vertebral bodies shows a well-demarcated, coarsely trabeculated red lesion, clearly distinct from normal cancellous bone.

Fig. 10.23 Photomicrograph of a hemangioma of bone reveals characteristic increased vascular channels of varying sizes. Note in the lower part of the photograph reactive bone formation at the rim of the lesion.

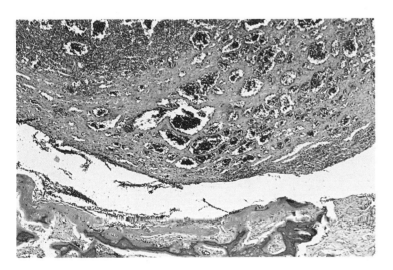

Skeletal Hemangiomatosis/Lymphangiomatosis
Cystic angiomatosis of bone, lymphangiectasis of bone

Systemic hemangiomatosis/lymphangiomatosis is a hamartomatous malformation involving the skeleton and, often, the visceral organs. The condition is usually diagnosed incidentally on radiologic examination, or following complications such as pathologic fractures, soft-tissue masses (rarely), or chylous or hemorrhagic effusions. The patients are usually in the first three decades of life at the time of diagnosis. The presence of hemangiomas or lymphangiomas in the skeleton is often seen in association with visceral hemangiomas and lymphangiomas, most often involving the spleen, pleura, and skin. There is no known familial tendency.

The roentgenographic features of skeletal hemangiomatosis/lymphangiomatosis are similar to those of solitary hemangiomas. The lesions usually have a fine peripheral rim of increased density (Fig. 10.24). Rare cases of diffuse blastic skeletal lesions may mimic metastatic cancer; however, upon closer scrutiny, the lesions reveal a central lytic area surrounded by dense sclerotic bone (Figs. 10.25 to 10.27).

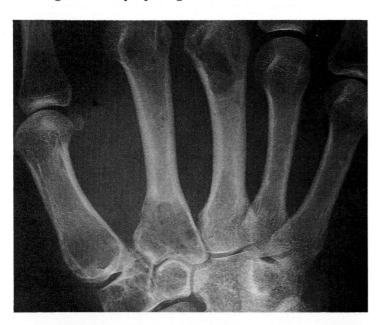

Fig. 10.24 Roentgenogram of a hand with multiple hemangiomas. Lucent zones well demarcated from surrounding bone are evident.

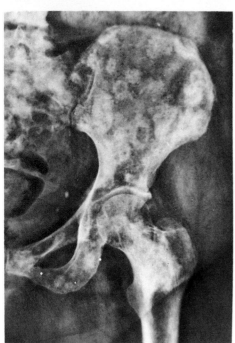

Fig. 10.25 Hemangiomas are characteristically lucent lesions, although the surrounding bone reaction may be sufficiently sclerotic to give the appearance of density. Sometimes this appearance is the dominant pattern, as seen in this clinical roentgenogram, with multiple densities throughout the skeleton mimicking a malignant bone-forming metastatic tumor.

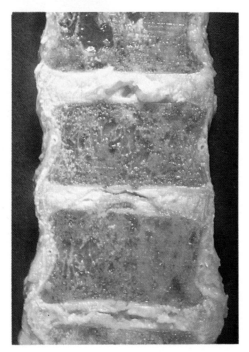

Fig. 10.26 Cross section of the spine removed at autopsy from the patient with hemangiomatosis shown in Fig. 10.25. Note the disruption of the normal cancellous architecture of the vertebral bone. Multiple areas of dense bone, often with dark reddish centers, can be seen adjoining areas of osteopenia in which the underlying yellow fat is readily evident.

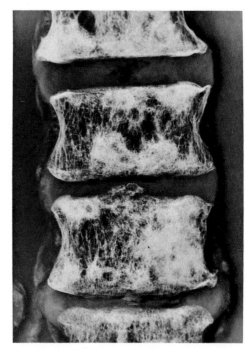

Fig. 10.27 Roentgenogram of the specimen shown in Fig. 10.26. Note that within the areas of density there are relatively lucent foci that represent the hemangioma.

Laboratory findings in patients with this condition are usually unremarkable, although increases in alkaline phosphatase activity have been noted.

On gross examination, lesions are cystic, with a reddish fluid indicative of blood, or a clear yellow fluid indicating a lymphatic origin. Combinations of both hemangiomas and lymphangiomas may occur. On microscopic examination, the lesions are seen to consist of thin-walled vascular spaces lined by flattened endothelial cells and separated by collagen septa (Fig. 10.28).

The prognosis of patients with this disorder is variable, although the condition usually is self-limiting.

MASSIVE OSTEOLYSIS

Disappearing bone disease, Gorham's disease, phantom bone

Massive osteolysis is a skeletal disorder characterized radiographically by progressive and extensive reduction in bone density, and morphologically by the replacement of osseous tissue with fibrous tissue and thin-walled dilated vascular channels. Generally detected initially in children or in young adults, the disorder usually affects the peripheral skeleton, and is often confined to a single bone or to two or more bones centered around a joint. The shoulder and hip are the most common sites of involvement. The clinical course is protracted but rarely fatal, with eventual stabilization the most common outcome. Patients may complain of a dull aching pain or the insidious onset of progressive weakness.

Roentgenographic examination reveals initial intramedullary and subcortical ill-defined lucent areas, with a subsequent loss of density extending from one end of the bone to the other. Reactive bone formation is not evident. Characteristic shrinking or tapering of the long bones may occur (Fig. 10.29).

Reported descriptions of whole surgical specimens have featured thin, tapered, soft bone, and, in specimens in which the mineralized bone has entirely disappeared, a fibrous band may be seen to have replaced the original bone. Biopsies of earlier lesions have revealed hypervascular, fibrous connective tissue replacing bone; the vessels are variably capillary, sinusoidal, or cavernous (Fig. 10.30).

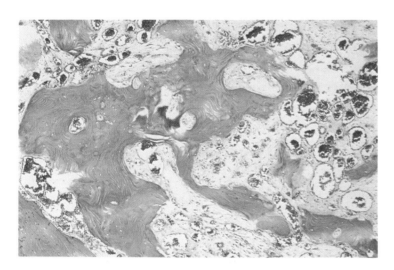

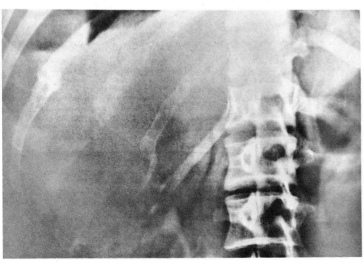

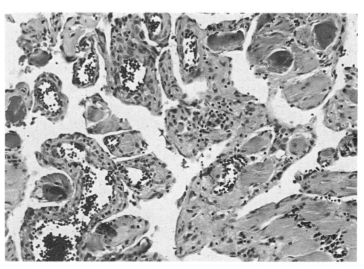

Fig. 10.28 Photomicrograph of one of the dense lesions illustrated in Figs. 10.26 and 10.27. Vascular channels of varying sizes and shapes can be seen. The thickened bone appears immature, with increased cellularity and irregular architecture.

Fig. 10.29 Roentgenogram of a patient with massive osteolysis shows marked loss of density and attenuation of 9th, 10th, 11th, and 12th ribs. In this type of case a hemothorax may complicate the disease, sometimes fatally.

Fig. 10.30 Photomicrograph of tissue obtained during biopsy from a patient with massive osteolysis (disappearing bone disease) reveals proliferating vascular channels with thrombi and extravasated blood.

10.11

SYNOVIAL HEMANGIOMA

A synovial hemangioma is a solitary, unilateral, benign lesion seen most commonly in the knees of children and adolescents. The patient may be asymptomatic, or he may have a swollen knee and experience mild pain or limitation of movement. Patients may report a history of recurrent episodes of joint swelling and pain of several years' duration.

A soft-tissue mass may be evident on roentgenographic examination, although arthrograms may be necessary to show it clearly (Fig. 10.31). In severe cases, a periosteal reaction or lucent zones in the adjacent bones may also be seen.

On gross examination, one may note a brown, soft, doughy mass with overlying villous synovium that is frequently stained mahogany brown (Fig. 10.32). When the mass is viewed microscopically, arborizing vascular channels of different dimensions are seen (Fig. 10.33). The overlying synovium is hyperplastic and, in chronic cases with repeated hemarthrosis, copious iron deposition can be noted.

Complete surgical excision (i.e., total synovectomy) may be difficult, which probably accounts for the reported cases of local recurrence.

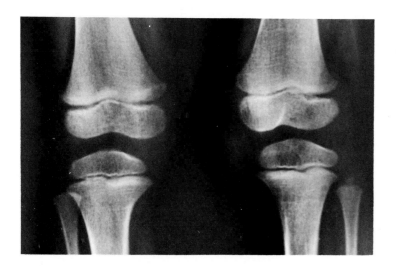

Fig. 10.31 Roentgenogram of the knee in a 3-year-old girl with a history of repeated joint effusions. Note the soft-tissue swelling on the medial side of the joint.

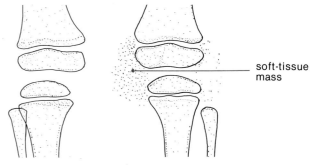

soft-tissue mass

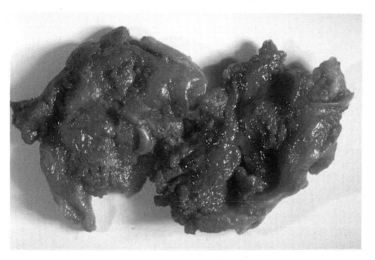

Fig. 10.32 Gross specimen removed from the knee of a patient with a history of recurrent hemorrhages into the joint. Marked hemosiderin staining of the tissues has occurred, but the synovium does not show either the villous appearance seen in association with hemophilia or the papillary appearance usually seen in patients with pigmented villonodular synovitis.

Fig. 10.33 Photomicrograph of part of the synovial tissue shown in Fig. 10.32 demonstrates the vascular malformation present in this patient's synovium. At the synovial surface, copious hemosiderin deposits and hyperplastic reactive tissue were evident.

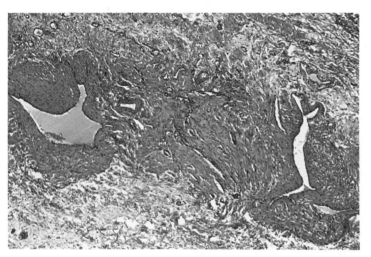

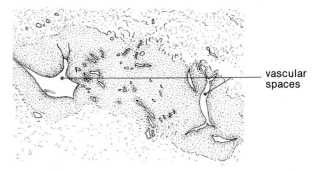

vascular spaces

FIBROUS DYSPLASIA

Fibrous dysplasia is a relatively common, usually solitary (monostotic), slow-growing hamartomatous lesion composed mainly of bone and fibrous tissue, but occasionally with foci of cartilage. The condition is usually manifested in children and adolescents.

Generally the lesion is asymptomatic; therefore, it is usually discovered accidentally on roentgenographic examination. Occasionally a patient with fibrous dysplasia will have symptoms, i.e., a pathologic fracture or impingement. Most commonly the ribs are affected, but involvement of the jaw, skull, or long bones is also frequent. Any involvement of the craniofacial bones may result in marked asymmetry (unilateral cranial hyperostosis).

The classic appearance of fibrous dysplasia is fusiform expansion of a rib or long bone, with thinning of the cortex, and replacement of bone tissue by a firm, whitish tissue of gritty consistency, often containing cysts (Figs. 10.34 to 10.36).

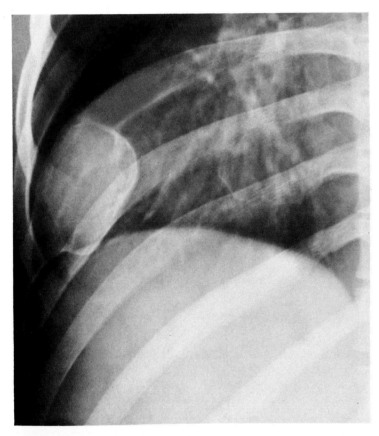

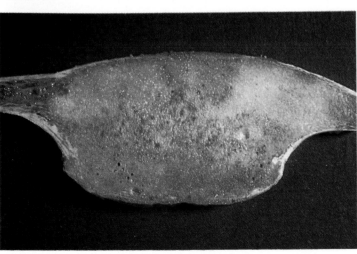

Fig. 10.34 Roentgenogram of the chest in a 20-year-old man who complained of a swollen area on the seventh right rib. Note the uniform density of the expanded tumor; this presentation is referred to as a "ground glass" appearance.

Fig. 10.35 In this gross photograph of fibrous dysplasia in a rib, one may note a well-circumscribed expansile lesion with a solid white and tan appearance. Note the normal cancellous and cortical bone of the rib on both sides of the lesion. In such a lesion, the cut surface has a gritty consistency.

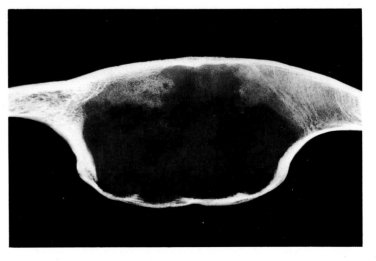

Fig. 10.36 Roentgenogram of the specimen shown in Fig. 10.35 reveals a relatively lucent expanded zone with marked thinning of the cortex. Throughout the lesion there is a "ground glass" appearance due to diffusely distributed fine spicules of bone.

Roentgenographic examination reveals that the lesion is well defined, although the rim is not sclerotic, and it often has a "ground glass" appearance. On histologic examination, one observes irregular foci of woven (nonlamellar) bone trabeculae in a cellular but otherwise unremarkable fibrous stroma (Figs. 10.37 to 10.39). Osteoblastic rimming of bone is minimal, if present, which distinguishes this lesion from a so-called ossifying fibroma. (In that lesion, the bone spicules are lined by a thin layer of lamellar bone, with prominent osteoblastic rimming.)

In patients with fibrous dysplasia, secondary reactive changes may result from a pathologic fracture. These changes include areas of multinucleated giant cells (Fig. 10.40), foamy histiocytes, and fracture callus (Fig. 10.41). If only these areas are sampled, the lesion may be mistaken on histologic examination for a primary neoplasm or even a metastatic carcinoma.

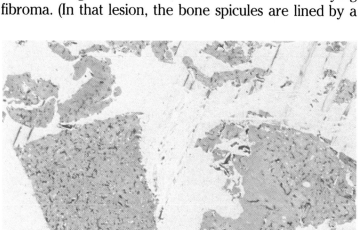

Fig. 10.37 Low power view of curetted fragments from a patient with fibrous dysplasia shows a fibrous tissue stroma with a sprinkling of immature tissue throughout.

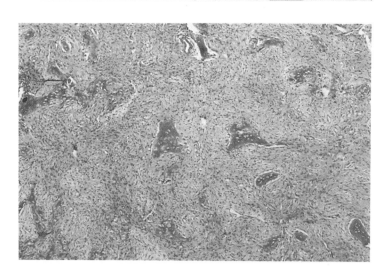

Fig. 10.38 Photomicrograph of fibrous dysplasia shows a background of collagenized fibrous tissue, within which are irregularly shaped spicules of immature bone. Note that although bone production is readily evident, there are relatively few osteoblasts rimming the bone spicules. This finding suggests a direct metaplasia of bone from the underlying fibrous tissue.

Fig. 10.39 The same tissue seen in Fig. 10.38 viewed with polarized light demonstrates the woven appearance of the collagen within the bone matrix. (This photograph should be compared with the appearance of an ossifying fibroma in Figs. 10.44 to 10.46.)

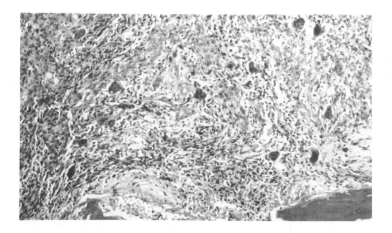

Fig. 10.40 Photomicrograph taken through an area of fracture in a patient with fibrous dysplasia demonstrates a spindle cell stroma with numerous giant cells and a sprinkling of chronic inflammatory cells. A biopsy taken through such an area may be confusing in differential diagnosis.

The classic "Shepherd's crook" deformity of the upper end of the femur is the result of multiple sequential fractures, after each of which some residual deformity remains (Fig. 10.42).

Polyostotic involvement by fibrous dysplasia is decidedly rare. Usually the multiple lesions affect predominantly one side of the body or a single limb (Fig. 10.43). The histologic features of polyostotic lesions are identical to those of monostotic lesions. The condition may cause severe deformities, and it is occasionally associated with patchy skin pigmentation and precocious puberty, mostly in females (Albright's syndrome).

The clinical course of fibrous dysplasia is most consistent with that of a developmental abnormality, and no familial association is known.

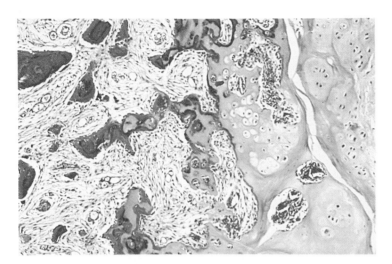

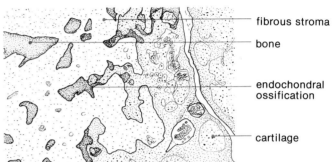

Fig. 10.41 Photomicrograph from a patient with fibrous dysplasia demonstrates areas of cartilage within the lesion. In some cases of fibrous dysplasia, cartilage formation may be considerable, and may lead to confusion with a cartilage tumor in differential diagnosis.

fibrous stroma
bone
endochondral ossification
cartilage

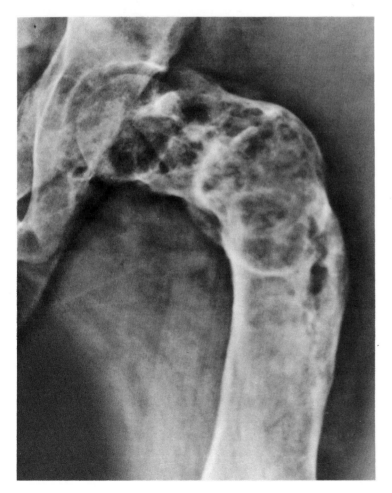

Fig. 10.42 Roentgenogram of the upper end of the femur in a patient with fibrous dysplasia shows marked varus ("Shepherd's crook") deformity. This typical deformity in patients with polyostotic fibrous dysplasia results from repeated fractures through the involved section of the proximal femur, with additional deformity occurring after each fracture.

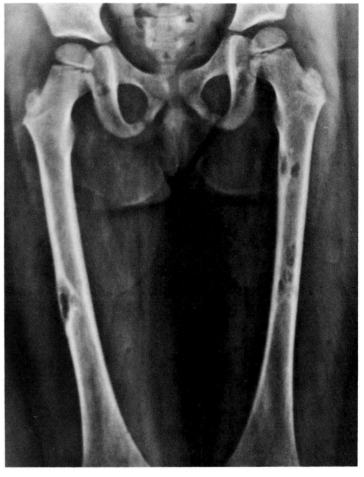

Fig. 10.43 Roentgenogram of a 4-year-old girl with multiple cystic lesions in the femur and ischium that proved, on histologic examination, to be fibrous dysplasia.

OSSIFYING FIBROMA
Osteofibrous dysplasia

Ossifying fibroma is a fibro-osseous lesion seen characteristically in the jaw, and only rarely in the long bones. Considered by some to be a variant of fibrous dysplasia, the lesion is thought by others to be truly neoplastic, with aggressive local behavior. In long bones, the lesion has a predilection for the tibia, and patients tend to be young children with enlarging but usually painless masses. The deformity of the involved leg may be quite dramatic.

Seen on radiologic films, the lesion is extensive and involves either the diaphysis or the metaphysis in long bones; the epiphysis is generally not affected. Characteristic eccentric intracortical osteolysis, with distortion and thinning of the cortex, is evident (Fig. 10.44). The cortical bone may actually be absent in places. Anterior bowing of the tibia is common, as is the appearance of multiloculation. The periosteum is usually well preserved.

The histologic appearance of the affected tissue is similar to that seen in fibrous dysplasia, with irregular spicules of trabecular bone, and unremarkable spindle cells producing a collagenous stroma. However, in contrast to fibrous dysplasia, the bone spicules are characteristically lined by osteoblasts that produce a rim of lamellar bone, even though the center of these spicules of bone may have a woven appearance (Figs. 10.45 and 10.46). The finding of woven bone with juxtaposed lamellar bone laid down by prominent plump osteoblasts is characteristic of ossifying fibroma, and distinguishes it from fibrous dysplasia. Foci of hemorrhage and foamy histiocytes, as well as an occasional area of cartilage (usually in the vicinity of a fracture), may be observed.

The natural history of this lesion is the subject of much debate, but it appears that ossifying fibroma behaves in a less aggressive manner as the affected child gets older. Metastases do not occur.

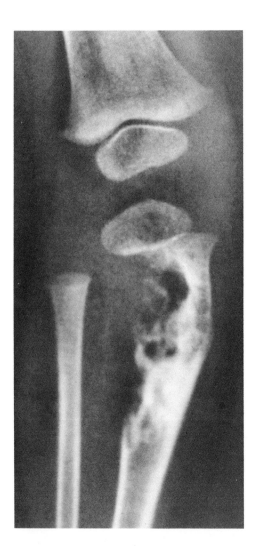

Fig. 10.44 Roentgenogram of a 15-month-old boy with a large, lytic, eccentric defect in the upper end of the tibia which proved, on histologic examination, to be an ossifying fibroma.

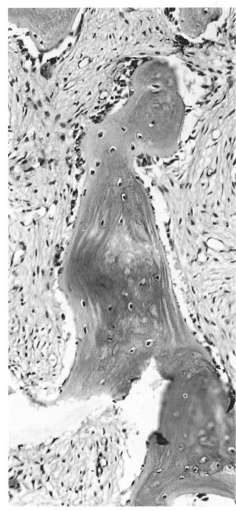

Fig. 10.45 Photomicrograph of tissue obtained from a patient with ossifying fibroma reveals a cellular spindle cell stroma, with spicules of bone rimmed by plump osteoblasts.

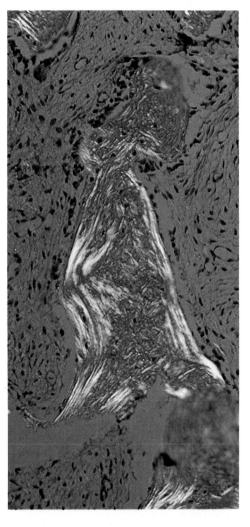

Fig. 10.46 The field shown in Fig. 10.45 viewed under polarized light shows lamellar bone on the surface of the bone spicule, with a core of woven bone. This finding of peripheral maturation to lamellar bone is regarded as characteristic of an ossifying fibroma.

NONOSSIFYING FIBROMA

Fibrous cortical defect, benign fibrous histiocytoma

A nonossifying fibroma is a benign, eccentric, solitary (or, rarely, multiple), well-circumscribed lesion in the long bones of children. Most commonly the femur or tibia is involved, and the lesions usually spontaneously regress. Most cases are detected as incidental findings on roentgenographic examination, although occasionally a pathologic fracture through a large lesion will cause the patient to seek medical attention.

Upon gross inspection, the lesions are found to be formed of soft, somewhat friable, yellow or brown tissue (Fig. 10.47). The microscopic findings include a cellular tissue of unremarkable spindle cells arranged in an interlacing whorled pattern, interspersed with multinucleated giant cells and foamy pale histiocytes (Figs. 10.48 to 10.51). Histologically, these characteristics may cause diagnostic confusion of a nonossifying fibroma with a giant-cell tumor. However, the site of involvement is different in the two lesions, as is the age at presentation.

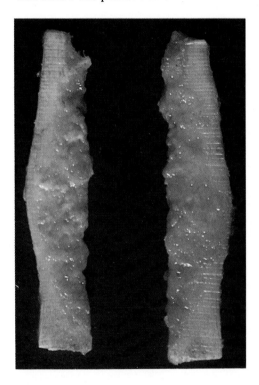

Fig. 10.47 A transected specimen of a nonossifying fibroma removed intact from the distal end of a fibula. Characteristically, the lesion has an orange-tan color and a firm consistency. It can be seen from this photograph that the lesion is eroding the overlying cortex.

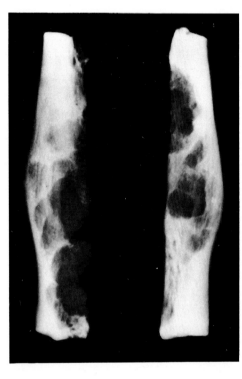

Fig. 10.48 Roentgenogram of the specimen shown in Fig. 10.47 shows the well-defined scalloped margin with a thin rim of bone sclerosis.

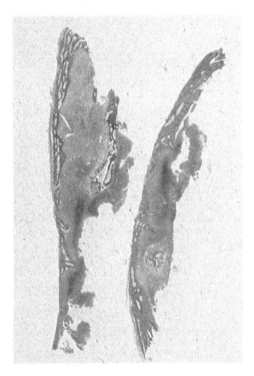

Fig. 10.49 Low power photomicrograph of a histologic section through the lesion shown in Figs. 10.47 and 10.48 demonstrates the variegated appearance of a nonossifying fibroma. In some areas, the lesion is more cellular; in others, it has a pink collagenous stroma.

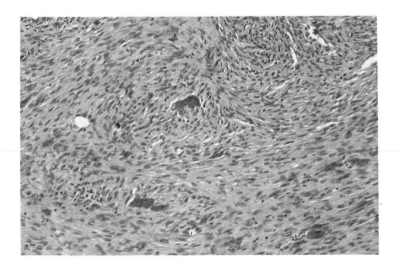

Fig. 10.50 Low power photomicrograph of a nonossifying fibroma shows the spindle cell stroma with occasional giant cells and mitoses. Note that the stromal cells are crowded, with little collagen formation.

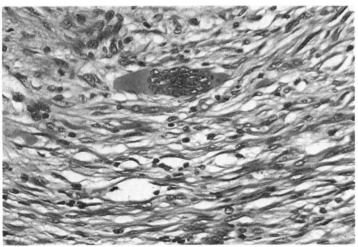

Fig. 10.51 High power photomicrograph of the stromal cells shows a foamy cytoplasm in some of the cells and one multinucleated giant cell.

Radiologic surveys have shown a 35 per cent incidence of fibrous cortical defect in normal children. The lesions range in size from a few millimeters to several centimeters, and they are characterized on roentgenograms by their cortical, eccentric position, and their appearance as well-demarcated lucent zones surrounded by scalloped, sclerotic margins (Fig. 10.52). Often a nonossifying fibroma is elongated in the longitudinal axis of the bone. Serial roentgenograms have demonstrated the migration of the defect away from the epiphyseal plate.

Lesions that are histologically indistinguishable from nonossifying fibroma may be seen roentgenographically as either lucent or more sclerotic lesions in adults (Fig. 10.53). Patients may experience mild pain or remain asymptomatic. On histologic examination, the spindle cell stroma appears in a whorled or "storiform" pattern (Fig. 10.54). The underlying cell, a fibroblast, is mixed with polygonal cells having more vacuolated cytoplasm (a histiocyte or macrophage). Iron deposits, multinucleated giant cells, sparse chronic inflammatory cells or lipid-laden cells may be evident. In adults, such a lesion is often reported as a benign fibrous histiocytoma or a fibroxanthoma.

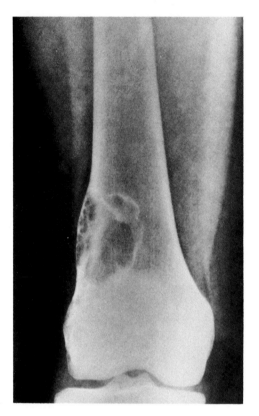

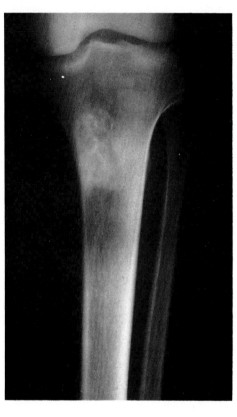

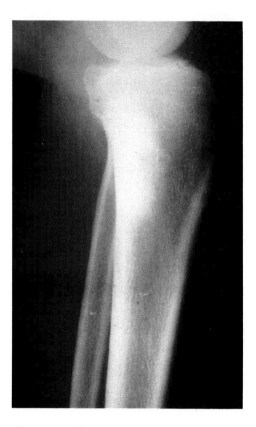

Fig. 10.52 Clinical roentgenogram of a nonossifying fibroma in a 16-year-old boy. These lesions are most prominent in the metaphysis of the upper tibia, lower femur, and lower tibia. Multiple views reveal that the entity is eccentric, extends to the cortex of the bone, and has well-defined sclerotic margins that are usually scalloped.

Fig. 10.53 Anteroposterior (left) and lateral (right) roentgenograms of the tibia in a 64-year-old man who had had a bone scan for suspected metastatic disease. The lesion in the tibia was discovered incidentally, and the roentgenograms show a dense lesion in the metaphysis that is well defined and shows no periosteal reaction.

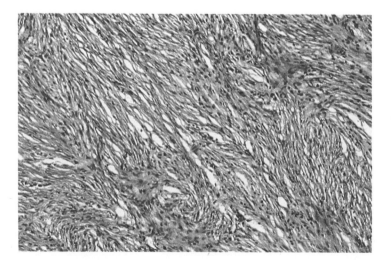

Fig. 10.54 Photomicrograph of tissue removed from the patient shown in Fig. 10.53. The lesion was formed of a benign but cellular spindle cell stroma, with scattered chronic inflammatory cells and giant cells and a matted storiform pattern. This histologic appearance is similar to that seen in the typical nonossifying fibroma in children; in an adult, this lesion is sometimes referred to as a fibroxanthoma or a benign fibrous histiocytoma.

11 Skeletal Hamartomas and Other Benign Tumorous Conditions II

PERIOSTEAL "DESMOID"

Periosteal desmoid is a common periosteal fibrous lesion that affects boys in the first two decades of life, characteristically with local bone destruction in the posteromedial aspect of the lower metaphysis of the femur. On roentgenographic examination, one may note an erosion of the cortex with a sclerotic base (Fig. 11.1). The lesions are composed of dense collagenized tissue with uniform unremarkable fibroblasts and reactive bone formation (Fig. 11.2).

The lesion probably occurs posttraumatically. It is characteristic in location and does not warrant a biopsy.

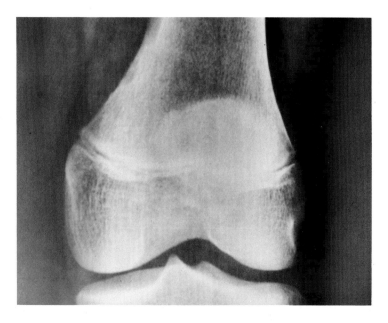

Fig. 11.1 A scalloped periosteal defect with a sclerotic base in the medial metaphysis of the femur is the characteristic roentgenographic appearance of a periosteal desmoid tumor.

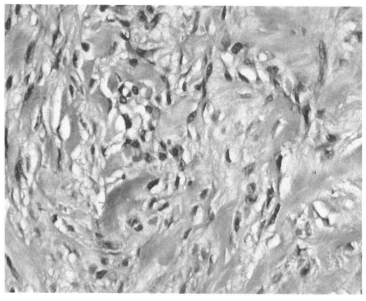

Fig. 11.2 Photomicrograph of the dense fibrous tissue removed from the lesion illustrated in Fig. 11.1. Abundant collagen production by poorly organized but unremarkable fibroblasts has occurred.

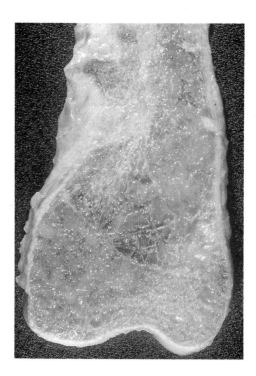
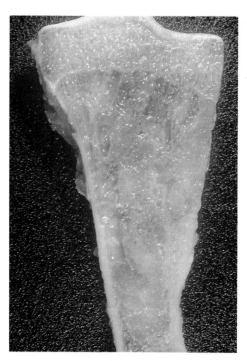
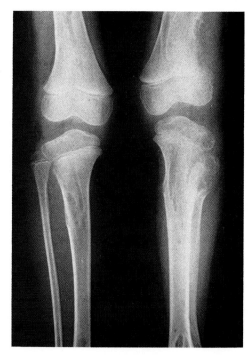

Fig. 11.3 In the coronal section of a femur (left) and tibia (right) involved by enchondromatosis, note the replacement of the cancellous portion of the bone with circumscribed grayish-blue nodules. In addition to the metaphysis and diaphysis, the epiphysis and periosteal surface are also affected by the disease.

Fig. 11.4 Roentgenogram of the lower limbs in a patient with multiple enchondromas. Typically, the lytic lesions are seen most prominently in the metaphysis, and they have a striated appearance. However, the lesions also affect the epiphysis and the periosteal surfaces, and may result in bone shortening and deformity of the articular ends.

ENCHONDROMATOSIS

Ollier's disease

Ollier's disease is a rare, nonhereditary developmental abnormality in which multiple cartilaginous tumors, ranging from microscopic foci to bulky masses, may appear throughout the epiphyses, metaphyses, and diaphyses of the skeleton (Fig. 11.3). The distribution of these tumors is most often unilateral and confined to one limb. On roentgenographic examination, one finds multiple lucent lesions, often within deformed or shortened bone (Fig. 11.4). Stippled calcification is common. The histologic features of these lesions resemble those of solitary enchondromas (see Chapter 12), but in enchondromatosis the tumors are more cellular (Figs. 11.5 to 11.7). Malignant transformation may occur in some cases.

Maffucci's syndrome is the occurrence of multiple enchondromas in association with hemangiomas, including visceral hemangiomas (Fig. 11.8).

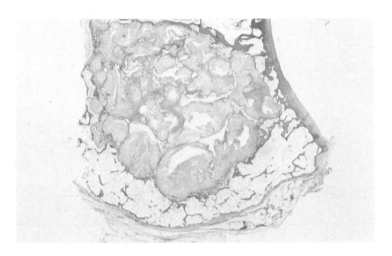

Fig. 11.5 Low power photomicrograph of the articular end of a bone demonstrates a cartilaginous nodule extending up to the articular surface. Note the lobular arrangement of the cartilage and the lesion's bony rim.

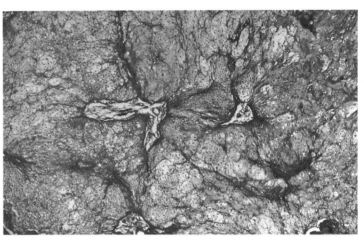

Fig. 11.6 Photomicrograph of a portion of the lesion shown in Fig. 11.5 demonstrates the lobular and cellular appearance of the cartilaginous nodules in enchondromatosis. These lesions generally tend to show more cellularity than is seen in solitary enchondromas.

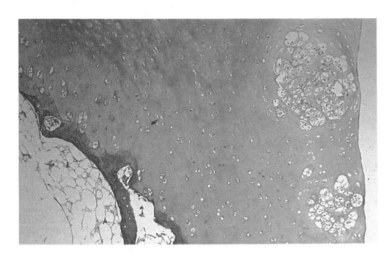

Fig. 11.7 Histologic section of the cartilaginous end of a bone in a young child with enchondromatosis. Proliferating clones of markedly atypical chondrocytes are seen within the cartilaginous epiphysis, thus demonstrating that this condition arises from abnormal clones of chondrocytes within the cartilage anlagen of the affected limb.

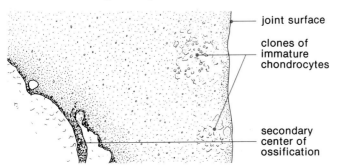

joint surface

clones of immature chondrocytes

secondary center of ossification

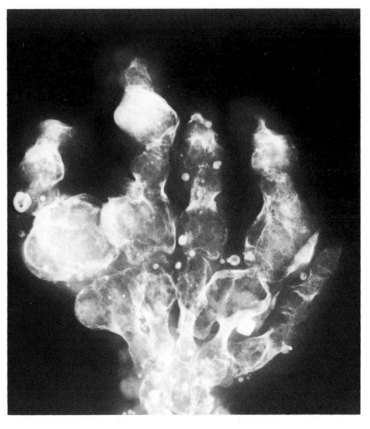

Fig. 11.8 Roentgenogram of a hand in a patient with multiple enchondromas reveals numerous calcified phleboliths in association with soft-tissue hemangiomas. This combination of soft-tissue hemangiomatosis and enchondromatosis is known as Maffucci's syndrome.

11.3

OSTEOCHONDROMA

Exostosis

An osteochondroma is a common developmental aberration thought to result from the herniation and separation of a fragment of epiphyseal growth plate cartilage through the periosteal bone cuff that normally surrounds the growth plate (Fig. 11.9). Persistent growth of the herniated cartilage fragment and its subsequent endochondral ossification results in a cartilage-capped subperiosteal bony projection from the bone surface. On roentgenograms these projections appear as either a flattened (sessile) or stalklike protuberance (exostosis) from the bone shaft in a juxtaepiphyseal location (Figs. 11.10 to 11.14). This bony protuberance is seen to be contiguous with the adjacent cortical bone. The most common sites of occurrence of osteochondromas are the lower end of the femur and upper end of the tibia.

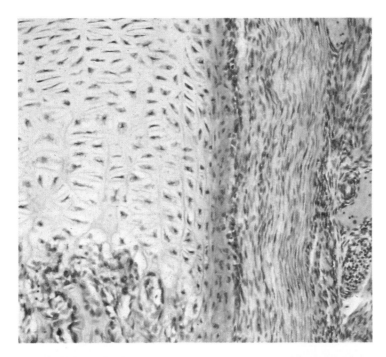

Fig. 11.9 Histologic section taken from a normal 12-week- old fetus. One can see the cartilaginous epiphysis on the left, and the underlying bony metaphysis. To the right of the epiphysis is a thin layer of periosteal bone that forms a cuff around the cartilaginous epiphysis. The perichondral bone cuff is important to the mechanical integrity of the epiphyseal growth plate cartilage.

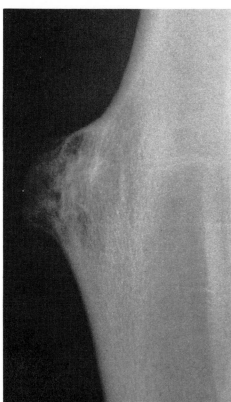

Fig. 11.10 Roentgenogram of the metaphyseal end of a femur shows an eccentric irregularity on the cortex with a lucent cap. The margins of the lesion are continuous with the surrounding cortex of the femur.

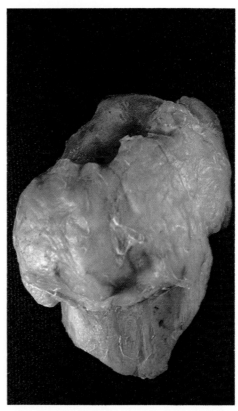

Fig. 11.11 Photograph of a specimen removed from the femur seen in Fig. 11.10. An irregular, cauliflowerlike, bluish-gray cartilage mass is seen lying over the cortical bone.

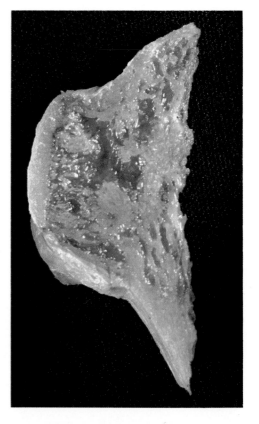

Fig. 11.12 Cross section of the specimen shown in Fig. 11.11 demonstrates that the lesion seen radiologically is continuous with the surrounding cortex, but capped by a thin layer of bluish-gray cartilage.

The lesion generally manifests clinically before the third decade, with the patient complaining of pain or a mass. The pathologist usually receives an irregular bony protuberance with a bluish-gray, irregular, cauliflowerlike, cartilaginous cap, and the base of the lesion consists of cortical bone contiguous with the normal shaft. The histologic examination reveals a somewhat disorganized cartilaginous cap covered by a thin layer of fibrous periosteum (Figs. 11.15 and 11.16). The older the patient, the thinner the cartilaginous component becomes. Following adolescence and closure of the growth plates, no further growth of the osteochondroma usually occurs. The lesion may recur if it is inadequately excised. In rare circumstances, a malignant tumor—usually a chondrosarcoma—may be engrafted onto the lesion.

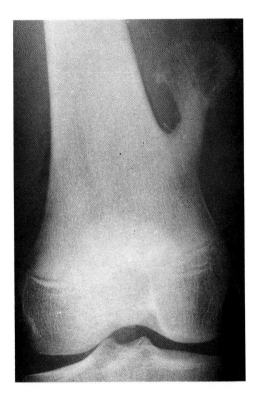

Fig. 11.13 Clinical roentgenogram of a pedunculated osteochondroma in the distal femur. Characteristically, the stalk points away from the adjacent joint surface, and the cortex of the osteochondroma is continuous with the cortex of the femur.

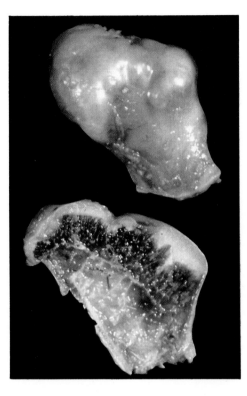

Fig. 11.14 Surface and cross section of the osteochondroma removed from the patient seen in Fig. 11.13. The cartilage cap varies considerably in thickness, and islands of calcified cartilage can be seen within the stalk of the osteochondroma underlying the cartilage cap.

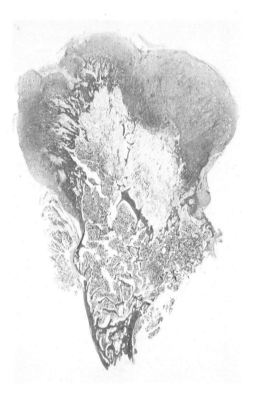

Fig. 11.15 A histologic preparation of a pedunculated osteochondroma shows a thick proliferating cartilage cap overlying poorly organized cancellous bone. The irregular endochondral ossification at the base of the cartilage cap is evident

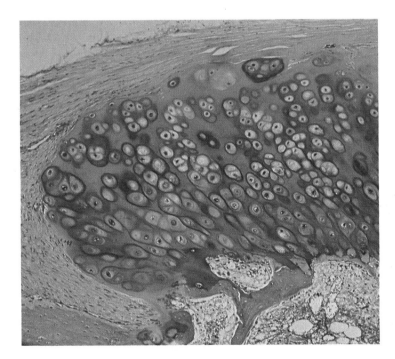

Fig. 11.16 Photomicrograph of the cartilage cap at a higher power demonstrates the reflected layer of periosteum over the exostosis and, in addition, the irregularity of the chondrocytes within the cartilage cap. Endochondral ossification is apparent at the base of the cap.

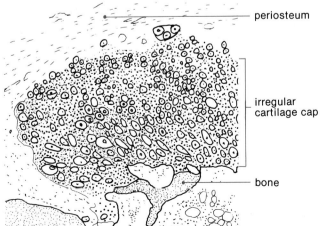

periosteum

irregular cartilage cap

bone

11.5

MULTIPLE OSTEOCARTILAGINOUS EXOSTOSES

Hereditary multiple exostoses

The occurrence of multiple osteocartilaginous exostoses is rare. Inherited as an autosomal-dominant condition, it is usually associated with short stature and other bone deformities (Figs. 11.17 and 11.18). The patients present with disfigurement, or with pain induced by pressure on surrounding soft-tissue structures. Individual lesions are roentgenographically, grossly, and microscopically similar

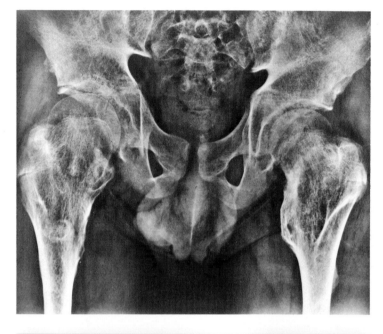

Fig. 11.17 Roentgenogram of an adolescent boy with hereditary multiple exostoses. Note the short, wide, deformed femoral neck, on which can be seen several exostoses.

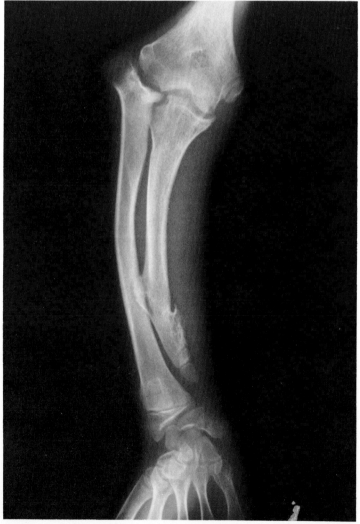

Fig. 11.18 Roentgenogram of the forearm of the patient shown in Fig. 11.17. Note multiple exostoses, with shortening and deformity of the forearm associated with malformation of the distal ulna.

to solitary osteochondromas, although frequently the multiple lesions are more disorganized in structure.

The significance of this disorder for the surgeon lies in the management of the multiple lesions; however, the pathologist must consider the incidence of malignant transformation, compared with that in solitary osteochondromas (1 to 20 per cent, depending on the stringency of the criteria). A lesion with a suspected malignant transformation is shown in Figures 11.19 to 11.22.

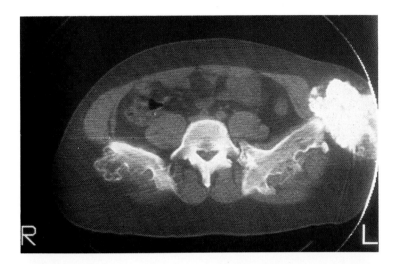

Fig. 11.19 In this CT scan of the pelvis in a 36-year-old man with known multiple exostoses, a large mass is seen on the wing of the ilium. The patient's history revealed that this mass had been increasing in size.

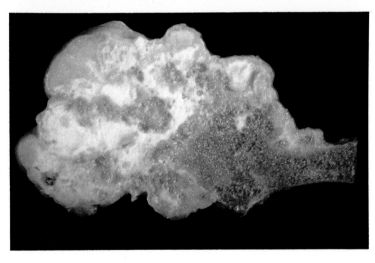

Fig. 11.20 The transected specimen removed from the patient shown in Fig. 11.19. Note the thick cartilage cap on the surface and the extensive calcification (calcified cartilage) within the irregular bosselated lesion.

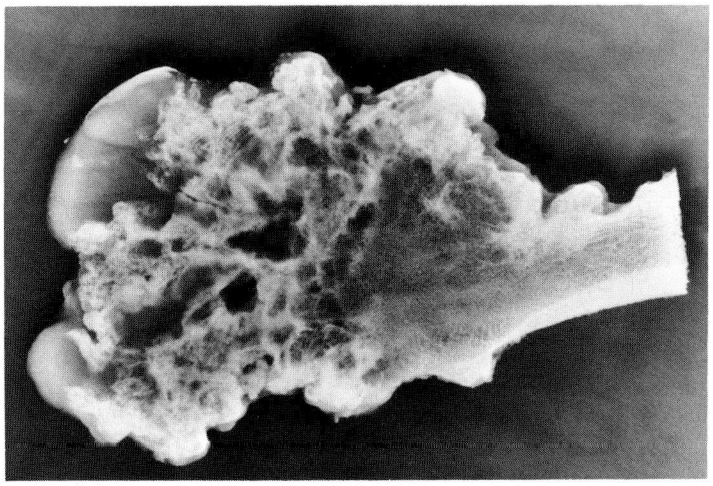

Fig. 11.21 Roentgenogram of the specimen shown in Fig. 11.20 again reveals the thick cartilage cap and the extensive calcification of the cartilage matrix.

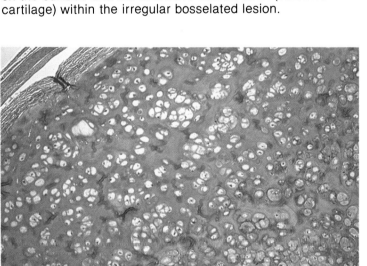

Fig. 11.22 Photomicrograph of the cartilage cap in the specimen shown in the previous three figures. The cartilage cap is covered by a dense fibrous capsule, and the cartilage matrix is filled by crowded viable chondrocytes. The finding of a thick, active cartilage cap on an exostosis in a skeletally mature individual (especially if the lesion has a history of recent growth) must alert the clinician and the pathologist to the possibility of malignant transformation in such a case.

DYSPLASIA EPIPHYSEALIS HEMIMELICA
Osteochondroma of the epiphysis, Trevor's disease

Dysplasia epiphysealis hemimelica is a skeletal developmental disorder, usually manifested in young children in whom unilateral irregular enlargement of the epiphysis occurs (Fig. 11.23). The disorder most commonly involves the lower femur or upper tibia, and sometimes the tarsal bones.

When excised and examined microscopically, the lesion is reminiscent of an osteochondroma, with a cartilage cap and an underlying zone of endochondral ossification, and normal progression of cancellous bone formation.

The lesion has no known genetic transmission. Although it is a benign condition, varus or valgus deformities of the limb may ensue. Surgical excision is the treatment of choice.

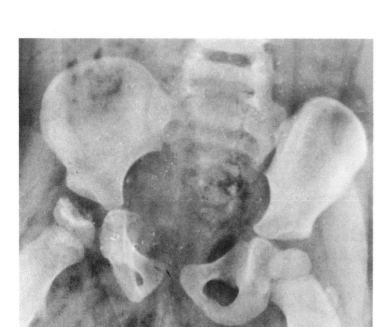

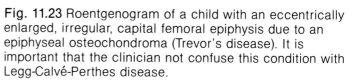

Fig. 11.23 Roentgenogram of a child with an eccentrically enlarged, irregular, capital femoral epiphysis due to an epiphyseal osteochondroma (Trevor's disease). It is important that the clinician not confuse this condition with Legg-Calvé-Perthes disease.

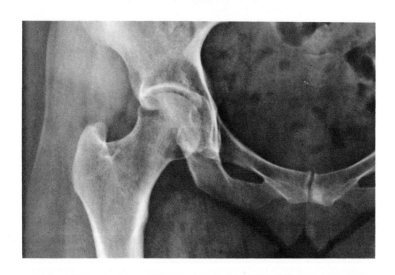

Fig. 11.24 Clinical roentgenogram shows an incidental finding of a bone island in the wall of the acetabulum. A well-circumscribed dense lesion is seen. In this film, the lesion appears to be in the joint space, but a CT scan *(below)* shows that the lesion is confined to the bone.

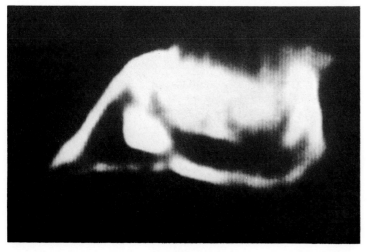

BONE ISLAND
Solitary enostosis
A solitary fleck of density in a bone is not an uncommon incidental finding on roentgenograms. Usually these lesions are only a millimeter or two in diameter, but occasionally they may measure a centimeter or two (Fig. 11.24). The lesions are called bone islands or enostoses, and they are probably developmental; they are significant only in differential diagnosis (e.g., of osteoid osteoma when they are small, or of sclerosing osteosarcoma if they are large).

On gross examination, these foci are found in the intramedullary spongy bone and are formed of compact bone that merges with the surrounding trabecular bone. Microscopic examination of a specimen of this tissue reveals mature lamellar bone with well-developed haversian and interstitial lamellar systems (Figs. 11.25 to 11.28). No endochondral ossification or calcified cartilage can be seen.

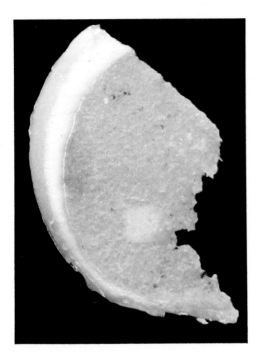

Fig. 11.25 Coronal section through a femoral head reveals a whitish circumscribed piece of bone, clearly demarcated from the surrounding cancellous bone.

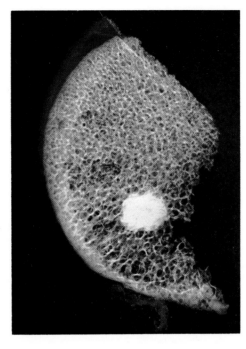

Fig. 11.26 Roentgenogram of the specimen illustrated in Fig. 11.25 demonstrates the marked density of the solitary bone island.

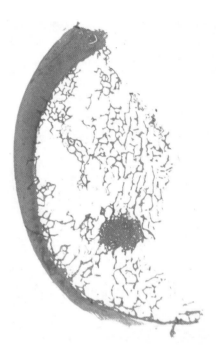

Fig. 11.27 The bone island consists of normal bone distinctly separated from the surrounding cancellous bone spicules, but note that the spicules merge with the nodule in a radial fashion. This bone is found to be lamellar when viewed under polarized light.

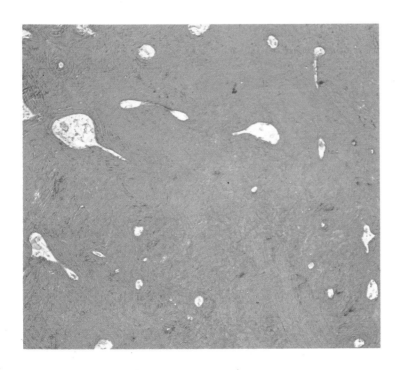

Fig. 11.28 High power view of the bone island illustrated in Fig. 11.27 shows the mature, dense appearance of the bone.

OSTEOPOIKILOSIS

Osteopoikilosis is a rare, symptomless, and clinically benign condition. It is inherited as an autosomal-dominant trait. On roentgenograms of patients with this disorder, the bones show multiple discrete or clustered foci of radiopacity with uniform density, giving the bone a spotted appearance. The disorder is usually symmetrical, affecting both the epiphyseal and metaphyseal zones. It most commonly involves the small bones of the hands and feet, and the ends of the long bones of the extremities (Fig. 11.29). The microscopic features of the lesions are similar to those of solitary bone islands (Fig. 11.30).

Osteopoikilosis has also been reported in patients with cutaneous nodules, which usually prove upon microscopic examination to be fibrous tissue (e.g., fibromatosis, scleroderma-like lesions, and keloids). This finding suggests a general mesenchymal defect in these patients.

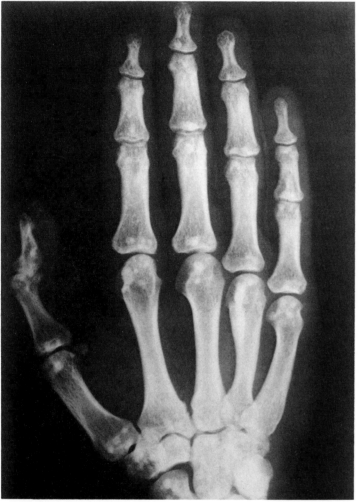

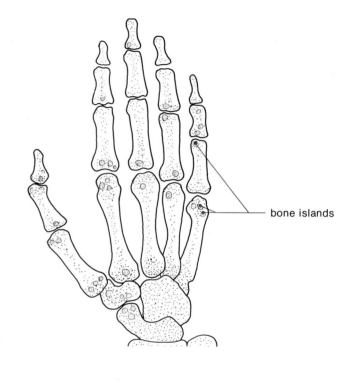

Fig. 11.29 Roentgenogram reveals circumscribed dense foci distributed throughout the hand in a patient with osteopoikilosis.

bone islands

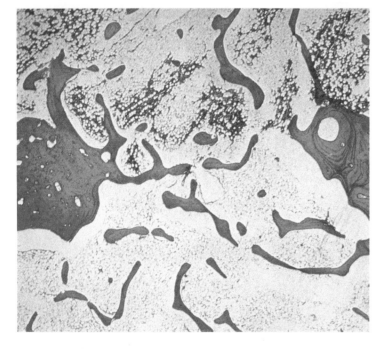

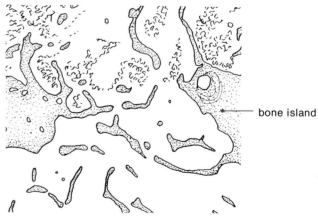

Fig. 11.30 Nodules of bone with connected spicules of cancellous bone are evident in this specimen from a patient with osteopoikilosis.

bone island

OSTEOPATHIA STRIATA

Voorhoeve's disease

Osteopathia striata is a benign, asymptomatic disorder characterized roentgenographically by usually symmetrical, axially oriented, dense striations. Its presence in association with sclerosis of the base of the skull has been determined to be genetically transmitted as an autosomal-dominant condition.

When osteopathia striata is seen in association with osteopoikilosis and/or melorheostosis, the condition is referred to as "mixed sclerosing bone dystrophy" (Figs. 11.31 to 11.33).

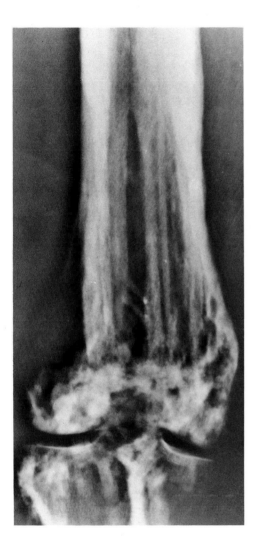 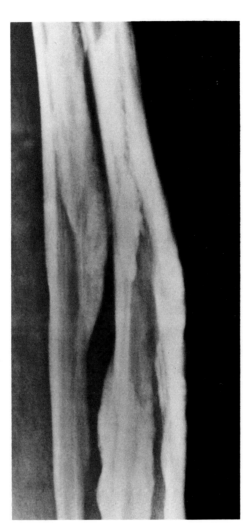 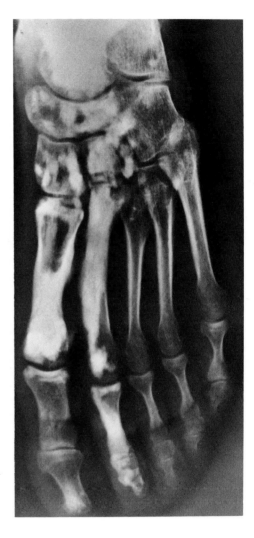

Fig. 11.31 In this 35-year-old man with generalized mild bone pain, roentgenograms here and in the following two figures revealed a mixed pattern of disease. In this roentgenogram of the lower femur, the striated pattern of Voorhoeve's disease can be clearly seen.

Fig. 11.32 Roentgenogram of the patient in Fig. 11.31 shows the thickened endosteal and periosteal bone "candle-dripping" appearance of melorheostosis.

Fig. 11.33 Numerous bone islands and evidence of melorheostosis can be seen in the foot of the patient shown in Figs. 11.31 and 11.32. This rare pattern of mixed sclerosing bone dystrophy was generalized throughout the skeleton.

MELORHEOSTOSIS

Melorheostosis is a rare, nonfamilial, usually unilateral lesion of long bones in which the affected bones display a peculiar irregular cortical hyperostosis similar in appearance to melting wax dripping down the sides of a candle (see Fig. 11.32). The lesions occur on both the periosteum and the endosteum. Associated cutaneous lesions, including vascular malformations and focal subcutaneous and para-articular fibrosis, are common.

In affected children, the skeleton is characterized by hyperostoses of the bones of the extremities and pelvic girdle, by inequality in the length of the extremities, and by contractures resulting in joint deformity. On roentgenograms, the lesions may be found to involve the epiphysis, and osseous tissue may be seen crossing the growth plate. In children, prominent soft-tissue fibrosis may predate osseous abnormalities. Attempts at surgical management of the contractures have been unrewarding.

In adult melorheostosis, the patients present with pain, deformity, or limitation of joint motion. The lesion may involve one or multiple bones. Ectopic bone may be present in para-articular locations. The involvement of one side of a bone (or row of bones, in some cases) has suggested a sclerotome distribution.

On gross examination, the affected bones are irregular on both their periosteal and endosteal surfaces, and they show thickened trabeculae. The marrow cavity is narrowed. A histologic examination reveals that the new bone may be woven or lamellar (Figs. 11.34 and 11.35). When the tissue is lamellar, it is architecturally irregular, and the affected cortical bone is often quite cellular, with a distinct differentiation between the normal and the melorheostotic bone.

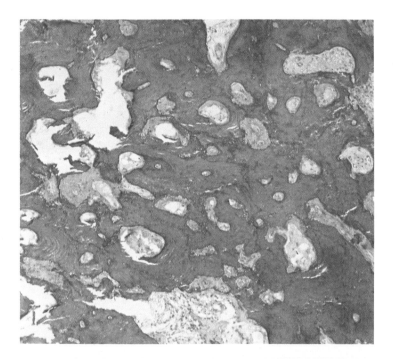

Fig. 11.34 Biopsy of cortical bone from a patient with melorheostosis reveals markedly irregular bone with relatively little cellular activity on the endosteal surfaces. The marrow may show mild fibrosis.

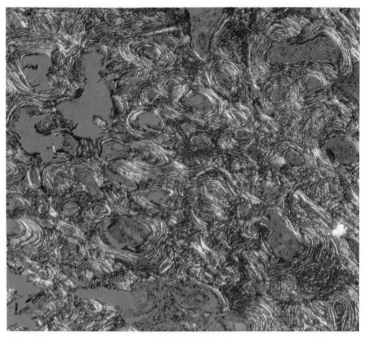

Fig. 11.35 The same histologic field shown in Fig. 11.34, photographed with polarized light. Note the irregular mixture of lamellar and woven bone.

OSTEOID OSTEOMA

Osteoid osteomas are small (generally less than a centimeter in diameter), solitary, benign but painful lesions of bone characteristically seen in children and adolescents. The most commonly involved site is a lower extremity, and lesions tend to occur near the end of the diaphysis.

The characteristic clinical presentation of osteoid osteoma is nocturnal pain that is usually relieved by aspirin. One may see local swelling, and the lesion may be exquisitely tender; mild leukocytosis may also be present. When the lesion is close to or within a joint, the patient may present with joint effusion and symptoms of synovitis, and this type of presentation may be seen in approximately one-fifth of the cases. Individuals with lesions in the vertebral column may present with scoliosis.

On roentgenograms, the typical lesion is located within the cortex of a long bone, and shows a central lucent zone (or nidus) and surrounding bone density (Figs. 11.36 to 11.41). Osteoid osteomas located subperiosteally or in the cancellous portion of the bone show much less surrounding sclerosis. On bone scans, these lesions show up as very active foci ("hot spots").

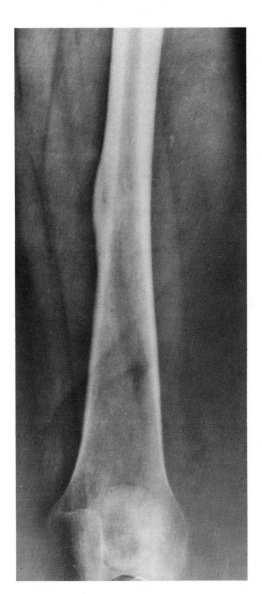

Fig. 11.36 A 20-year-old man complained of pain in the midshaft of the right femur. Roentgenogram shows an area of cortical thickening, in the center of which is a lucent defect with an opaque central nidus. An osteoid osteoma in cortical bone produces a considerable amount of reactive bone tissue, as can be seen in this case. (However, in the cancellous area of the bone it may be difficult to see the lesion because of a lack of reactive bone sclerosis.)

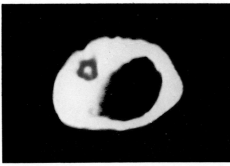
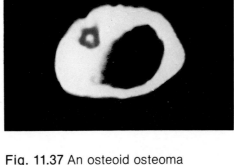

Fig. 11.37 An osteoid osteoma located in the cortex of the tibia is well demonstrated on this CT scan.

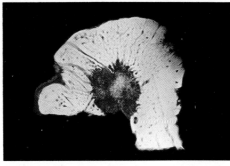

Fig. 11.39 Roentgenogram of a slice taken through the nidus shown in Fig. 11.38. The nidus is formed of fine bone spicules and, corresponding to the hyperemic zone, a lucent zone lies between the nidus and the surrounding sclerotic cortical bone.

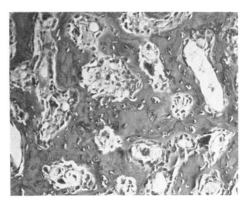

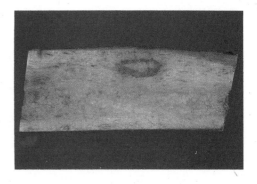

Fig. 11.38 Gross photograph of a segment of cortical bone containing an osteoid osteoma nidus. Note the dense center in the nidus and the surrounding hyperemia.

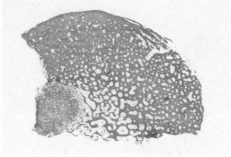

Fig. 11.40 Photomicrograph of the osteoid osteoma shown in Figs. 11.38 and 11.39 shows the central nidus formed of irregular trabeculae of immature woven bone surrounded by a fibrous hyperemic zone and sclerotic cortical bone.

Fig. 11.41 High power photomicrograph of the central nidus of an osteoid osteoma shows interconnecting trabeculae of immature woven bone with an extremely vascular stroma. Numerous osteoclasts and active osteoblasts line the bone trabeculae.

At surgery, the area of involvement may be difficult to ascertain, although there may be a mild pinkish cast to the overlying cortical bone. The lesion itself may be seen as a well-demarcated nodule, often cherry red (Figs. 11.42 and 11.43), but occasionally very dense and white. Osteoid osteomas are characterized microscopically by a maze of small spicules of immature bone, most often lined by prominent osteoblasts and osteoclasts. The intervening stroma is sparsely cellular, with readily apparent vascular spaces (Figs. 11.44 to 11.46). Cartilage is not evident. Striking amounts of periosteal new bone may appear in the overlying cortex.

The minute size of the lesion often makes it difficult for both the surgeon and the pathologist to locate. A fine-

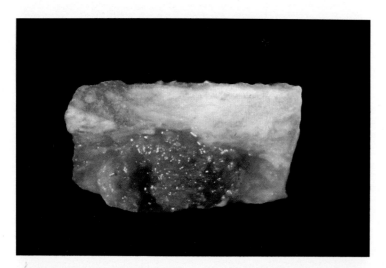

Fig. 11.42 Gross photograph of an excised osteoid osteoma that appeared on roentgenograms as a lucent lesion. Note the hyperemic appearance of the tissue.

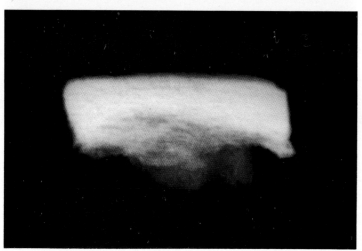

Fig. 11.43 Roentgenogram of the specimen shown in Fig. 11.42 demonstrates the relative lucency of the nidus. However, there are fine bone trabeculae coursing through the lesion.

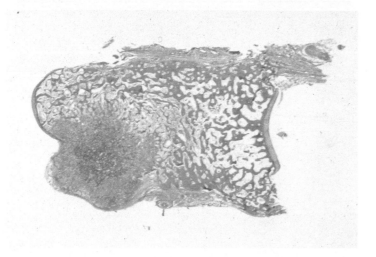

Fig. 11.44 Low power photomicrograph of the middle phalanx of a finger. A subperiosteal osteoid osteoma is seen adjacent to the joint margin.

grain roentgenogram may be helpful in determining the location of the nidus of an osteoid osteoma in tissue submitted for microscopic examination (Fig. 11.47). However, even with this technique and multiple samples, the lesion may be difficult to localize. Preoperative technetium isotope injections with intraoperative localization of radioactivity and postoperative localization by specimen autoimaging on undeveloped film may be of considerable help.

The etiology of this bizarre condition remains obscure. The radiologic differential diagnosis includes a small focus of osteomyelitis or a stress fracture.

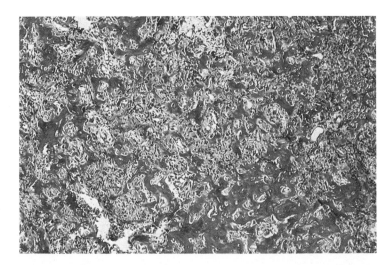

Fig. 11.45 Higher power view of the osteoid osteoma shown in Fig. 11.44 demonstrates immature bone formation and a vascular fibrous stroma with considerable osteoblastic and osteoclastic activity.

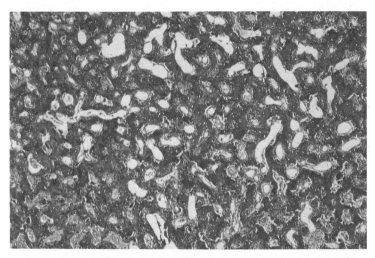

Fig. 11.46 Photomicrograph of the nidus of a more mature osteoid osteoma with more dense interconnecting trabeculae of bone and less cellular activity than is seen in Fig. 11.45.

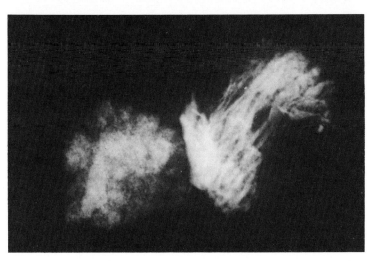

Fig. 11.47 Roentgenogram of curetted tissue taken during surgery in a patient with a suspected osteoid osteoma. Roentgenograms of the specimen were taken immediately, and in this portion of the specimen one can discern a piece of bone with a very fine trabecular pattern typical of an osteoid osteoma (*left*), and a fragment of more normal cancellous bone (*right*). When numerous specimens are received from a patient with an osteoid osteoma, roentgenograms of the specimens not only help the pathologist to inform the surgeon whether he has removed the lesional tissue, they also enable the pathologist to select the proper pieces for histologic examination.

OSTEOMAS OF THE CRANIUM AND FACIAL BONES

These lesions are asymptomatic, benign, slow-growing, tumorlike lesions that occur in the calvarium and facial bones. The histologic features of the calvarial lesions differ from those of the facial lesions.

Osteomas appear on the outer surface of the calvarium as circumscribed ivorylike excrescences formed of mature lamellar bone (Figs. 11.48 and 11.49). The lesions on the facial bones are often seen in relation to the sinuses, and these lesions are formed of immature bone, often with active osteoblasts and osteoclasts (Figs. 11.50 to 11.53).

The etiology of osteomas is obscure. The lesion does not recur if it is surgically excised, and it is not associated with malignant change.

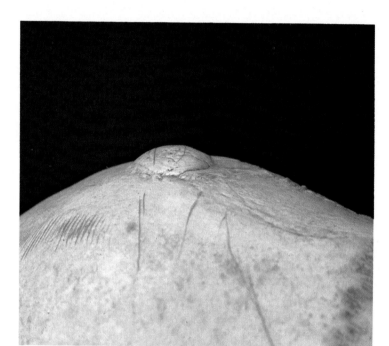

Fig. 11.48 Gross photograph of an osteoma (or ivory exostosis) of the calvarium shows a well-circumscribed nodular growth distorting the smooth contour of the skull.

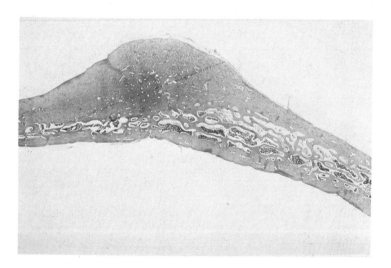

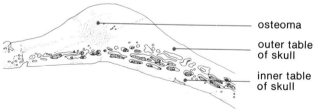

Fig. 11.49 Photomicrograph of the lesion shown in Fig. 11.48 demonstrates that the lesion is composed of mature lamellar bone.

osteoma

outer table of skull

inner table of skull

It should be remembered that osteomas of the facial bones may be seen in association with colonic polyps (Gardner's syndrome). Other disorders characteristically grouped with this syndrome are odontomas, supernumerary and unerupted teeth, and soft-tissue tumors including fibromas and epidermal inclusion cysts. Gardner's syndrome is an autosomal-dominant genetic disorder, and it is of particular importance because of the associated malignant change seen in the adenomatous lesions of the intestine.

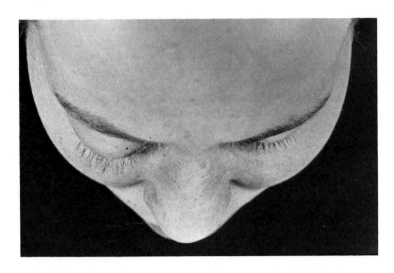

Fig. 11.50 The protrusion of the orbit seen in this patient results from an osteoma arising from the bone in the frontal sinus.

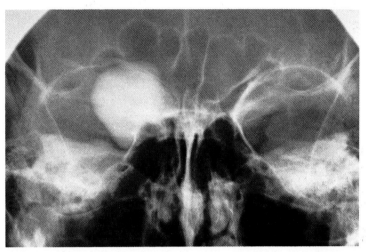

Fig. 11.51 Roentgenogram of the patient shown in Fig. 11.50 demonstrates a well-circumscribed dense lesion that is distorting the frontal sinus (the cause of the orbital protrusion in the clinical photograph).

Fig. 11.52 Histologic section through the lesion excised from the frontal sinus of the patient shown in Figs. 11.50 and 11.51. The lesion consists of dense immature bone with a small focal area of fibrous modeling.

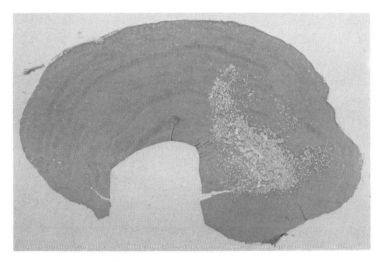

Fig. 11.53 Close-up of the area of fibrous modeling shown in Fig. 11.52 shows irregular bone trabeculae with fibrous marrow and osteoclastic resorption of the bone.

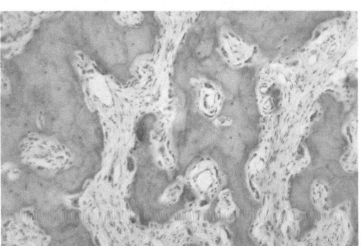

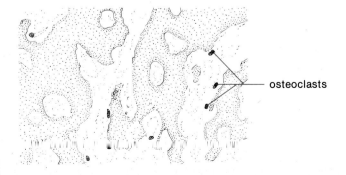

osteoclasts

HOFFA'S DISEASE

Hoffa's disease is a condition characterized by enlargement of the infrapatellar fat pad on either side of the patellar tendon, with resulting pain or deep aching in the anterior compartment of the knee. The pain is aggravated by physical activity or extension of the knee. Swelling or recurrent effusions are consequences of synovial injury. The treatment of Hoffa's disease is surgical reduction in the volume of extrasynovial fat.

When the lesion is examined macroscopically (Fig. 11.54), the synovium is seen to have a marked papillary appearance; microscopically, a mild hyperplasia of the synovial lining cells overlying abundant unremarkable fat can be discerned.

EOSINOPHILIC GRANULOMA
Histiocytosis X

The entity known as eosinophilic granuloma may be seen as a unifocal lesion or as multifocal osseous lesions, sometimes with systemic involvement. Classically, eosinophilic granuloma presents in males in the first decade of life. Patients may complain of pain or local tenderness. Laboratory tests are usually unremarkable, though the erythrocyte sedimentation rate may be elevated. The most commonly affected parts of the skeleton are the proximal femoral metaphysis, the skull (Fig. 11.55), mandible, ribs, and vertebral column (Fig. 11.56). An eosinophilic granuloma may occur in soft tissue, including the skin, oral mucosa, lymph nodes, and lungs. When the

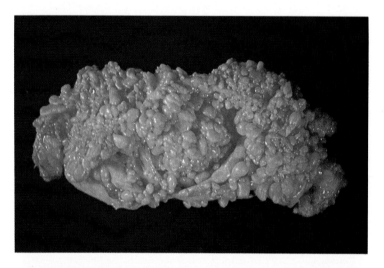

Fig. 11.54 Gross photograph of the synovium resected from a patient with Hoffa's disease. Note the fatty appearance of the tissue and the papillomatous folds into which the surface has been thrown.

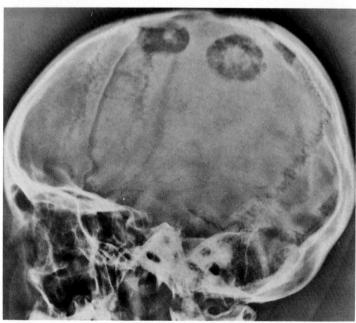

Fig. 11.55 Roentgenogram of the skull in a child with eosinophilic granulomas. Several lytic lesions are evident, and in the largest, one can appreciate the beveled edge that is typical of this presentation of eosinophilic granuloma.

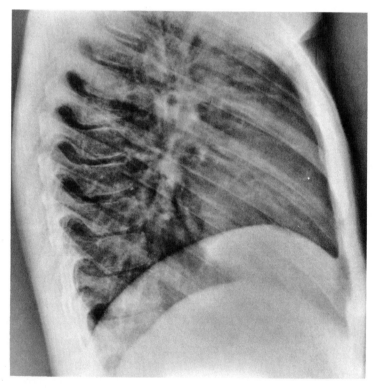

Fig. 11.56 Roentgenogram of the thoracic spine shows the collapse and wedging of T6 associated with eosinophilic granulomas. Note the absence of any disc involvement (as would be seen in an infection). This type of presentation may progress to a complete collapse or vertebra plana (described by Calvé). Such lesions may resolve spontaneously, or as a result of low dosage radiation. The vertebral body consequently regains its height.

lung is affected, patients may develop progressive fibrosis with impaired pulmonary function.

On roentgenographic examination, one or more sharply circumscribed lytic defects may be evident in the bone. These defects usually lack sclerotic rims. Sometimes a more destructive permeative lesion with periosteal new bone formation can be seen.

The lesion is usually examined by the pathologist in the form of multiple curetted specimens, usually of a glisten-ing reddish tissue with flecks of opaque yellow material throughout (Fig. 11.57).

Eosinophilic granuloma is characterized microscopically by a mixture of eosinophils, plasma cells, histiocytes, and peculiar large mononuclear and multinucleated giant cells (Langerhans cells) with abundant pale-staining cytoplasm (Figs. 11.58 to 11.60). Many of the large mononuclear cells have indented or cleaved nuclei. Varying degrees of necrosis and fibrosis may be evident, as

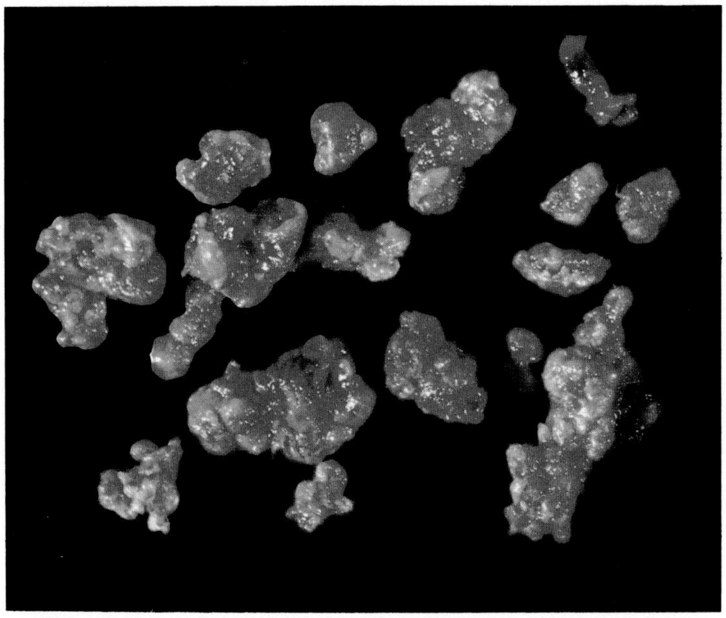

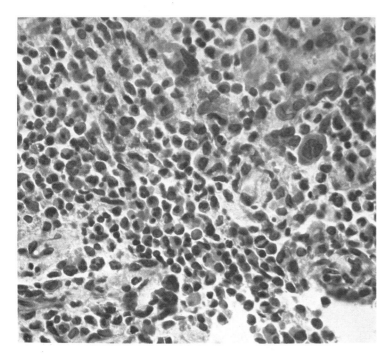

Fig. 11.57 Gross photograph of curetted tissue obtained from a patient with an eosinophilic granuloma shows typically scant reddish-gray fragments of tissue flecked with dense yellow areas. These yellow areas represent foci of lipid accumulation or necrosis.

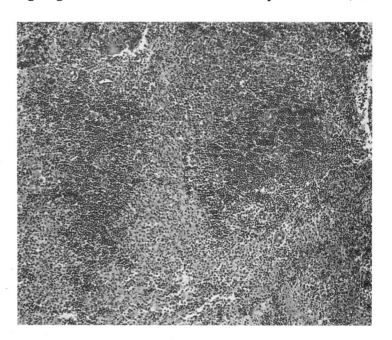

Fig. 11.58 Low power view of tissue curetted from a patient with an eosinophilic granuloma demonstrates the lesion's variegated hypercellular appearance. One should not confuse this tissue with inflammatory tissue from a patient with osteomyelitis.

Fig. 11.59 In this photomicrograph, the mixed cellular appearance of an eosinophilic granuloma can be appreciated. In addition to plasma cells and eosinophils, large histiocytes and giant cells are present. Occasionally, if this tissue is scarred, confusion with Hodgkin's disease may be a problem.

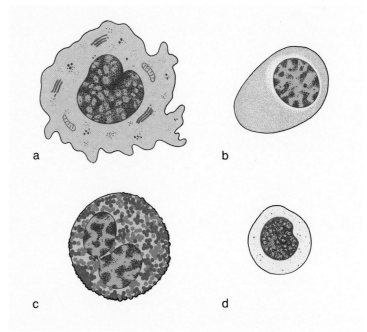

Fig. 11.60 Diagram of the various cells seen in eosinophilic granuloma (drawn to scale). (a) Histiocyte, (b) plasma cell showing a cartwheel nucleus, (c) eosinophil, (d) lymphocyte.

11.19

may reactive cells such as foamy macrophages. Mitotic activity is minimal. The Langerhans cell shows on electron microscopy peculiar racket-shaped inclusion bodies in the cytoplasm (Birbeck granules).

Patients with unifocal lesions may show spontaneous regression, or they may be treated with minimal chemotherapy. In general, if a second lesion does not appear within one year, the prognosis is good. In those patients who present with a more systemic illness characterized by fever and organomegaly, as well as multiple osseous lesions, the course of the disease is likely to be protracted. Both the clinical course of this disease and its histopathology indicate that this disease is not neoplastic in nature. The presence of eosinophils and the occasional occurrence of skin lesions suggest the possibility that this is a peculiar immunoallergic phenomenon.

Eosinophilic granuloma has been considered one of a group of disorders known as the histiocytoses, which includes (in addition to eosinophilic granuloma) Hand-Schüller-Christian disease and Letterer-Siwe disease. However, Hand-Schüller-Christian disease is probably better thought of as a multiple eosinophilic granuloma, and Letterer-Siwe disease (a rare disease of infants with a characteristically fulminant course) is probably an unrelated neoplastic condition.

12 Neoplasms I

Neoplastic lesions seen in bone are usually metastases (often carcinomatous) from another site. It is important to realize that a solitary bone metastasis may be the initial clinical presentation for a number of patients with occult cancer.

Primary tumors of bone are, with the exception of myelomas, rare, and they range from benign lesions to highly malignant neoplasms. They will be described in essential detail in the following two chapters.

OSTEOBLASTOMA

An osteoblastoma is a solitary, benign, osteoid- and bone-forming neoplasm that contains numerous well-differentiated osteoblasts and osteoclasts, and usually has a vascular stroma. In most cases, the vertebrae or bones of the limbs are the sites of involvement. In long bones, the lesion may occur in either the metaphysis or the diaphysis. Osteoblastomas are usually painful lesions that manifest predominantly in young adults; swelling and tenderness may prompt the patient to seek medical attention. In cases of spinal involvement, neurologic symptoms related to spinal cord compression may occur.

On roentgenographic examination, the lesion characteristically appears as a lucent defect with varying degrees of central density; it is usually well circumscribed, without extensive surrounding bone sclerosis or any periosteal reaction (Fig. 12.1).

At surgery, an osteoblastoma is found to be composed of hemorrhagic, granular, friable, and calcified tissue. On microscopic examination, the lesion can be seen to con-

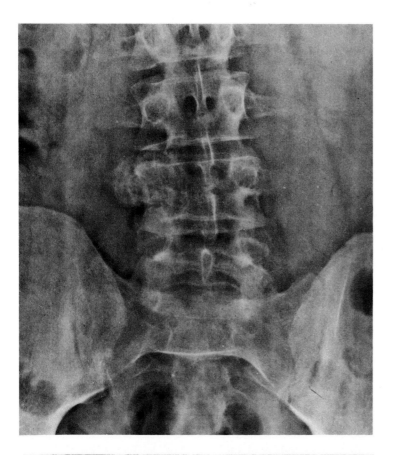

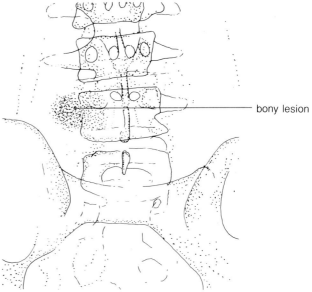

Fig. 12.1 A 20-year-old man complained of low back pain and was admitted to the hospital with an expanding, destructive lesion affecting the pedicle and transverse process on the right side of L4. On roentgenographic examination, the margin of the lesion is well defined, and there is a patchy increase in density. An excisional biopsy of the lesion proved it to be a benign osteoblastoma.

bony lesion

Fig. 12.2 Low power photomicrograph of an osteoblastoma demonstrates irregular trabeculae of woven bone, with a vascular cellular fibrous stroma between the trabeculae. Several osteoclasts can be seen on the surface of the bone.

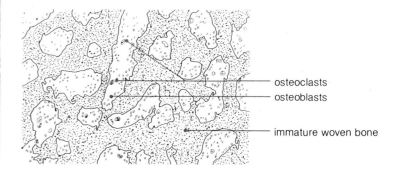

osteoclasts
osteoblasts

immature woven bone

sist of a vascular spindle cell stroma with abundant irregular spicules of mineralized bone and osteoid (Figs. 12.2 and 12.3). Osteoblasts and multinucleated giant cells are readily evident on the bone surfaces, but no cartilage can be seen in the lesional tissue. Treatment consists of curettage or en bloc excision.

Microscopically, it may be difficult to differentiate an osteoblastoma from an osteoid osteoma. However, the tissue pattern appears less regular in an osteoblastoma than in an osteoid osteoma. Furthermore, osteoid osteomas rarely exceed 1 cm in diameter, while osteoblastomas may be several centimeters in diameter and have a tendency to grow in size. Nevertheless, the lesions are similar enough for osteoblastomas to occasionally be referred to in the literature as giant osteoid osteomas.

On rare occasions, osteoblastomas have been noted to act aggressively, with significant bone destruction and extension into adjacent soft tissues. Retrospective analyses of these lesions have revealed more cellular atypia with large, plump osteoblasts (Fig. 12.4). These lesions do not metastasize, so they should be considered aggressive variants of osteoblastoma; however, it may on occasion be difficult to differentiate an aggressive osteoblastoma from osteosarcoma. Changes characteristic of an aneurysmal bone cyst may be present within these lesions and add to diagnostic problems.

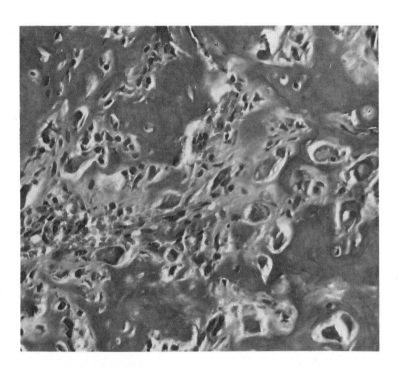

Fig. 12.3 High power photomicrograph of an osteoblastoma shows plump osteoblasts and osteoclasts on the surface of the woven bone trabeculae.

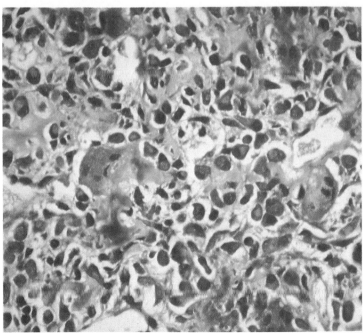

Fig. 12.4 Photomicrograph of an atypical osteoblastoma with crowded, large, epithelioid stromal cells; small irregular foci of woven bone are present. It is important for the pathologist to recognize that an osteoblastoma may be cellular, and to distinguish this pattern from osteosarcoma, a histologic differentiation that can at times be very difficult.

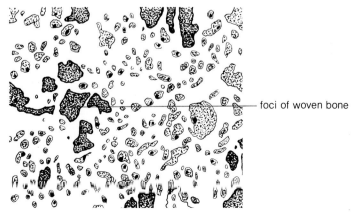

foci of woven bone

OSTEOSARCOMA
Osteogenic sarcoma

Osteosarcoma is a malignant, bone-producing neoplasm in which the bone matrix is formed by malignant cells, and therefore the bone cells (osteoblasts and osteocytes) themselves are malignant. This lesion must be differen-tiated from other neoplasms in bone (e.g., giant-cell tumor) which may also contain bone, but that bone is reactive and the bone cells are benign.

Osteosarcoma constitutes about 20 per cent of all primary malignant tumors of bone. It generally affects children (before the closure of the growth plate), and oc-

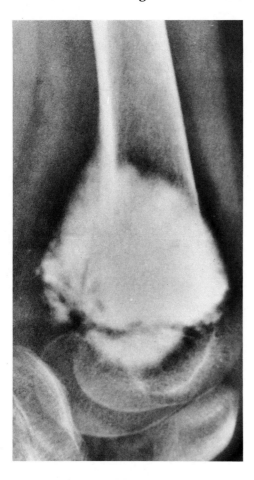

Fig. 12.5 A 10-year-old boy presented with complaints of pain around the knee joint. On physical examination, some fullness was felt in the lower femur, which was noted to be warmer than the surrounding tissue. Roentgenogram shows a radiodense tumor involving the metaphyseal end of the femur, with extension of the tumor both anteriorly and posteriorly into the soft tissue. It is difficult to determine whether or not the epiphyseal end of the bone is involved because of the two-dimensional radiologic image of the three-dimensional bone. (This roentgenogram should be compared with Fig. 12.14, a gross photograph of the specimen resected from this patient.)

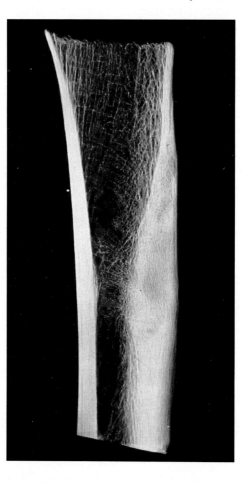

Fig. 12.6 A teenage boy complained of pain in the shin. Roentgenogram shows marked cortical thickening with a dense intracortical lesion, and a biopsy of this lesion revealed evidence of an osteosarcoma.

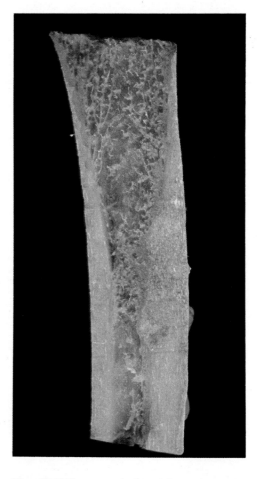

Fig. 12.7 The resected specimen from the patient in Fig. 12.6 demonstrates tumor confined to the cortical area of the bone.

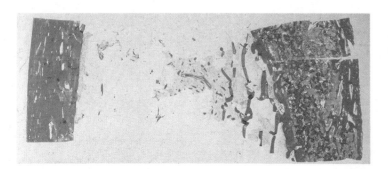

Fig. 12.8 Histologic section through the shaft of the femur shown in Fig. 12.7 shows an osteosarcoma confined to the cortex of the bone.

curs more often in boys than in girls. Most osteosarcomas are located in the medulla of the bone (Fig. 12.5); very rarely, they may develop in the cortex of the bone (Figs. 12.6 to 12.8) or in the soft tissues (Figs. 12.9 to 12.11).

In affected children, over 90 per cent of the lesions occur at the ends of long bones, especially around the knee joint. Localized swelling, often accompanied by pain (and sometimes by a fracture), develops in children who are otherwise in good health. The level of alkaline phosphatase in these patients is two to three times that found in normal individuals.

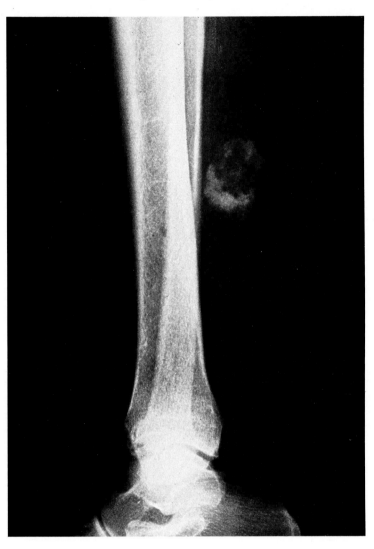

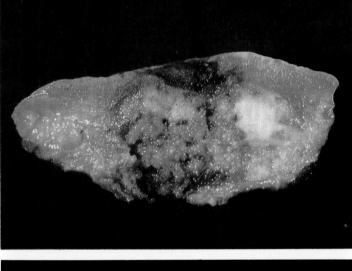

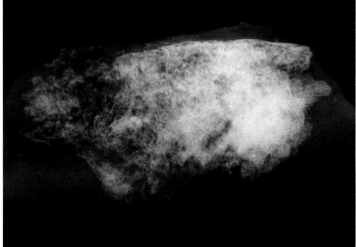

Fig. 12.9 Roentgenogram of a 50-year-old man who presented with a small painful mass in the calf region. A well-defined ossified lesion is evident in the soft tissue.

Fig. 12.10 Gross lesion resected from the patient in Fig. 12.9 *(upper)* and roentgenogram of the specimen *(lower)*. In the roentgenogram, one can appreciate the formation of mineralized tissue throughout the lesion. There is no evidence of maturation of the bone toward the periphery, a finding in contrast to those in myositis ossificans, a lesion that can be mistaken for a soft-tissue osteosarcoma.

Fig. 12.11 Photomicrograph of a portion of the tumor shown in Figs. 12.9 and 12.10 demonstrates the hypercellular, anaplastic nature of the lesion, and the microscopic foci of osteoid that are being formed by the tumor cells. This is in marked contrast to the histologic picture found in cases of myositis ossificans circumscripta (see Figs. 14.42 to 14.45).

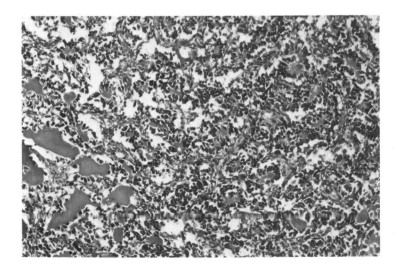

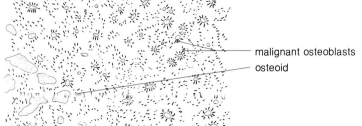

malignant osteoblasts

osteoid

12.5

Roentgenographic examination reveals a sclerotic (in about 35 per cent), lytic (in about 25 per cent), or mixed lesion in the metaphysis, often with abundant periosteal new bone formation (which sometimes shows a sunburst pattern). At the edge of the tumor, elevation of the periosteum may result in a triangle visible on radiologic films and referred to as Codman's triangle. The margins of the triangle are the periosteum, the underlying cortex,

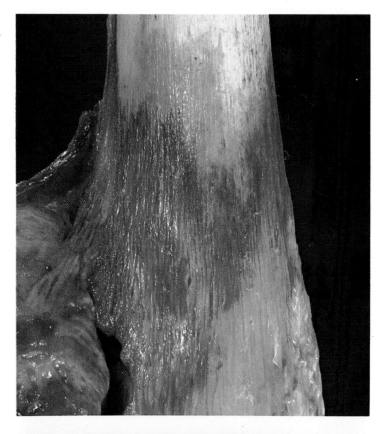

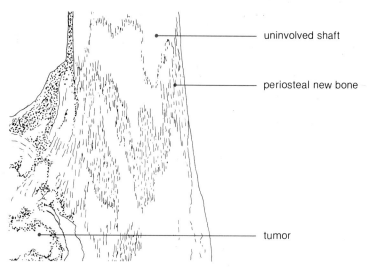

Fig. 12.12 Gross photograph of part of an osteosarcoma of the lower end of the femur. At the upper end of the photograph a portion of the uninvolved femoral shaft can be seen, and at the lower end of the photograph the tumor may be observed breaking through the cortex of the bone. Between the tumor and the normal cortex there is a hyperemic zone that has an irregular margin with the cortical bone. This hyperemic zone is composed of reactive bone formed by the periosteum, and would appear on a roentgenogram as Codman's triangle.

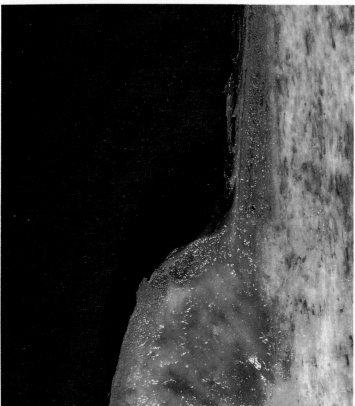

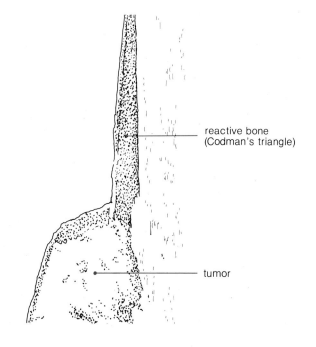

Fig. 12.13 A slice taken through the specimen shown in Fig. 12.12 demonstrates the reactive periosteal bone above and the tumor below. If this reactive periosteal bone is the site of biopsy, it will fail to produce any evidence of malignant tumor histologically.

and, along the narrow margin, the tumor mass. However, the triangle itself is formed of benign reactive bone, and this tissue may result in diagnostic problems if the surgeon obtains biopsy specimens only in this area (Figs. 12.12 and 12.13).

The gross appearance of osteosarcoma varies, depending on the type of matrix (bony, fibrous, or cartilaginous) produced by the lesion (Figs. 12.14 to 12.17). Penetration of the cortex is common, and of the epiphysis less common, but the joint space is rarely involved.

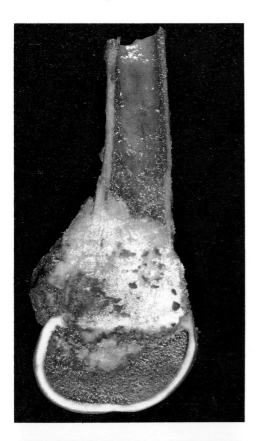

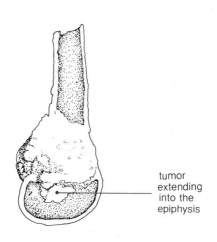

Fig. 12.14 Gross photograph shows a dense osteoblastic osteosarcoma in the lower end of the femur. It has extended through the cortex into the soft tissue, and is also present in the epiphysis. Although epiphyseal extension is rarely seen on clinical roentgenograms, it is commonly present when the resected specimen is examined grossly (compare with Fig. 12.5).

tumor extending into the epiphysis

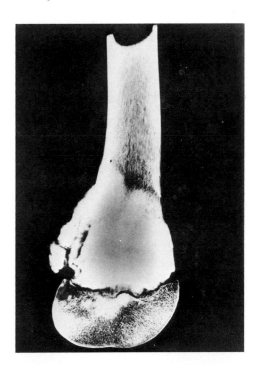

Fig. 12.15 Specimen roentgenogram of the lesion shown in Fig. 12.14 reveals extensive bone formation by the tumor (an osteoblastic osteosarcoma).

Fig. 12.17 Specimen roentgenogram of the lesion shown in Fig. 12.16 demonstrates that in the anterior part of the tumor, the lesion is purely lytic, without bone formation. Posteriorly, bone formation has occurred, and the newly formed bone spicules are oriented at right angles to the surface of the bone, producing a sunburst pattern. A well-defined Codman's triangle is apparent at the upper end of the lesion.

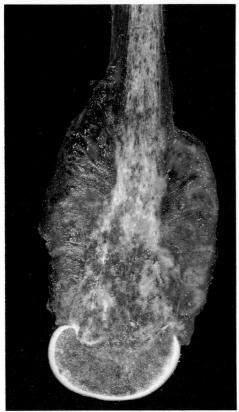

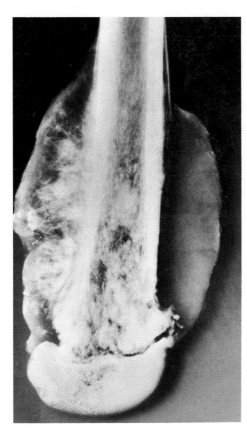

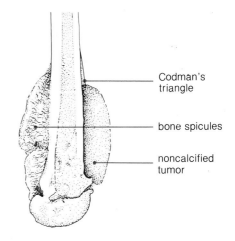

Codman's triangle

bone spicules

noncalcified tumor

Fig. 12.16 Gross photograph shows a bulky and more vascular osteosarcoma. Again, extensive soft-tissue extension and involvement of the epiphysis may be observed.

Most osteosarcomas have in common a pleomorphic and anaplastic cell population that produces bone matrix (Figs. 12.18 to 12.20). However, the pluripotential nature of the neoplasm may be noted in the abundant fibrosarcomatous or chondrosarcomatous tissue matrix present in many lesions. Roughly 50 per cent of all osteosarcomas are osteoblastic; the rest are chondrosarcomatous or fibroblastic. Heterogeneity may lead to confusion of this lesion with a number of entities, including fracture callus (especially following a stress fracture, without clinical history of injury), aneurysmal bone cyst, chondrosarcoma, and even giant-cell tumor. These diagnostic problems may be increased if a pathologic fracture through the lesion is also present.

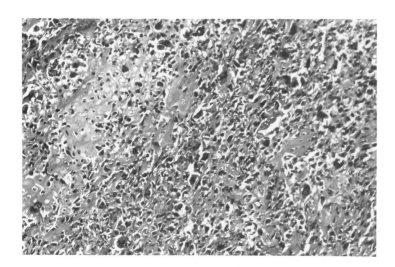

Fig. 12.18 Low power photomicrograph of tissue from an osteosarcoma shows a cellular pleomorphic tumor that is producing a collagenous matrix; focally, this matrix has the appearance of primitive bone. (In an osteosarcoma, one may see primitive bone or cartilage matrix formation, together with areas of malignant spindle cell tumor and giant-cell tumor.)

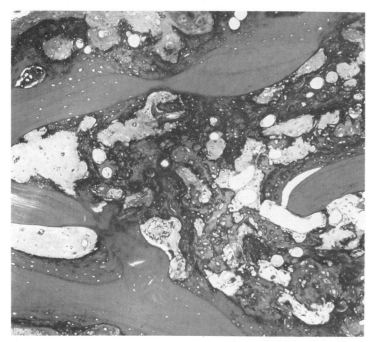

Fig. 12.19 A characteristic feature of osteosarcoma is the observation of a malignant tumor, which forms an abundant mineralized matrix and infiltrates through the marrow spaces between the existing trabeculae of the bone. The malignant tumor tissue becomes firmly applied to the surface of the existing bone, as seen in this photomicrograph.

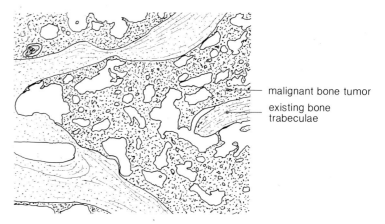

malignant bone tumor

existing bone trabeculae

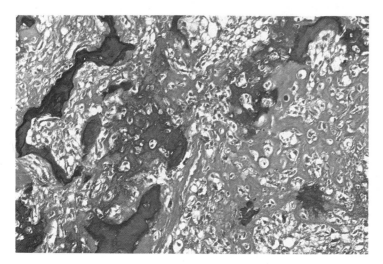

Fig. 12.20 Photomicrograph of a sclerotic osteoblastic osteosarcoma shows extensive primitive bone matrix formation that is focally calcified. Sometimes, as seen here, it may be difficult to distinguish cartilage matrix formation from bone matrix formation, since the primitive matrix being formed has features of both.

Osteosarcomas metastasize, primarily hematogenously, most commonly to the lungs. Favorable prognostic factors include small and distal lesions.

A telangiectatic osteosarcoma is characterized roentgenographically by a large lytic defect, grossly by its blood-filled cavity (Fig. 12.21), and microscopically by dilated vascular channels lined by multinucleated giant cells and an anaplastic sarcomatous stroma with evident bone formation (Figs. 12.22 and 12.23). This lesion may be difficult to distinguish from an aneurysmal bone cyst.

Periosteal (peripheral) osteosarcoma is a rare, predominantly cartilage-forming osteosarcoma, recently described and characterized on roentgenograms by ill-defined swelling and periosteal new bone formation (Fig. 12.24). The lesion usually occurs at the midshaft of the femur or tibia in children.

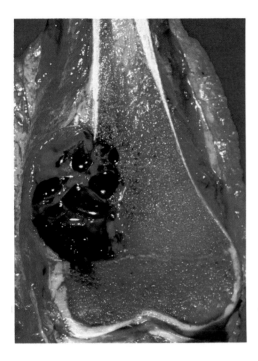

Fig. 12.21 Gross photograph of a telangiectatic osteosarcoma at the lower end of the femur. Note the extremely hemorrhagic appearance of this tumor, which on roentgenographic examination appeared completely lytic.

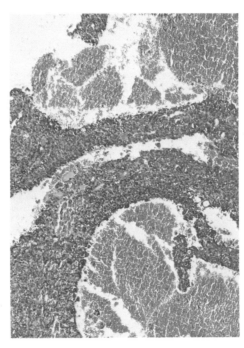

Fig. 12.22 Low power photomicrograph of a telangiectatic osteosarcoma. Septa of cellular tissue are separated by large blood-filled spaces. At this magnification the lesion can easily be confused with an aneurysmal bone cyst.

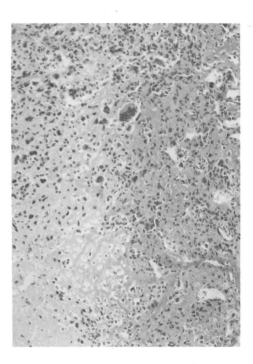

Fig. 12.23 Higher power view of one portion of the tumor illustrated in Fig. 12.22 demonstrates the anaplastic, malignant quality of the tumor tissue. Such tissue may be difficult to find in a telangiectatic osteosarcoma and must be carefully looked for in this type of hemorrhagic tumor.

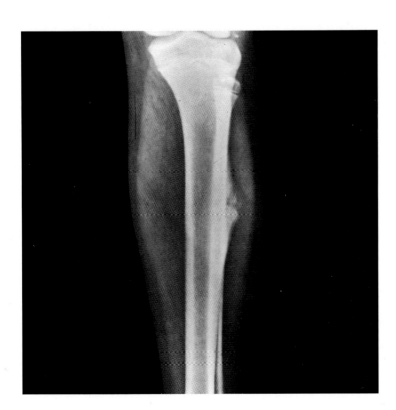

Fig. 12.24 Roentgenogram of a 14-year-old boy who complained of pain in the upper part of the leg. In the upper part of the diaphysis there is a peripheral lesion apparently confined to the surface of the bone. It is composed of an irregular bone-forming lesion, and there is reactive periosteal new bone both superiorly and inferiorly. On histologic examination, this proved to be a cartilage-rich periosteal osteosarcoma.

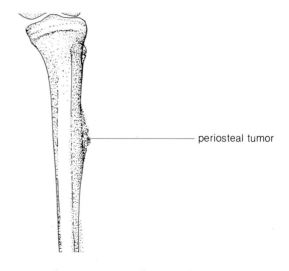

periosteal tumor

JUXTACORTICAL OSTEOSARCOMA
Parosteal osteogenic sarcoma

Juxtacortical osteosarcoma is usually a histologically low grade, slow-growing osteosarcoma that occurs on the external surface of a bone, most commonly on the back of the lower end of the femur (the popliteal region) in patients over 20 years of age (Figs. 12.25 to 12.28). This lesion generally has a much better prognosis than the classic intramedullary osteosarcoma. However, some fully malignant osteosarcomas may present as juxtacortical lesions.

On roentgenographic films, the entity appears as a large, well-circumscribed, dense, juxtacortical mass. The mass may be separated from the cortical bone by a fine, relatively lucent line.

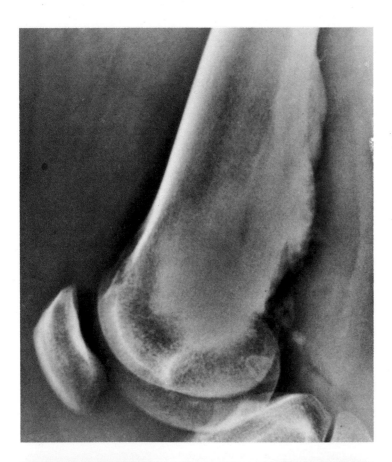

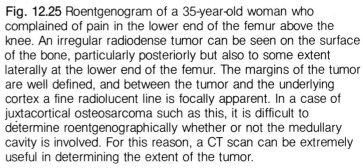

Fig. 12.25 Roentgenogram of a 35-year-old woman who complained of pain in the lower end of the femur above the knee. An irregular radiodense tumor can be seen on the surface of the bone, particularly posteriorly but also to some extent laterally at the lower end of the femur. The margins of the tumor are well defined, and between the tumor and the underlying cortex a fine radiolucent line is focally apparent. In a case of juxtacortical osteosarcoma such as this, it is difficult to determine roentgenographically whether or not the medullary cavity is involved. For this reason, a CT scan can be extremely useful in determining the extent of the tumor.

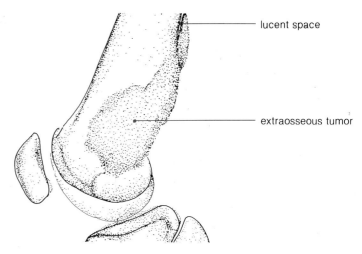

Fig. 12.26 Gross photograph of the lower end of the femur resected from a patient with a juxtacortical osteosarcoma. A large mass is present on the cortex of the bone just above and between the two femoral condyles. This location is typical for juxtacortical osteosarcoma.

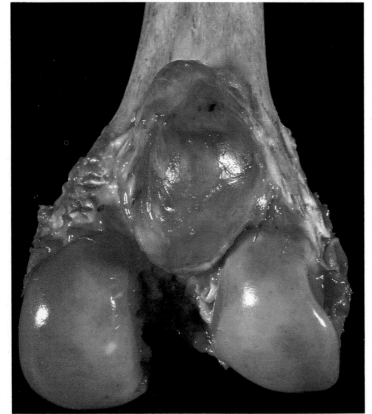

When examined microscopically, the lesion is found to be a well-defined, lobulated mass with extensive bone and (occasionally) cartilage formation. Most tumors contain a bland, well-differentiated fibrosarcomatous stroma (Figs. 12.29 and 12.30). The treatment of choice is surgical removal of the mass.

On occasion, a juxtacortical lesion will be a fully malignant tumor, so it should not be assumed that because the lesion is juxtacortical it has a better prognosis. Although it is very rare, an intramedullary sclerosing osteosarcoma with a histologic pattern identical to that seen in the classic low grade juxtacortical osteosarcoma will sometimes present. In such a case, the prognosis is much better than that of the classic high grade intramedullary osteosarcoma.

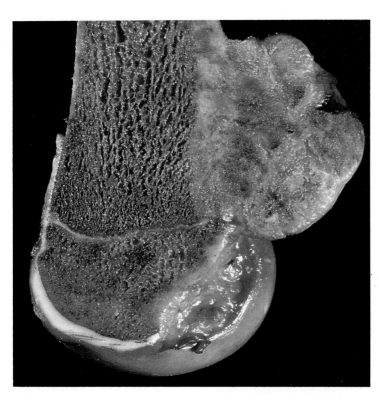

Fig. 12.27 Gross photograph of a sagittal section through the lesion shown in Fig. 12.26 demonstrates that the lesion is well encapsulated and formed of bone-producing tissue. As in the case shown here, the lesion frequently extends for a short distance through the cortex into the medullary cavity. For this reason, when planning surgical treatment of a juxtacortical osteosarcoma, medullary extension should be carefully sought and taken into account if local recurrence is to be prevented.

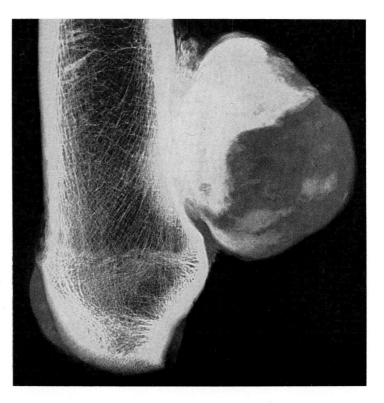

Fig. 12.28 Roentgenogram of the specimen in Fig. 12.27. In a juxtacortical osteosarcoma, as seen here, one may find a large area of tumor which is either purely fibrous or purely cartilaginous, and therefore radiolucent.

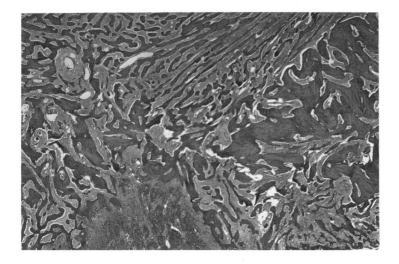

Fig. 12.29 Low power photomicrograph of a juxtacortical osteosarcoma shows the typical appearance of a heavily collagenized fibrous matrix with irregular trabeculae of bone.

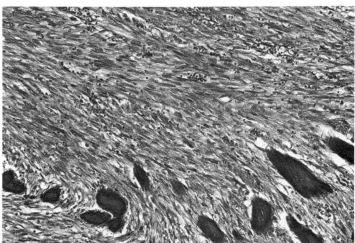

Fig. 12.30 Higher power photomicrograph shows the cellular, though unremarkable, fibrous stroma of a juxtacortical osteosarcoma with islands of bone tissue.

12.11

PAGET'S SARCOMA

Rarely, patients with Paget's disease also develop sarcoma. Most often, the patients who develop sarcoma are those with advanced polyostotic Paget's disease (Figs. 12.31 and 12.32). However, on rare occasions, sarcoma may occur in patients with monostotic disease; for example, in a single vertebral body. The tumor most frequently associated with Paget's disease is osteosarcoma (Figs. 12.33 and 12.34), though occasionally one may see other patterns of sarcoma (chondrosarcoma, malignant fibrous histiocytoma, etc.), and, rarely, a benign giant-cell tumor occurs. The prognosis for sarcomas arising in patients with Paget's disease is very poor.

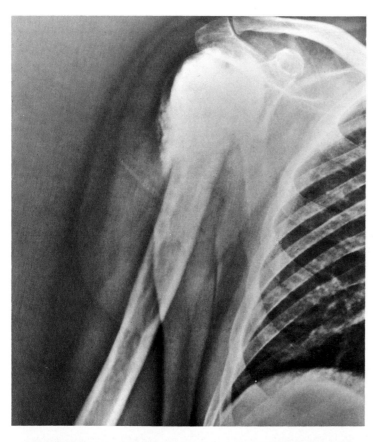

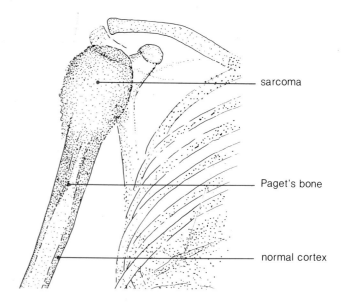

Fig. 12.31 Roentgenogram of a 65-year-old man who presented with severe pain in the upper end of the right humerus shows a large destructive and sclerotic tumor which has developed in the upper end of the humerus and extends into the soft tissue. Note that the cortex of the bone below the tumor is thickened and indistinct, characteristic of Paget's disease.

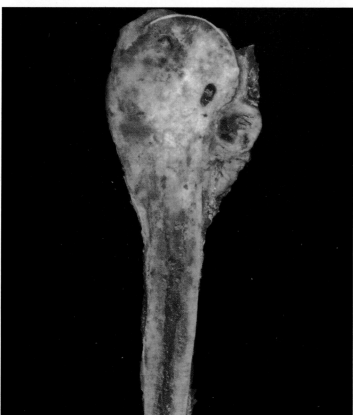

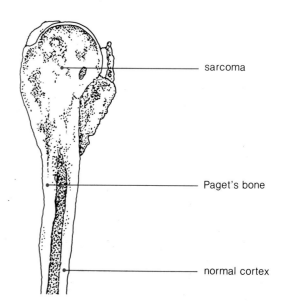

Fig. 12.32 Sagittal section through the humerus of the patient with Paget's disease in Fig. 12.31 shows that a large destructive tumor has developed at the upper end. The tumor has extended through the cortex into the soft tissue. (Often, sarcoma in Paget's disease will occur in the midshaft of the bone, and this finding is in contrast to those of primary osteosarcoma which are more frequently seen in the metaphysis.) Note the thickened hyperemic cortical bone involved by Paget's disease.

ENCHONDROMA

An enchondroma is a common, usually asymptomatic, benign, intramedullary cartilaginous neoplasm. Enchondromas are commonly seen in the short tubular bones of the hands and feet of adults, but may also occur in the long bones. Enlarging lesions may fracture, and this complication is the usual reason for clinical presentation.

The roentgenographic appearance of an enchondroma is usually of a well-delineated solitary lucent defect in the metaphyseal region of the bone, though in the small tubular bones the whole shaft is usually involved. The cortex is generally intact unless a fracture has occurred through the weakened bone. Calcification is usually present in the lesion in the form of a fine, punctuate stippling (Fig. 12.35). When calcification is pronounced, the lesion may be suggestive of a bone infarct (Fig. 12.36).

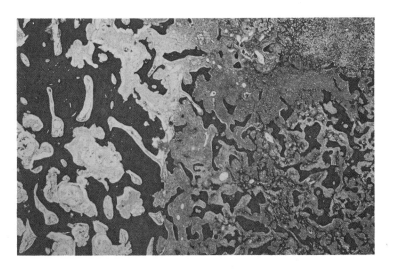

Fig. 12.33 Photomicrograph of tissue removed from the patient in Fig. 12.32. On the left, one can see pagetoid bone; on the right, a cellular bone-forming tumor.

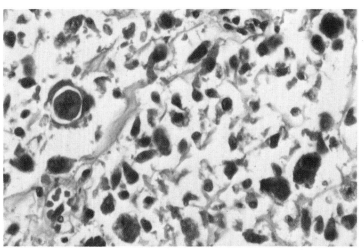

Fig. 12.34 High power view of the cellular tumor in the patient in Fig. 12.33 demonstrates an anaplastic and pleomorphic sarcoma with several malignant giant cells, as well as collagen production.

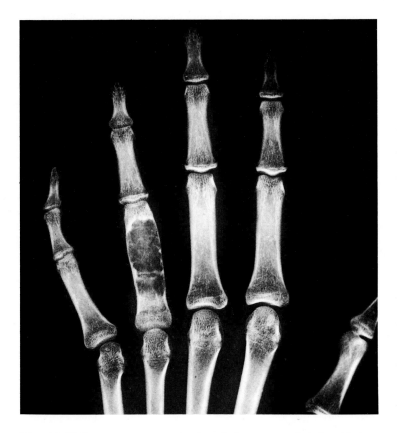

Fig. 12.35 Roentgenogram of a hand shows a well-defined lytic lesion with small punctate calcifications in the proximal phalanx of the ring finger. At the proximal end of the lesion there is a line of density, suggesting a fracture through the tumor. This appearance is characteristic of an enchondroma.

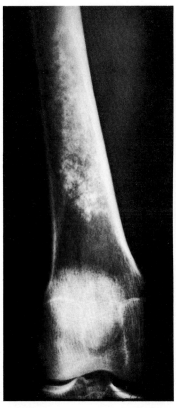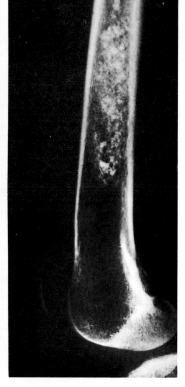

Fig. 12.36 Anteroposterior *(left)* and lateral *(right)* roentgenograms of a 52-year-old man with pain in the knee joint reveals a heavily calcified intramedullary lesion in the lower end of the femur. There were no apparent symptoms related to this lesion. Histologic examination revealed a heavily calcified cartilage tumor, interpreted as an enchondroma.

Gross inspection of the lesion reveals bluish-gray lobules of translucent, firm tissue (Fig. 12.37). On microscopic examination, these lobules are found to be proliferating nests of cartilage cells without obvious atypia. Foci of calcification are usually present (Fig. 12.38), and one may see bone rimming the cartilage nodules (Fig. 12.39). However, invasive infiltration of the bone marrow spaces is not a characteristic of benign enchondromas, and this finding helps to distinguish the lesion from a chondrosar-

coma. Rarely, one may see a chondrosarcoma develop in a preexisting enchondroma, usually in long tubular bones (Fig. 12.40).

Although it may be difficult to differentiate an enchondroma from a low grade chondrosarcoma on histologic examination, small peripheral cartilage tumors generally tend to be benign, and large axial tumors tend to be malignant in their behavior.

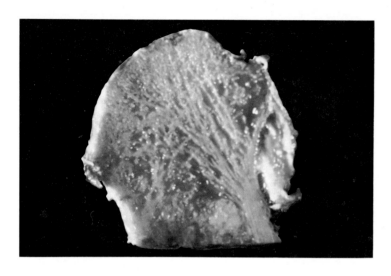

Fig. 12.37 Gross photograph of a femoral head resected for osteoarthritis. A small cartilage tumor is present in the neck of the femur. Note the glistening, lobulated, bluish-white appearance of the cartilaginous tissue.

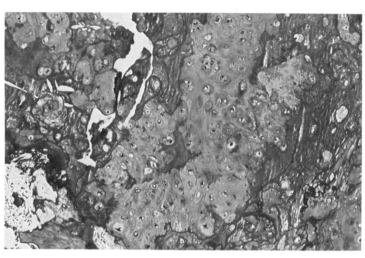

Fig. 12.38 Photomicrograph of the lesion shown in Fig. 12.37 reveals a calcified cartilaginous lesion. The cartilage cells are uncrowded and unremarkable.

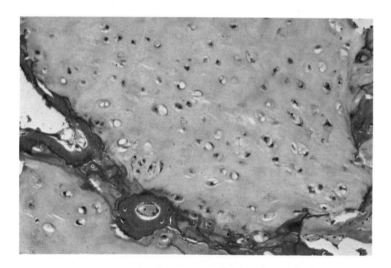

Fig. 12.39 Frequently, in an enchondroma, the cartilage lobules are surrounded by a narrow rim of bone, as seen in this photomicrograph.

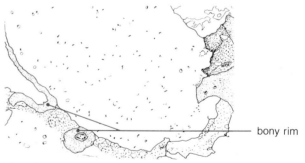

bony rim

Fig. 12.40 Photomicrograph demonstrates the development of a chondrosarcoma in a patient with preexisting enchondroma. In the lower center part of the photomicrograph a heavily calcified enchondroma is apparent. In the upper left and right part a cellular myxoid chondrosarcoma is present.

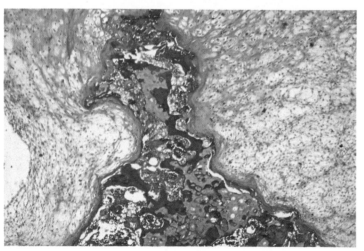

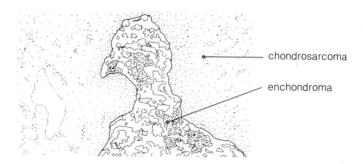

chondrosarcoma

enchondroma

Juxtacortical Chondroma

Periosteal chondroma

A juxtacortical chondroma is a benign cartilaginous lesion characterized by its location in the metaphyseal cortex of both long and short tubular bones. A cup-shaped or scalloped cortical defect is evident on typical roentgenograms, and the lesion is surrounded by a sclerotic bone, often with overhanging edges (Fig. 12.41). Calcified material and, in some instances, a visible soft-tissue mass may be seen. On gross inspection, a juxtacortical chondroma is seen as a well-circumscribed lesion that is par-tially embedded in cortical bone and covered by the periosteum. Examination of its cut surface reveals a grayish-white or bluish lobulated appearance. When examined microscopically, proliferating chondrocytes show minimal pleomorphism and nuclear abnormalities (Fig. 12.42). Focal calcification and ossification within the cartilage may occur.

The treatment of a juxtacortical chondroma is en bloc resection.

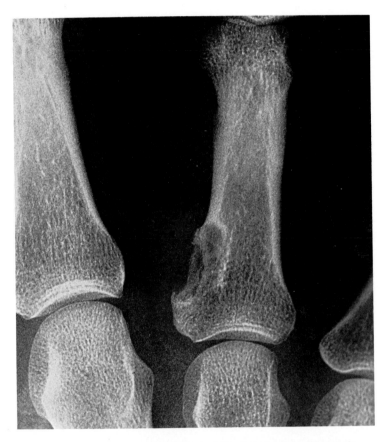

Fig. 12.41 Roentgenogram of a hand shows a well-defined saucerlike depression of the cortex at the proximal end of one phalanx. This roentgenographic picture is typical of a juxtacortical chondroma.

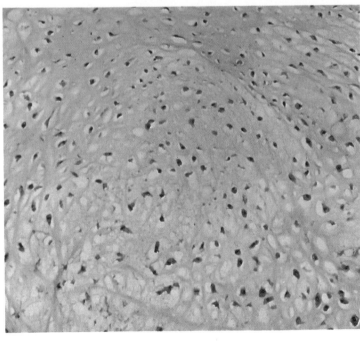

Fig. 12.42 Photomicrograph of the lesion illustrated in Fig. 12.41 shows a cellular but benign cartilaginous lesion.

CHONDROBLASTOMA

A chondroblastoma is an uncommon, benign cellular neoplasm located in the epiphysis of long bones, and usually noted in the patient's second decade of life. On rare occasions, these lesions may be seen in older individuals and in odd locations such as the spine.

The roentgenographic signs of a chondroblastoma include a well-demarcated lucent defect with mottled calcification, located in the epiphysis and sometimes ex-

tending into the metaphysis of long bones (Fig. 12.43). The cortical bone may be intact or expanded. The lesion has a predilection for the upper end of the humerus, upper and lower ends of the femur, and upper end of the tibia.

The gritty, grayish-pink tissue of this lesion is characterized microscopically by round and ovoid cells, often mixed with a scattering of giant cells. Focally, an intercellular chondroid matrix is produced in which a

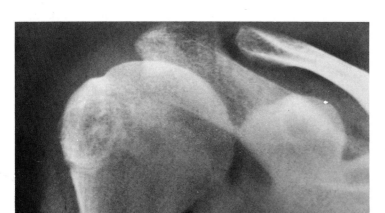

Fig. 12.43 Roentgenogram of an 11-year-old boy who complained of pain and limitation of motion in the right shoulder. An eccentric lytic lesion with patchy calcification can be seen involving the epiphysis of the humerus laterally. Curettage of this lesion proved it to be a chondroblastoma. The roentgenographic appearance and location shown here are typical. Occasionally, the lesion may be seen extending into the metaphysis.

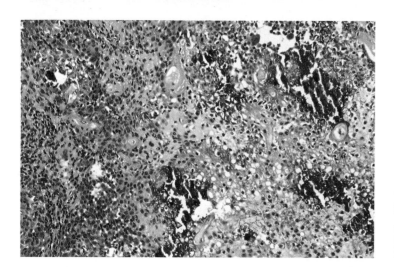

Fig. 12.44 Low power photomicrograph of a chondroblastoma demonstrates the varied appearance of such a lesion. Cellular areas mixed with areas of cartilage matrix formation and calcification can be seen.

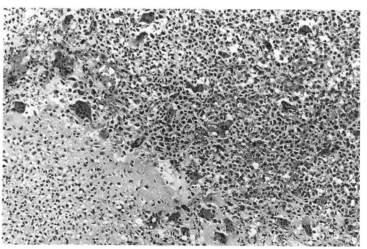

Fig. 12.45 Higher power photomicrograph reveals the juxtaposition of an area of chondroid matrix on the lower left, with a more cellular area of polyhedral cells and admixed giant cells on the right.

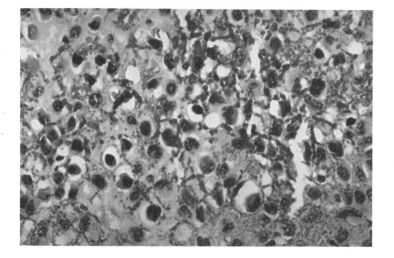

Fig. 12.46 High power photomicrograph of the cartilaginous area in Fig. 12.45 shows the fine stippled calcification that is characteristic of chondroblastoma and frequently extends around the individual chondroblasts, producing a "chicken wire" appearance.

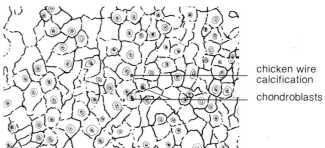

chicken wire calcification

chondroblasts

lacelike deposit of calcium granules may typically be noted (so-called "chicken wire" calcification) (Figs. 12.44 to 12.46). On occasion, lesions can be cystic and hemorrhagic (cystic chondroblastoma), and these findings give rise to the confusion of chondroblastomas with aneurysmal bone cysts. (The presence of cartilage and giant cells in chondroblastomas may lead to the diagnostic confusion of the lesion with either chondrosarcomas or giant-cell tumors of bone.)

Either curettage or local excision is the treatment of choice. In very rare cases, lung metastases have occurred; when present, they are usually rimmed with bone. These metastases should be surgically removed.

CHONDROMYXOID FIBROMA

A chondromyxoid fibroma is a rare, benign bone neoplasm discovered most often during the patient's second and third decades of life. The lesion occurs most frequently in the femur and upper metaphysis of the tibia, but it also develops occasionally in other bones. Patients may experience pain and local swelling. On roentgenograms, the lesion is usually characterized by an eccentric lucent defect with a thin, well-defined, scalloped border of sclerotic bone (Fig. 12.47).

The inspection of intact gross specimens reveals that the lesion is sharply demarcated and covered on its outer surface by a thin rim of bone or periosteum. Examination of the cut surface reveals a firm, lobulated, grayish-white mass, sometimes with small cystic foci and areas of hemorrhage (Fig. 12.48).

On microscopic examination, a chondromyxoid fibroma is found to have a lobulated pattern with sparsely cellular lobules alternating with more cellular zones. The sparsely cellular lobules show spindle and stellate cells without distinct cytoplasmic borders in a myxoid or chondroid matrix. Running between the lobules are areas of increased cellularity with multinucleated giant cells. Some nuclear pleomorphism may be evident, but mitotic figures are rare (Fig. 12.49).

Since recurrences of the lesion after curettage are frequent, en bloc excision is the preferred treatment.

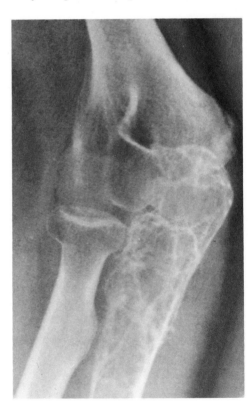

Fig. 12.47 Roentgenogram of the elbow joint in a young adult man who complained of pain shows a well-defined, trabeculated lytic lesion, with cortical thinning but no obvious soft-tissue extension. This soap-bubble appearance is rather typical of chondromyxoid fibromas, although these lesions are so rare that the diagnosis is usually not made until histologic examination has been undertaken.

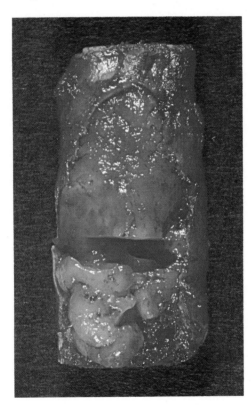

Fig. 12.48 Gross photograph of a segment of resected fibula with a chondromyxoid fibroma. Note the well-demarcated lesion and the glistening fleshy appearance.

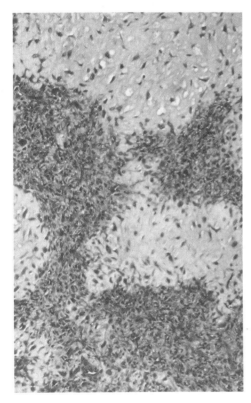

Fig. 12.49 Photomicrograph of a chondromyxoid fibroma shows the typical lobulated and variegated appearance of the lesion. Lobules of chondromyxoid tissue and septa of cellular fibrous tissue are evident, with occasional multinucleated giant cells running between the lobules.

FIBROMYXOMA

A fibromyxoma is, on microscopic examination, superficially similar to a chondromyxoid fibroma, but it is rarer and occurs in older individuals than does chondromyxoid fibroma. In addition, a fibromyxoma lacks both the lobular pattern and chondroid matrix which typify a chondromyxoid fibroma.

Occurrence is so rare that no roentgenographic characteristics have been substantiated. The roentgenogram in Figure 12.50 was thought to show a giant-cell tumor. However, the histologic specimen in Figure 12.51 showed it to be a fibromyxoma. Follow-up on the few cases described in the literature has revealed no local recurrence or metastases.

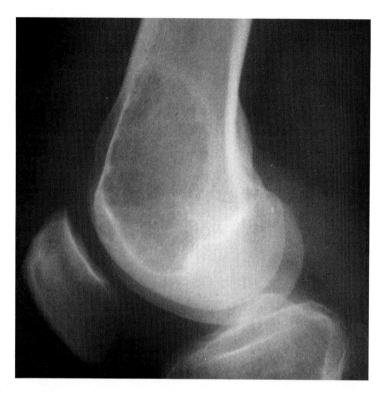

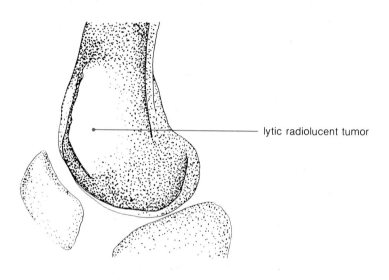

Fig. 12.50 Roentgenogram of the lower end of the femur in a 38-year-old man who complained of pain in the knee joint. A lytic destructive lesion can be seen to involve both the epiphysis and the metaphysis of the femur; on roentgenograms, this lesion resembles a giant-cell tumor.

lytic radiolucent tumor

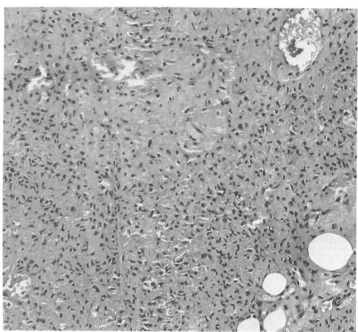

Fig. 12.51 Photomicrograph of the lesion shown in Fig. 12.50 shows a loose fibromyxomatous tissue without lobulation and without obvious chondroid areas. A few such cases have been reported, usually in older people, and these lesions have been designated as fibromyxomas.

CHONDROSARCOMA

A chondrosarcoma is a malignant neoplasm whose cells produce cartilage matrix. It is characteristically seen in adults, most frequently occurring in the medullary cavity of the femur and humerus, and on the surface of the pelvis and spine (Figs. 12.52 to 12.55). Patients initially complain of mild pain and local swelling.

Seen on roentgenograms, chondrosarcomas in the long bones are located in the metaphysis, and often extend into the diaphysis to produce a fusiform lucent defect with a scalloped inner cortex. Frequently occurring punctate or stippled calcifications are characteristic and occasionally extensive, thereby giving rise to the radiologic confusion of chondrosarcoma with a bone infarct.

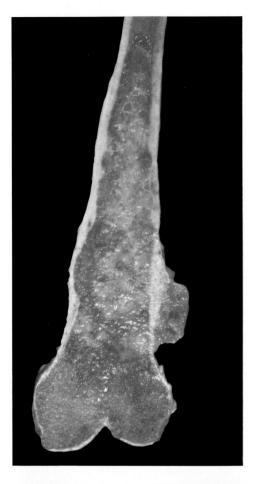

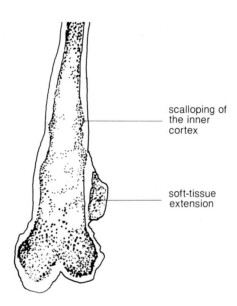

scalloping of the inner cortex

soft-tissue extension

Fig. 12.52 Gross photograph of a transected femur with a large intramedullary chondrosarcoma at the lower end. The tumor has a bluish-white lobulated appearance, and it can be seen to have caused expansion and scalloping of the inner cortex of the bone. Focally, the tumor has extended through the cortex into the soft tissue.

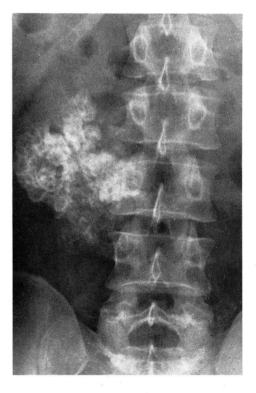

Fig. 12.53 In this roentgenogram, a large calcified mass is present adjacent to the lumbar spine. This lesion proved to be a chondrosarcoma.

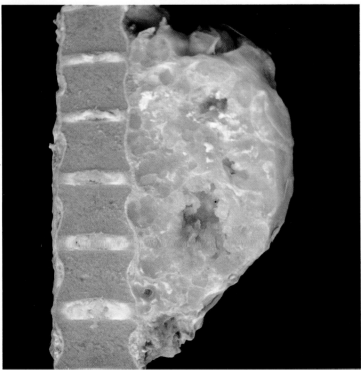

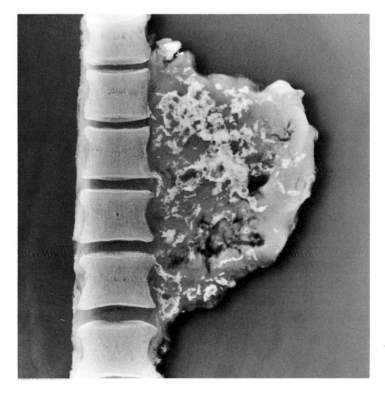

Fig. 12.54 Gross photograph of a chondrosarcoma arising from the vertebral column.

Fig. 12.55 Roentgenogram of the specimen shown in Fig. 12.54 demonstrates irregular areas of calcification within the lesion.

Chondrosarcomas are lobulated, grayish-white or blue, focally calcified masses, often with areas of mucoid degeneration or necrosis. The lesions are distinguished histologically from benign cartilage tumors by their increased cellularity and pleomorphism (Figs. 12.56 and 12.57). Attempts to grade chondrosarcomas have been based on the degree of differentiation, variation in nuclear size, the presence of double nuclei and multinucleated giant cells, and the frequency of mitoses. (Adequate sampling of cartilage tumors is necessary to discern these features.)

Low grade chondrosarcomas are difficult to differentiate from benign enchondromas on microscopic examination. However, it is generally true that lesions occurring in the axial skeleton and the proximal portions of the appendicular skeleton are more likely to have a malignant course than tumors in the distal skeleton. Furthermore, in chondrosarcomas, infiltration of the marrow spaces occurs, so one finds trabeculae of normal bone embedded in the tumor. In assessing low grade chondrosarcomas, this finding can be a useful way of distinguishing the lesion from an enchondroma (Fig. 12.58).

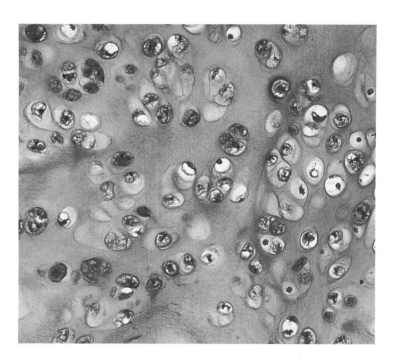

Fig. 12.56 Photomicrograph of a histologic section obtained from a low grade chondrosarcoma that had extended through the cortex of the bone into the soft tissues. Despite the locally aggressive nature of the lesion, the appearance of the cells is fairly innocuous. There is, however, some crowding of the chondrocytes and slight variation in the appearance of the cells. In the interpretation of such a lesion, careful clinical and radiologic correlation must be made in order to arrive at the correct diagnosis.

Fig. 12.57 Photomicrograph of a fully malignant, anaplastic chondrosarcoma shows marked cellular atypia and crowding (in contrast to Fig. 12.56).

Fig. 12.58 A useful microscopic finding that helps to distinguish chondrosarcoma from enchondroma is that the tumor tissue invades the marrow spaces and becomes applied to the surfaces of existing trabeculae, as seen in this photomicrograph. This feature, which is characteristic of malignant tumors, does not generally occur in benign lesions.

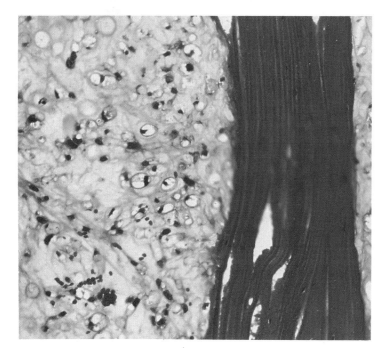

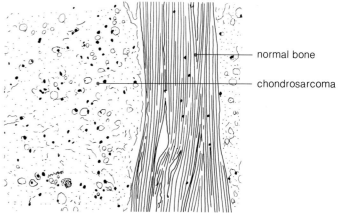

— normal bone

— chondrosarcoma

The course of a chondrosarcoma depends on several factors. In general, well-differentiated tumors rarely metastasize, but they recur locally after incomplete excision. Anaplastic, fully malignant tumors metastasize early, primarily to the lung.

Complete surgical excision of the tumor is the treatment of choice. (Cartilage lesions do not, in general, respond to chemotherapy or radiation therapy.)

About 10 per cent of all chondrosarcomas undergo dedifferentiation in one area or another and become highly malignant sarcomas with spindle cells and bizarre giant cells (features of fibrosarcoma or malignant fibrous histiocytoma) (Figs. 12.59 to 12.61). These dedifferentiated tumors carry a poor prognosis and often metastasize widely, the metastases frequently showing only the fibrosarcomatous component of the tumor. Roentgenograms may reveal a poorly defined and destructive lucent zone in an otherwise typical chondrosarcoma with stippled calcification.

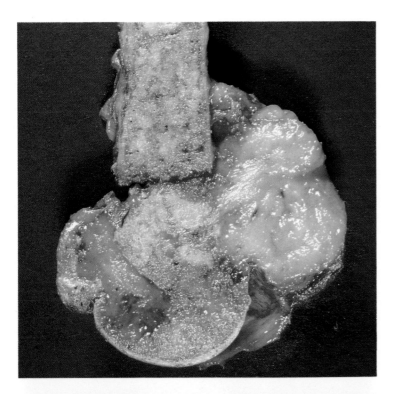

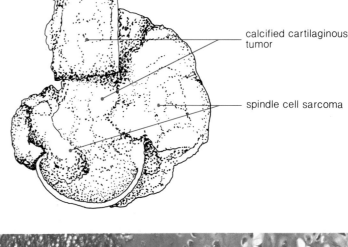

Fig. 12.59 Gross photograph of the lower end of a femur removed from a patient with a long-standing cartilaginous tumor that had begun to grow rapidly. In the transected specimen, one can see a lobulated bluish-gray tissue filling the medullary cavity of the bone. However, at the lower end of the femur, filling the medulla and extending to the soft tissue, a fleshy yellow-tan tumor can be seen. This area of the tumor proved to be a malignant spindle cell tumor.

calcified cartilaginous tumor

spindle cell sarcoma

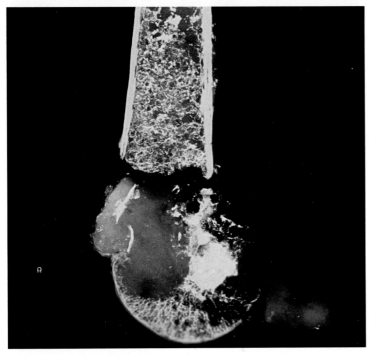

Fig. 12.60 Specimen roentgenogram of the malignant spindle cell tumor shown in Fig. 12.59. Note that although the cartilaginous portion of the tumor is heavily calcified, the dedifferentiated spindle cell component is entirely radiolucent.

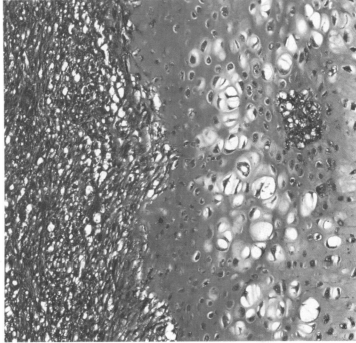

Fig. 12.61 Photomicrograph of the dedifferentiated spindle cell tumor that developed in the chondrosarcoma illustrated in Figs. 12.59 and 12.60. The spindle cell tumor has the pattern of a malignant fibrous histiocytoma and is seen here abutting the chondrosarcoma.

12.21

MESENCHYMAL CHONDROSARCOMA

A mesenchymal chondrosarcoma is a rare, malignant bone tumor which has been seen most commonly in the ribs and jaws of individuals in the second and third decades of life. Approximately one-third of the lesions have been found in soft tissue. Patients may experience pain and/or swelling.

An ill-defined osteolytic lesion with irregular calcifications may be noted on roentgenograms, and this radiologic appearance corresponds to the grayish-white or yellow tumor mass with evident foci of cartilage and calcification found on gross examination (Figs. 12.62 to 12.64). On microscopic examination, the tumor is found to be composed of sheets of small, poorly differentiated cells that resemble those of Ewing's tumor, but a mesenchymal chondrosarcoma has focal admixed areas of cartilaginous or chondroid matrix arranged in a lobular pattern (Fig. 12.65).

Mesenchymal chondrosarcoma metastasizes primarily to the lungs, but osseous and soft-tissue metastases have been documented.

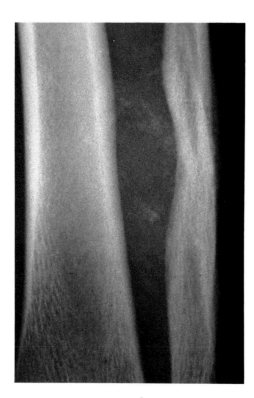 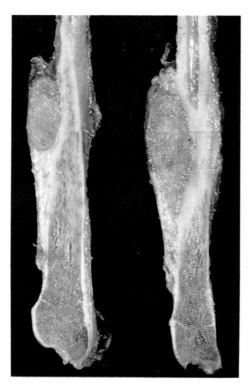 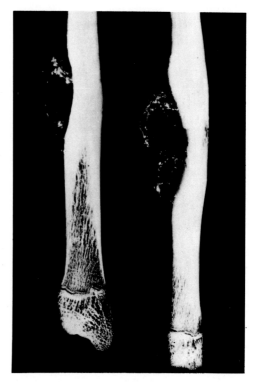

Fig. 12.62 Clinical roentgenogram of a young man who presented with pain and swelling in a leg. A soft-tissue mass can be seen eroding the adjacent bone between the fibula and the tibia. Focal calcification is evident within the tumor mass. In this case, the differential diagnosis would include synovial sarcoma.

Fig. 12.63 Gross photograph of the resected specimen from the patient in Fig. 12.62 shows a soft-tissue tumor eroding the cortex of the adjacent fibula.

Fig. 12.64 Specimen roentgenogram of the lesion shown in Fig. 12.63. Focal calcification is seen, particularly at the periphery of the lesion.

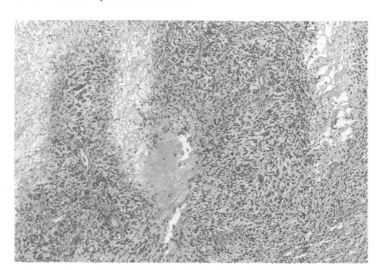

Fig. 12.65 Photomicrograph of the lesion shown in Fig. 12.64 reveals the typical biphasic pattern of a mesenchymal chondrosarcoma. Large areas of undifferentiated small-cell tumors (which resemble Ewing's sarcomas) are seen interspersed with a cellular chondroid tumor, which may show focal calcification or ossification.

CLEAR-CELL CHONDROSARCOMA

Clear-cell chondrosarcoma, considered by some an aggressive variant of chondroblastoma, is a very rare, destructive, low grade malignant tumor in adults, affecting the epiphyseal ends of long bones, most often the upper femur. On roentgenograms, these tumors are seen to be well-circumscribed lucent defects, often with a thin sclerotic border (Fig. 12.66).

On histologic examination, a clear-cell chondrosarcoma is found to contain numerous cells with abundant, clear, vacuolated cytoplasm. Frequently, one may observe scattered giant cells and, between the cells, a scant chondroid matrix (Fig. 12.67). The vacuolated clear cells may suggest the presence of a renal cell carcinoma, but the scattered giant cells and the scant chondroid matrix should help to differentiate that lesion from a clear-cell chondrosarcoma.

Clear-cell chondrosarcomas are locally aggressive, and metastases have been reported.

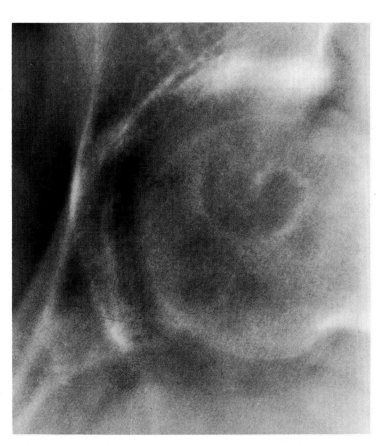

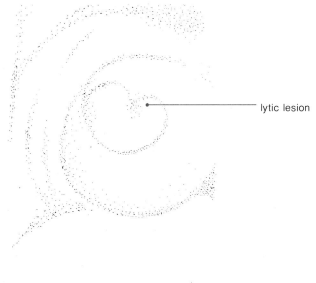

lytic lesion

Fig. 12.66 Tomogram of the femoral head in a 30-year-old man who complained of pain in the hip. While plain roentgenograms of the hip joint were inconclusive, this tomogram shows within the substance of the femoral head a lytic lesion having a faintly sclerotic margin. On curettage, this lesion proved to be a clear-cell chondrosarcoma.

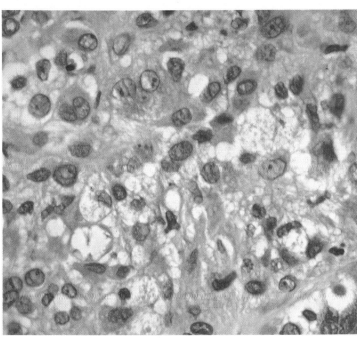

Fig. 12.67 Photomicrograph of an area within a clear-cell chondrosarcoma shows numerous vacuolated cells, some nuclear variation, and occasional giant cells.

DESMOPLASTIC FIBROMA

A desmoplastic fibroma is a rare, intraosseous, collagen-producing fibrous tumor that is well differentiated, and characterized clinically by pain. Usually the tumor is seen in patients during the first three decades of life, and it most commonly develops in a long bone or the pelvis. On roentgenograms, a lucent defect is evident in the metaphysis, often with cortical destruction simulating a malignant tumor (Fig. 12.68). A desmoplastic fibroma's histologic similarity to certain fibrous lesions elsewhere (such as palmar fibromatosis and desmoid tumors) suggests that it is an intraosseous counterpart of those lesions (Figs. 12.69 and 12.70). The tumor has a tendency to recur locally, but it does not metastasize. The lack of bone production in this lesion distinguishes it from fibro-osseous lesions of bone, including fibrous dysplasia and ossifying fibroma.

FIBROSARCOMA

A fibrosarcoma is a rare, malignant, spindle cell neoplasm that produces a collagen matrix, and demonstrates an overall herringbone pattern in its organization. (It has no other matrix differentiation.) The lesion usually occurs in the metaphyseal ends of the long bones in adults, especially around the knees. Pain or swelling in the affected area is frequently exacerbated by a pathologic fracture.

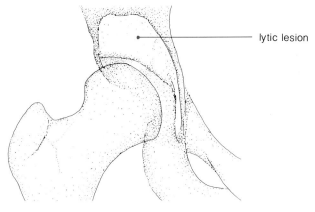

Fig. 12.68 Roentgenogram of a young adult patient who complained of pain in the hip joint reveals a large lytic defect in the ilium, just above the acetabulum. The margins of the lesion are fairly well defined, without obvious sclerosis. On curettage, this lesion proved to be a densely fibrous tumor, characterized microscopically as a desmoplastic fibroma.

lytic lesion

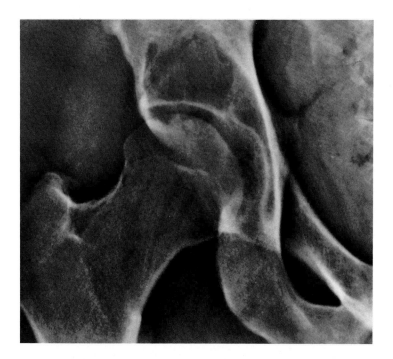

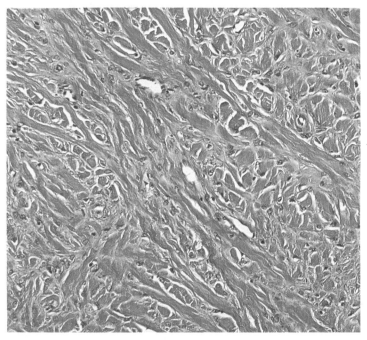

Fig. 12.69 Low power photomicrograph of a desmoplastic fibroma shows the dense, collagenized matrix of this lesion.

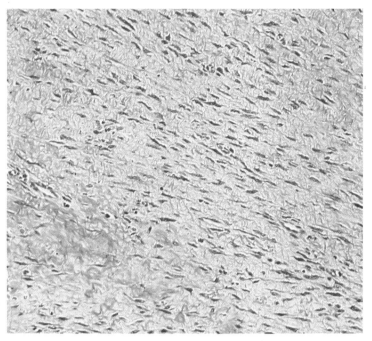

Fig. 12.70 Photomicrograph of another area of desmoplastic fibroma that is somewhat more cellular than that seen in Fig. 12.69. Note the innocuous appearance of the fibroblasts and the extensive collagen production.

On roentgenographic examination, fibrosarcomas are seen to be lucent lesions, often with cortical destruction and extension into soft tissue. The involved bone often has a mottled or moth-eaten pattern (Fig. 12.71).

The tumor is usually discrete, grayish-white, and rubbery (Fig. 12.72). Bone margins are irregular. On microscopic examination, fibrosarcomas are found to be either well or poorly differentiated. The well-differentiated lesions have homogeneous, spindle-shaped fibroblasts with ovoid nuclei, relatively little pleomorphism, and infrequent mitoses (Fig. 12.73). Poorly differentiated tumors are considerably more pleomorphic, with abundant mitotic activity and bizarre, hyperchromatic nuclei (Fig. 12.74). Whereas well-differentiated tumors grow slowly, a poorly differentiated fibrosarcoma metastasizes to the lung early in its course and requires radical surgery. Radiation therapy is ineffective.

The differential diagnosis of primary fibrosarcoma should include metastatic carcinoma, which may demonstrate a spindle cell pattern (e.g., carcinoma of the kidney), and metastatic melanoma.

It should be noted that sarcomas arising in patients with chronic, long-standing osteomyelitis, Paget's disease, irradiated bone, bone infarcts, or giant-cell tumors following radiation may have a predominantly malignant spindle cell appearance.

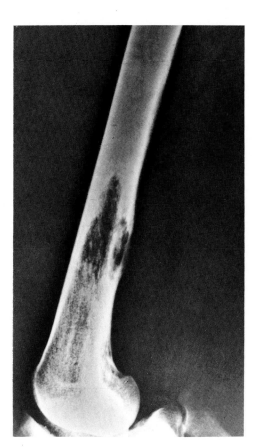

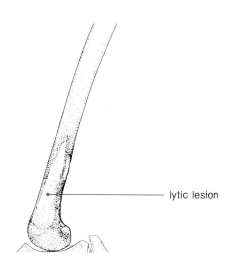

lytic lesion

Fig. 12.71 Roentgenogram of the lateral aspect of the femur in a 40-year-old man who complained of pain in the lower thigh shows an ill-defined, intramedullary lytic area extending into the posterior cortex. The margin is ill-defined, and the lesion has at its periphery a permeative appearance. On biopsy, this lesion proved to be a fibrosarcoma.

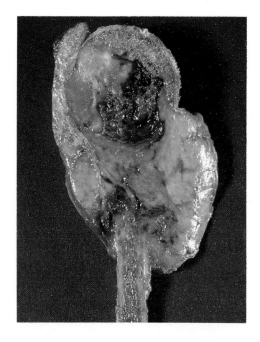

Fig. 12.72 Photograph of a transected humerus shows a solid tumor at the upper end of the humerus, extending into the soft tissue. Focal hemorrhage is evident. When examined histologically, this tumor proved to be a fibrosarcoma.

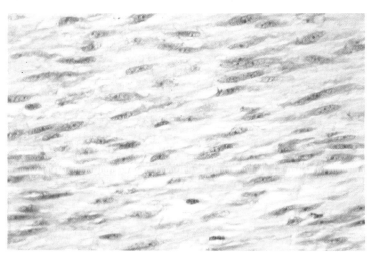

Fig. 12.73 Most fibrosarcomas of bone are well differentiated, as seen in this high power view. On low power, this type of lesion will show a characteristic herringbone pattern.

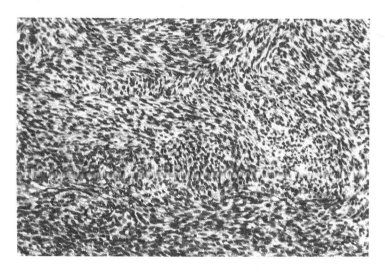

Fig. 12.74 Photomicrograph of a poorly differentiated fibrosarcoma shows the cellular crowding and pleomorphism associated with the less common, poorly differentiated fibrosarcoma.

MALIGNANT FIBROUS HISTIOCYTOMA

Malignant fibrous histiocytoma, when it occurs in bone, primarily affects adults, and is usually found in the lower femur or upper tibia. The lesion is a malignant sarcoma characterized by a heterogeneous population of pleomorphic spindle cells organized in a characteristic pattern.

On roentgenograms, malignant fibrous histiocytoma is found to be a poorly delineated lucent defect, often with cortical destruction. Minimal periosteal new bone formation may be evident. This tumor has, in many cases, been found in association with a preexisting bone infarct (Figs. 12.75 to 12.78).

The characteristic microscopic features of a malignant fibrous histiocytoma are bundles and whorls of pleomorphic spindle-shaped cells with patchy or extensive reticulin-fiber production. The cells and fibers often meet at right angles, and sometimes take on a pinwheel pattern (also known as a storiform or "starry night" pattern). Foci of rounded cells with foamy or vacuolated cytoplasm may be found, as well as giant-cell and multiple mitotic figures. One may often find evidence of phagocytosed intracytoplasmic material, including hemosiderin, hematin, and lipofuchsin pigments. The complicated microscopic appearance of the tumor is best understood in light of

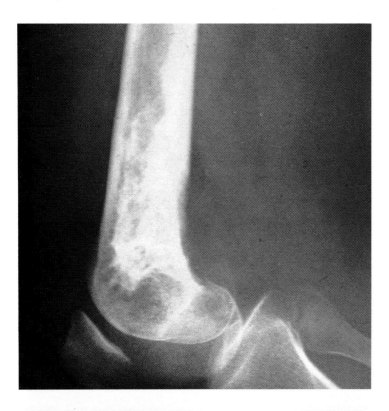

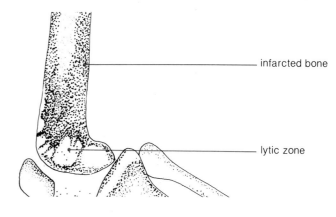

Fig. 12.75 Roentgenogram of the femur in a patient with a long-standing history of bone infarction resulting from his being a caisson worker. Recently, the patient had experienced severe pain in the lower end of the femur, and on the roentgenogram a lytic area can be discerned at the lower end of the infarcted zone.

infarcted bone

lytic zone

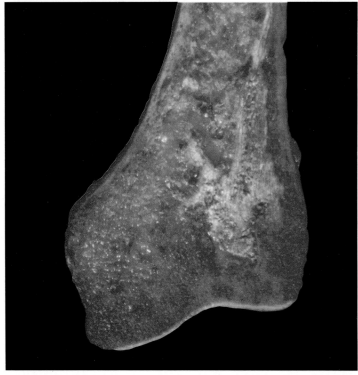

Fig. 12.76 Photograph of the transected specimen of the femur removed from the patient in Fig. 12.75. The infarcted bone, seen as an area of opaque yellow tissue, is clearly delineated from the surrounding normal bone. In the lower end of the femur, one may also see admixed, fleshy gray tissue that, on microscopic examination, proved to be a malignant tumor.

evidence supporting a pluripotential cell that has features of both a macrophage (thus, "histiocyte") and a collagen-producing cell (thus, "fibroblast").

Although a malignant fibrous histiocytoma is not as aggressive as an osteosarcoma, it is a fully malignant and metastasizing tumor, and radical treatment is recommended.

Rare instances of multicentricity have been reported.

GIANT-CELL TUMOR

A giant-cell tumor of bone is a locally aggressive neoplasm of the epiphyseal ends of long bones (most commonly the lower end of the femur, the upper end of the tibia, and the lower end of the radius). It occurs most commonly in the third and fourth decades of life, and individuals may complain of pain, show signs of local swelling, or have a pathologic fracture through the lesion.

Roentgenograms in these patients reveal a well-defined defect in the metaphysis and epiphysis that is usually eccentrically located and extends to the subchondral bone end plate of the articular surface. There is usually no evidence of sclerosis around the lesion (Fig. 12.79).

The unaltered lesional tissue can be seen to be rather homogeneous, with a tan color and a moderately firm consistency. However, in many lesions, foci of hemorrhage and/or necrosis may be seen (Fig. 12.80).

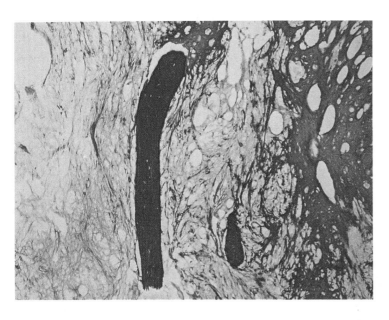

Fig. 12.77 Photomicrograph of the infarcted area of the lesion illustrated in Figs. 12.75 and 12.76.

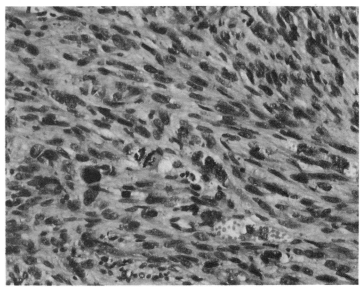

Fig. 12.78 Histologic section of the fleshy tumor illustrated in Figs. 12.75 to 12.77. This tumor is cellular, with marked variation in nuclear size and shape, and many giant cells. Focally, the tumor has a swirling pattern, characteristic of a malignant fibrous histiocytoma.

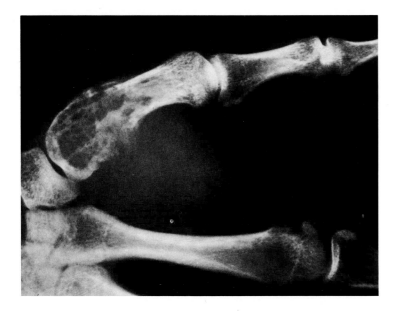

Fig. 12.79 Roentgenogram of a lytic lesion in the proximal end of the first metacarpal bone, through which there has been a pathologic fracture. On biopsy, this lesion proved to be a conventional giant-cell tumor.

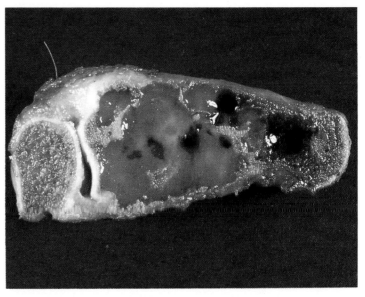

Fig. 12.80 Photograph of the transected specimen removed from the patient in Fig. 12.79. The pinkish tan soft tissue seen here is typical of a giant-cell tumor.

12.27

The microscopic features of the tumor include a background of proliferating, homogeneous, mononuclear cells with multinucleated giant cells that are dispersed evenly throughout (Figs. 12.81 and 12.82). In some cases, foci of reactive bone may also be present in the tumor, particularly at the periphery. Rare lesions have considerable cellular pleomorphism, with atypical mitoses and a fully malignant appearance (Fig. 12.83).

Multicentric lesions have been reported, but they are extremely rare. Malignant degeneration is also rare, but it follows in approximately 10 percent of all irradiated lesions after five to eight years. Following curettage, giant-cell tumors have a high local recurrence rate (50 per cent). Surgical excision is the treatment of choice.

In conventional giant-cell tumors, lung metastases may rarely appear. These lung nodules can be successfully treated by surgical excision. However, in the rare, fully malignant variety of giant-cell tumors, metastases are common, and the tumor runs a malignant course.

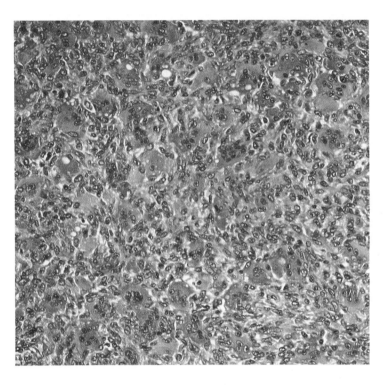

Fig. 12.81 Low power photomicrograph of a conventional giant-cell tumor reveals the cellular nature of the lesion, and the giant cells which are evenly distributed throughout.

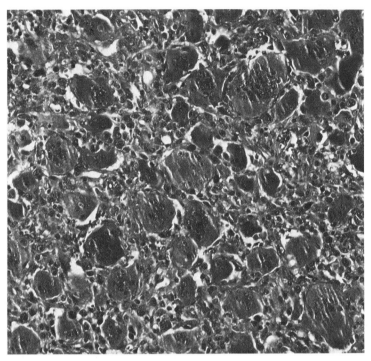

Fig. 12.82 High power photomicrograph demonstrates the homogeneous, mononuclear stromal cells and the evenly distributed multinucleated giant cells in a giant-cell tumor. (The presence of giant cells alone does not confirm the diagnosis of giant-cell tumor. Many lesions contain giant cells; it is the combination of mononuclear stromal cells and giant cells that is diagnostic of giant-cell tumor.)

Fig. 12.83 Photomicrograph of a malignant giant-cell tumor of bone shows marked pleomorphism and nuclear atypia, with sparse atypical giant cells scattered throughout the lesion.

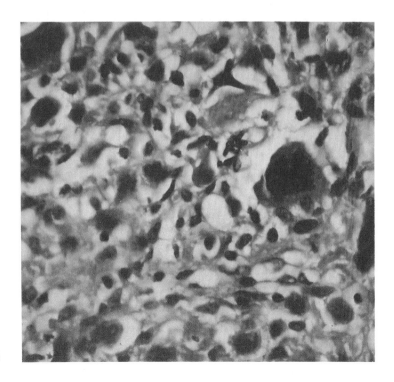

13 Neoplasms II

VASCULAR NEOPLASMS

Vascular neoplasms of bone are rare, and they include tumors arising from the endothelium (hemangioendothelioma or angiosarcoma) and tumors arising from the pericytes (hemangiopericytoma). Endothelial tumors vary from differentiated and locally aggressive lesions (hemangioendothelioma) to highly anaplastic, poorly differentiated, metastasizing neoplasms (angiosarcoma). The presence of multiple intraosseous lesions at the time of original diagnosis is a common finding in both well-differentiated and poorly differentiated tumors.

WELL-DIFFERENTIATED ENDOTHELIAL TUMORS: Hemangioendotheliomas are locally aggressive tumors that predominantly affect the long bones in adults. Complaints of pain or swelling are common. These tumors are osteolytic and may be poorly demarcated on roentgenograms (Fig. 13.1). Periosteal new bone formation is not typical of hemangioendotheliomas.

The tumor is characterized microscopically by anastomosing cords of vascular channels lined by plump endothelial cells that lack pleomorphism or significant mitotic activity. Solid foci of polygonal cells may also be seen (Figs. 13.2 to 13.4).

Wide resection is the treatment of choice. Although these tumors may recur, they rarely metastasize.

POORLY DIFFERENTIATED ENDOTHELIAL TUMORS: Angiosarcomas are fully malignant metastasizing neoplasms.

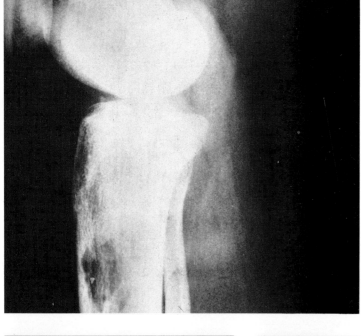

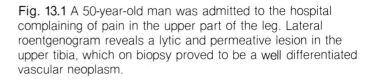

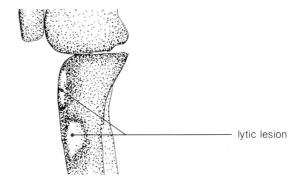

Fig. 13.1 A 50-year-old man was admitted to the hospital complaining of pain in the upper part of the leg. Lateral roentgenogram reveals a lytic and permeative lesion in the upper tibia, which on biopsy proved to be a well differentiated vascular neoplasm.

lytic lesion

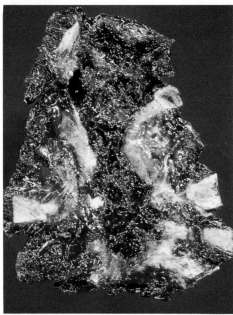

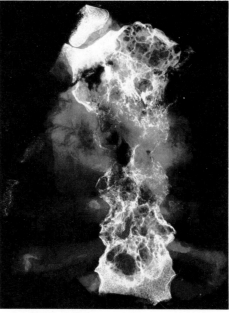

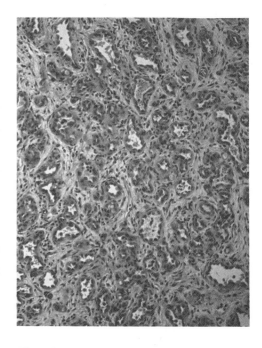

Fig. 13.2 Gross photograph of the sternum of a patient with a well-differentiated vascular tumor. The tumor has extensively involved the sternum, and extends into the adjacent soft tissue.

Fig. 13.3 Specimen roentgenogram of the tumor shown in Fig. 13.2. Note the lytic destructive character of the tumor.

Fig. 13.4 Photomicrograph of the tumor illustrated in Figs. 13.2 and 13.3 shows a fibrous stroma filled with proliferating vascular channels, lined by plump endothelial cells that lack obvious pleomorphism or significant mitotic activity.

They are characterized by rapid growth and extensive bone destruction, with erosion of the cortices and extension into soft tissues. Metastases to the lungs and other organs are common. The tumor consists of irregular, anastomosing vascular channels lined by malignant cells exhibiting prominent intravascular budding and striking cellular anaplasia with frequent mitoses (Fig. 13.5). Solid, undifferentiated areas are often present and may suggest a poorly differentiated carcinoma or an anaplastic lymphoma. As with other sarcomas, foci of necrosis are common.

Radical surgery is the treatment of choice.

HEMANGIOPERICYTOMA: A hemangiopericytoma is a rare, low grade vascular tumor that occasionally occurs as a primary intraosseous lesion. Patients may present with localized pain. Roentgenograms are nonspecific, and may show either lysis or focal sclerosis.

The intervascular stroma contains typical spindle-shaped mononuclear cells thought to arise from a perivascular cell (the pericyte) with the characteristics of smooth muscle. The key to the diagnosis of hemangiopericytoma is recognizing that the neoplastic cells surround the vascular spaces and are not formed from the endothelial lining cells. This finding may be confirmed by reticulum stains (Figs. 13.6 and 13.7).

Surgery is the treatment of choice; the prognosis should be guarded since metastases may occur.

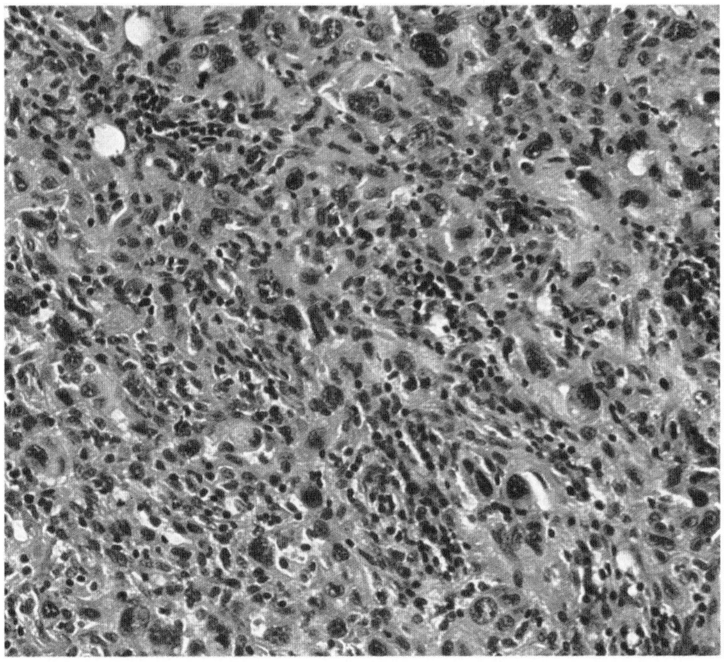

Fig. 13.5 Photomicrograph of a malignant angiosarcoma of the bone shows the striking pleomorphism of the lesion, with numerous malignant giant cells. In such a case, the true nature of the lesion may be difficult to determine, and the differential diagnosis would include poorly differentiated metastatic carcinoma as well as malignant lymphoma. A reticulum stain would assist in demonstrating the intraluminal position of the malignant cells.

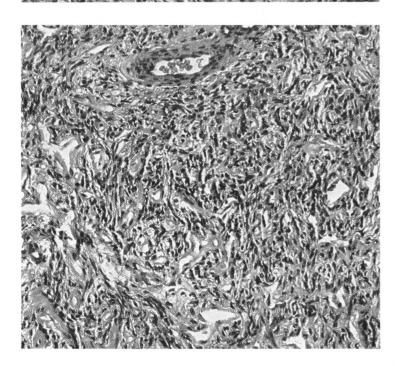

Fig. 13.6 Photomicrograph of a hemangiopericytoma of bone shows the vascular nature of the lesion. The tumor is formed of spindle cells that do not line the epithelial spaces, but are distributed around them.

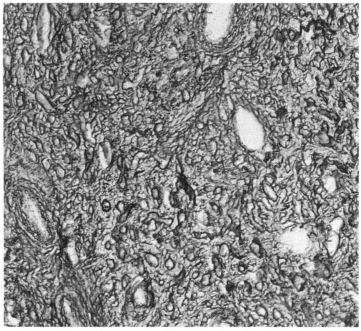

Fig. 13.7 The extravascular location of the tumor cells shown in Fig. 13.6 can be demonstrated histologically by the use of a reticulum stain, which shows the cells to be outside the vascular endothelium, and further shows a fine reticular network extending around the individual tumor cells.

EWING'S SARCOMA

Ewing's sarcoma is a small-cell malignant neoplasm of bone that develops in the diaphysis or metaphysis of long bones, as well as in the pelvis, scapulae, ribs, and other bones. It is essentially a tumor of childhood, with most patients under 20 years of age. Ewing's tumors may very rarely be found in soft tissues.

Patients usually complain of pain or tenderness of several weeks' or months' duration in the affected bone.

On physical examination, swelling and tenderness may be noted. Fever, anemia, leukocytosis, and elevated erythrocyte sedimentation rates often suggest a diagnosis of osteomyelitis and, because of the histologic appearance of the tumor, osteomyelitis is the most important differential in the diagnosis of Ewing's tumor.

On roentgenographic examination, one may observe a lytic, moth-eaten, mottled appearance (Fig. 13.8) or

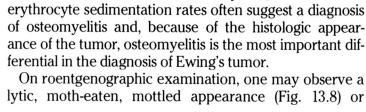

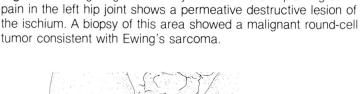

Fig. 13.8 Roentgenogram of a 9-year-old child complaining of pain in the left hip joint shows a permeative destructive lesion of the ischium. A biopsy of this area showed a malignant round-cell tumor consistent with Ewing's sarcoma.

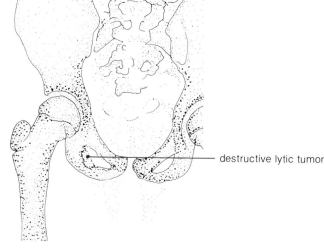

destructive lytic tumor

Fig. 13.9 Roentgenogram of the femur in a 13-year-old child complaining of pain in the thigh shows an extensive permeative lesion in the midshaft of the femur, with elevation of the overlying periosteum, and periosteal new bone formation which is present in several layers, giving an onion-skin appearance. Ewing's tumors are frequently located in the diaphysis, and in this respect are to be distinguished from osteosarcomas, the other common malignant primary tumor of bone in childhood which usually occurs in the metaphysis.

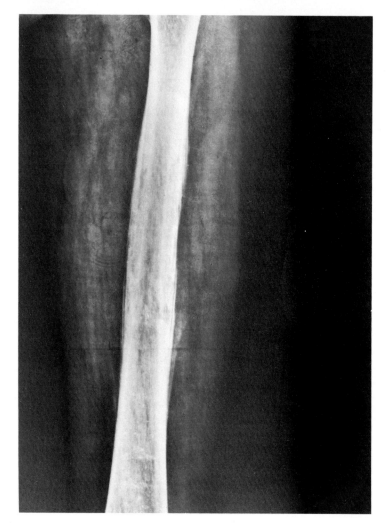

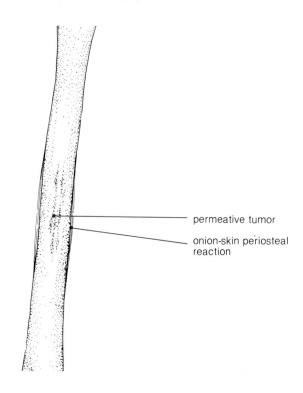

permeative tumor

onion-skin periosteal reaction

sometimes even sclerosis, and classically a laminated periosteal reactive bone likened by some to an onion peel (Fig. 13.9). (This onion peel appearance should, however, in no way be considered diagnostic of Ewing's tumor.) Bone destruction may be severe and, coupled with reactive bone changes, may suggest the radiologic diagnosis of an osteosarcoma.

Gross examination of intact specimens reveals poorly demarcated grayish-white tumor tissue with areas of hemorrhage, cystic degeneration, and necrosis. Actual bone destruction is usually greater than that evident on roentgenograms, and extension of the tumor into adjacent soft tissue is common.

A Ewing's sarcoma consists of a homogeneous population of densely packed small cells. Nuclei are regular and lack prominent nucleoli (Figs. 13.10 and 13.11). The cell wall is indistinct, but it may be visible on tissue touch imprints (Fig. 13.12). Mitoses are infrequent. Reticulin fibers

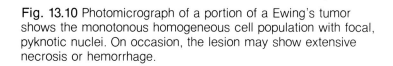

Fig. 13.10 Photomicrograph of a portion of a Ewing's tumor shows the monotonous homogeneous cell population with focal, pyknotic nuclei. On occasion, the lesion may show extensive necrosis or hemorrhage.

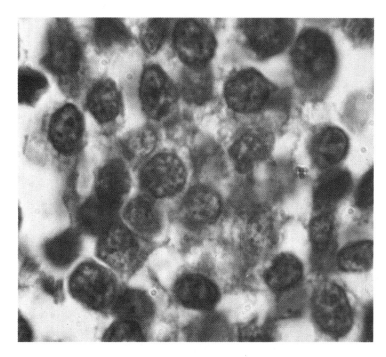

Fig. 13.11 High power view of a portion of a Ewing's tumor shows the small round cells and the indistinct lacy appearance of the cytoplasm. On tissue imprints, a thin rim of cytoplasm may be seen (see Fig. 13.12). Note the lack of prominent nucleoli in these cells.

Fig. 13.12 Photomicrograph of a direct imprint of fresh tumor tissue on a glass slide, subsequently stained with hematoxylin and eosin. By this technique, the cytologic detail of the cells is clearly demonstrated. A thin rim of delicate cytoplasm is seen around the vesicular nuclei, which lack any obvious nucleoli. A mitotic structure is noted in the upper part of the field.

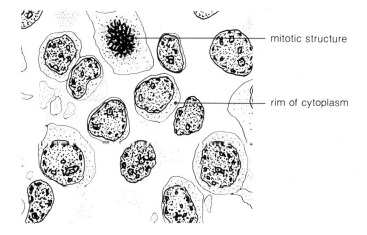

are scarce, but glycogen is evident after PAS staining and is usually found to be abundant on ultrastructural examination (Figs. 13.13 and 13.14). Areas of hemorrhage and necrosis are typically present. Although commonly referred to as a "small-cell tumor," Ewing's cells are actually two or three times larger than lymphocytes.

The differential diagnosis of Ewing's sarcoma includes osteomyelitis, eosinophilic granuloma, and the group of small-cell tumors that includes lymphoma, leukemia, and metastatic neuroblastoma (and, in the case of soft-tissue Ewing's sarcoma, embryonal rhabdomyosarcoma).

Ewing's sarcoma has a high incidence of early metastatic spread, usually to the lung or to other bones. Recent use of adjuvant chemotherapy with radiation and surgical resection has improved the outlook for patients with this tumor.

LYMPHOMA

In clinical cases of lymphoma, involvement of the bone is unusual; however, approximately one-fifth of all lymphomas reveal bone involvement as autopsy. Primary intraosseous lymphomas are uncommon, but it is important to recognize that patients with primary bone lymphomas and no systemic involvement have a substantially better prognosis than those with disseminated disease.

Most primary lymphomas of bone are undifferentiated tumors with a heterogeneous and pleomorphic reticulin-producing cell population. The tumor can occur at any age, but it is rare in patients during the first decade of life (cf., Ewing's sarcoma). Although patients are usually experiencing local pain at the time of presentation, the overall general health of the patient is good. Early changes on roentgenograms include vague, mottled, lucent areas. Considerable bone destruction may result from long-standing lesions.

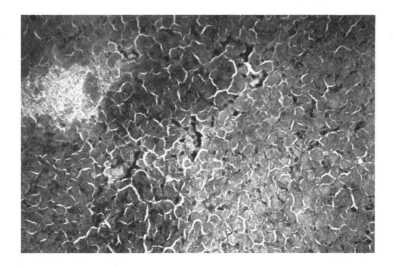

Fig. 13.13 Low power photomicrograph of a Ewing's tumor stained with PAS. The strong positivity of the tumor is due to the presence of glycogen in the tumor cells. If the PAS stain were followed by diastase digestion, the staining material would be digested, thus proving its glycogen character.

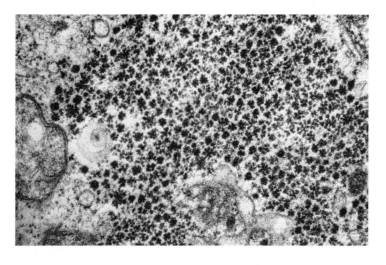

Fig. 13.14 Electron photomicrograph of a Ewing's sarcoma cell shows the packing of cytoplasm with glycogen granules.

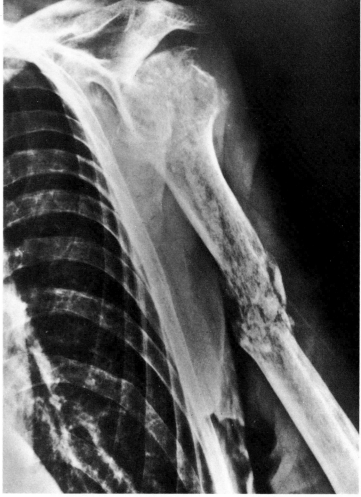

Fig. 13.15 A 45-year-old man complained of sudden onset of pain in the left arm. Roentgenogram shows a pathologic fracture through an area of permeative destruction of cortical and medullary bone. The fracture is quite recent, and there is little or no periosteal reaction either to the tumor itself or to the complicating fracture.

PRIMARY NON-HODGKIN'S LYMPHOMA (*Reticulum cell sarcoma of bone*): Primary non-Hodgkin's lymphomas of bone are usually poorly differentiated, and they generally involve the bones of the extremities. They occur mostly in patients over 20 years of age. The characteristic clinical picture is a patient in generally good health, with localized pain, swelling, or tenderness. No fever or marked weight loss can be noted in the typical case.

On roentgenograms, osteolysis can be seen as the predominant change, with the resulting appearance of a moth-eaten destructive lesion without a periosteal reaction (Fig. 13.15). Gross examination reveals grayish-white tissue infiltrating through the bone (Fig. 13.16).

Histologically, the tumor consists of sheets of poorly differentiated cells, some with distinct cytoplasmic borders (Figs. 13.17 and 13.18). The nuclei are irregular and often cleft, many showing prominent nucleoli. The differential diagnosis includes, in addition to Ewing's tumor, poorly differentiated metastatic carcinoma, melanoma, and, if the tissue is poorly preserved, osteomyelitis. The lack of glycogen (indicated by a negative PAS stain) and the abundance of reticulin fibers separating each cell help to differentiate reticulum cell sarcoma from Ewing's sarcoma (Fig. 13.19).

The treatment of choice is radiation, with wide local excision when possible.

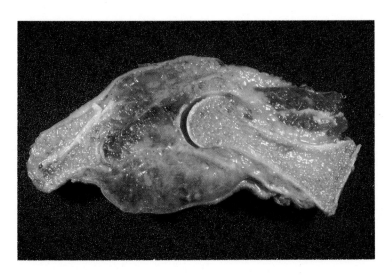

Fig. 13.16 An amputated toe from a patient with a primary non-Hodgkin's lymphoma of the bone. The proximal phalanx has been completely destroyed by a fleshy pink tumor which has extended both dorsally and ventrally into the soft tissue.

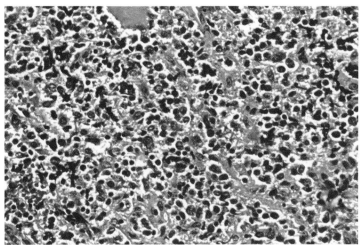

Fig. 13.17 Low power photomicrograph of an area of non-Hodgkin's lymphoma shows the crowded irregular cells. At high power, these cells frequently show nuclear indentation and clefts. When compared with the cells of Ewing's tumor, these cells are larger and the cytoplasmic borders are more distinct. Generally, the cells in a non-Hodgkin's lymphoma lack glycogen.

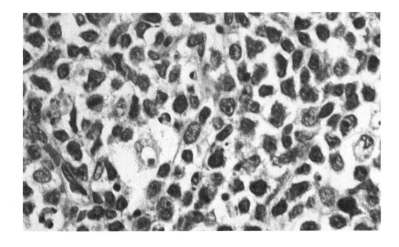

Fig. 13.18 High power photomicrograph of a non-Hodgkin's lymphoma, primary in the bone. The crowded cells are larger and more irregular in outline than those seen in Ewing's sarcoma.

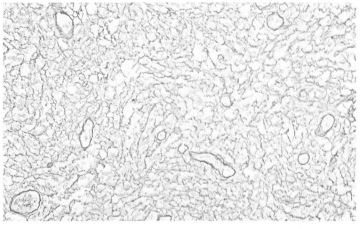

Fig. 13.19 Reticulum staining of the tumor shown in Figs. 13.17 and 13.18 reveals a fine network of reticulum separating small groups of cells as well as individual cells.

HODGKIN'S DISEASE: Hodgkin's disease is characterized by pain and tenderness, sometimes with a palpable mass. Unlike non-Hodgkin's lymphoma, which is more common in the long bones, Hodgkin's disease may appear anywhere in the skeleton. However, primary osseous involvement is rare. Lesions in the ribs and sternum may result in significant swelling and extension into soft tissues. Vertebral involvement may cause neurologic disorders.

The roentgenographic features of Hodgkin's disease are variable; lesions may be lytic, blastic, or mixed. The radiologic finding of a solitary, dense "ivory" vertebra is a classic presentation (Fig. 13.20).

Hodgkin's disease is characterized microscopically by a mixed cell population including plasma cells, lymphocytes, histiocytes, and eosinophils (Fig. 13.21). A large amount of fibrous stroma may complicate the diagnostic process, but the Sternberg-Reed cell is the necessary finding. The Sternberg-Reed cell is large, with sharply delineated, abundant cytoplasm and a mirror-image double nucleus with a large, prominent, central eosinophilic nucleolus (Fig. 13.22). (Large, irregular, mononuclear cells are also seen, with similar nuclear pleomorphism and prominent eosinophilic nucleoli.)

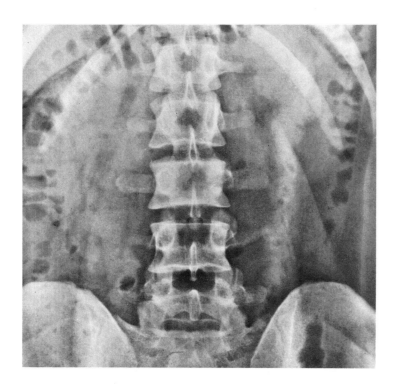

Fig. 13.20 Roentgenogram of the spine in a 28-year-old male who complained of back pain. One can note the increased density of the 3rd lumbar vertebra (also called "ivory" vertebra) without any change in bone contour as would be expected in Paget's disease. Biopsy proved this density to be due to Hodgkin's disease. Ivory vertebra is a classic, though rare, presentation of malignant lymphoma in bone.

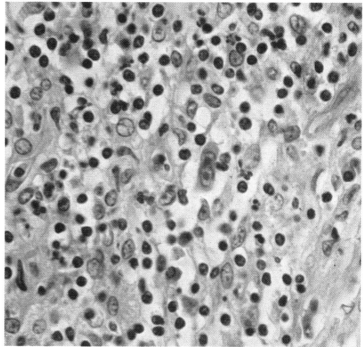

Fig. 13.21 Photomicrograph of an area of Hodgkin's disease in bone shows a fibrous stroma with a mixed cellular infiltrate of small round cells and larger histiocytes.

Fig. 13.22 High power photomicrograph demonstrates a binucleate Sternberg-Reed cell with prominent eosinophilic nucleoli.

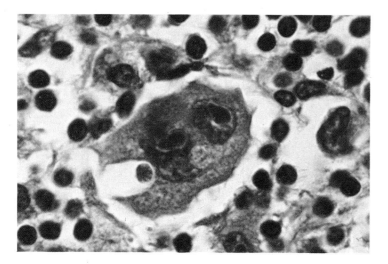

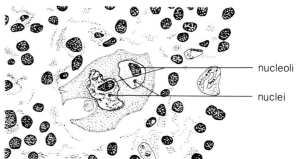

nucleoli

nuclei

MULTIPLE MYELOMA
Plasma cell myeloma
Multiple myeloma is the most common primary malignant tumor of bone, and it most often occurs in individuals over 40 years of age.

The tumor has a predilection for marrow-containing bones such as the skull, ribs, vertebrae, pelvis, and sternum. Multiple, roundish, osteolytic or "punched-out" lesions without sclerotic borders can be seen on roentgenograms (Fig. 13.23). In patients with diffusely disseminated disease, generalized osteoporosis may be evident. Osteoblastic lesions may occur very rarely. At the time of diagnosis, pathologic fractures of bone and, usually, anemia, weight loss, and general malaise may be noted in the patient. Vertebral involvement characteristically presents with pain and radiologic evidence of pathologic fractures, e.g., vertebral wedging or ballooning of the discs (Fig. 13.24).

The production of immunoglobulin by the tumor cells is the key to the diagnosis of myelomas. Analysis of serum and urine shows the monoclonal production of immunoglobulins, which produces a characteristic "spike" during immunoelectrophoresis. Light-chain subunits of immunoglobulins (Bence Jones proteins) are usually found in the urine. Laboratory analysis often reveals hypercalcemia and hypercalciuria.

On gross examination, one may observe discrete nodules in the bone, with replacement of original bone tissue by reddish-pink soft tissue (Figs. 13.25 and 13.26). In patients with the disseminated form of the disease, the tumor may be less apparent.

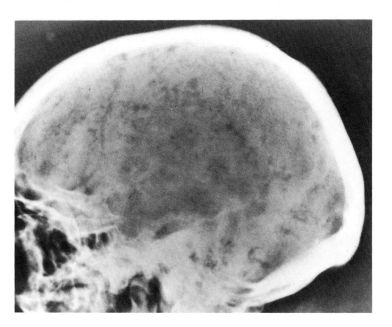

Fig. 13.23 Roentgenogram of the skull of a patient with multiple myeloma reveals multiple, round lytic defects in the bone. Frequently, these lytic defects will show a double or beveled margin.

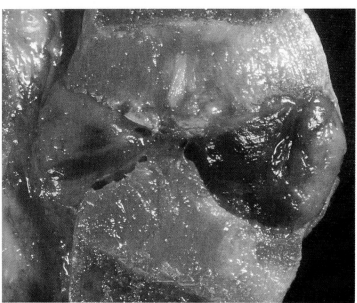

Fig. 13.24 Collapse of the fifth lumbar vertebra and replacement by a gelatinous, pinkish-gray tissue is seen in this gross photograph of the lower spine removed at autopsy from a patient with multiple myeloma.

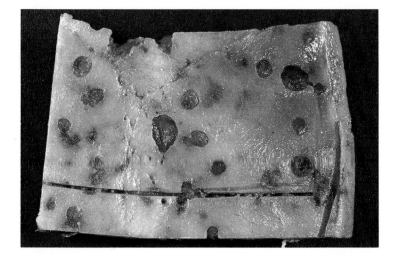

Fig. 13.25 A portion of the skull removed from a patient with multiple myeloma shows numerous round defects filled with pinkish-gray tissue.

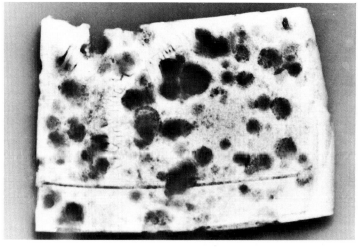

Fig. 13.26 Roentgenogram of the portion of skull shown in Fig. 13.25 demonstrates the clearly demarcated, lytic, punched-out lesions.

Diffuse replacement of the normal hematopoietic tissue by sheets of plasma cells with scant connective tissue stroma can be observed microscopically. The plasma cells may be well differentiated, but they are frequently larger than normal, variable in appearance, and may have double nuclei (Fig. 13.27).

Amyloid-like deposits can be noted in approximately one-fifth of the patients, and these deposits may be evident on gross inspection (Fig. 13.28).

Myelomas are strikingly aggressive tumors, generally resulting in the death of the patient within two years. Chemotherapy protocols have been effective in prolonging survival in some patients.

SOLITARY (LOCALIZED) MYELOMA

Plasmacytoma

The occurrence of a large solitary focus of plasma cell proliferation associated with radiologic evidence of bone destruction can be considered a distinct entity from multiple myeloma if the following criteria are met: There are no other radiographically evident lesions, a bone marrow biopsy from a site other than the solitary focus reveals no malignant cells, and no significant protein or immunoglobulin abnormality is discernible in serum and urine analyses (Figs. 13.29 and 13.30).

Patients who meet these criteria tend to be younger than those with multiple myelomas, and they have a

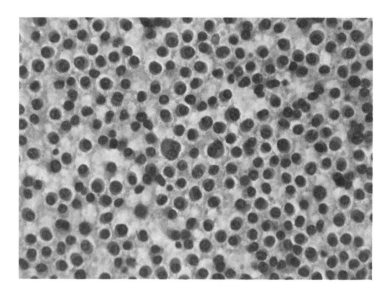

Fig. 13.27 Photomicrograph of a multiple myeloma shows closely packed plasma cells with some variation in shape and size, and an occasional double nucleus.

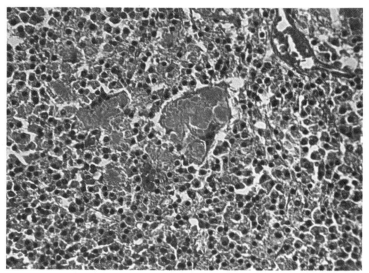

Fig. 13.28 In some cases of multiple myeloma, foci of smooth, homogeneous pink material (amyloid) may be found, as shown in this photomicrograph.

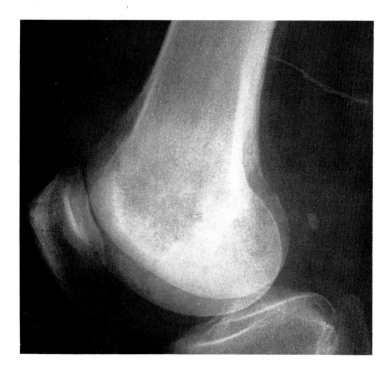

Fig. 13.29 Roentgenogram of a 54-year-old man who complained of severe pain in the knee shows a well-demarcated lytic lesion on the femur that, when biopsied, was found to contain only plasma cells.

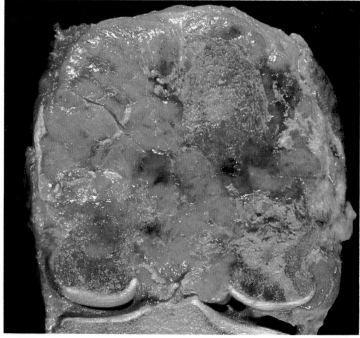

Fig. 13.30 Gross photograph of the specimen obtained from the patient shown in Fig. 13.29. At the time of resection, no other evidence of myeloma was present in this patient.

much better prognosis. The site of involvement is usually in a long bone or a vertebral body (or, in exceptional circumstances, confined to soft tissue). Long-bone lesions may be expansile, and vertebral involvement may lead to spinal cord compression and paraplegia.

The treatment of a solitary myeloma consists of radiotherapy, or an en bloc resection where feasible. Long-term follow-up is essential, since many of these solitary lesions may disseminate after long intervals.

ADAMANTINOMA OF LONG BONES

An adamantinoma is a slow-growing neoplasm of bone that is usually seen in the jaw bones but is sometimes found in long bones, most often the diaphysis of the tibia.

Patients with long-bone lesions are usually between 15 and 30 years of age. The principal clinical sign of an adamantinoma is the insidious onset of pain, sometimes developing over many years. The characteristic roentgenographic findings are a multicystic ("soap bubble") osteolytic lesion with surrounding sclerosis, cortical thinning, and expansion (Fig. 13.31).

The tumor is generally well circumscribed and rubbery in texture; however, focal areas of hemorrhage or necrosis may be evident on gross inspection. The biphasic histologic appearance of spindle-shaped collagen-producing cells alternating with sinewy cords or nests of epithelioid cells is characteristic (Figs. 13.32 and 13.33).

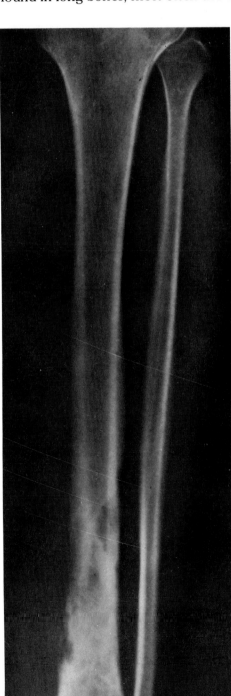

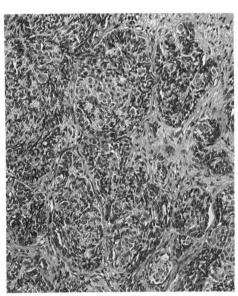

Fig. 13.31 Roentgenogram of the left leg in a young adult patient who complained of an aching pain in the leg shows multiple lytic lesions in the bone, particularly in the lower third of the diaphysis. Note that there is also a well-defined lytic lesion in the upper third of the diaphysis. The lytic, bubbly appearance of the tumor together with the presence of satellite lesions is characteristic of adamantinoma in the tibia. Occasionally, adamantinomas of long bones may also be seen in the fibula, and even more rarely in the long bones of the forearm.

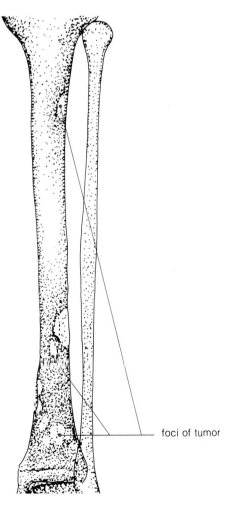

foci of tumor

Fig. 13.32 Photomicrograph of an adamantinoma of the tibia shows a fibrous, stroma with islands of basophilic epithelioid cells that may be sparse focally and show cleftlike spaces (as shown in Fig. 13.33).

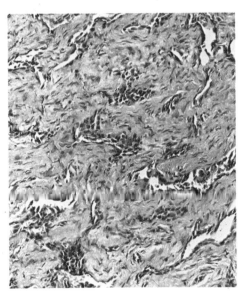

Fig. 13.33 Photomicrograph of an adamantinoma, with a dense fibrous stroma, and cleftlike spaces lined with epithelioid cells.

The histogenesis of this tumor is disputed. Epithelial, vascular, and synovial origins have been hypothesized, but an epithelial origin is favored.

Treatment of adamantinomas consists of adequate surgical excision; the margins of resection should be carefully planned if recurrence is to be avoided, because satellite lesions may occur at some distance from the major tumor mass (Fig. 13.34).

CHORDOMAS

Chordomas are rare, slow-growing, but locally invasive malignant tumors of the vertebral column and base of the skull. These lesions are thought to arise from notochordal remnants, and they have a distinct predilection for the spheno-occipital (≈10 per cent) and sacrococcygeal (≈70 per cent) regions. Patients with cranial chordomas usually complain of pain, headaches, or visual impairment,

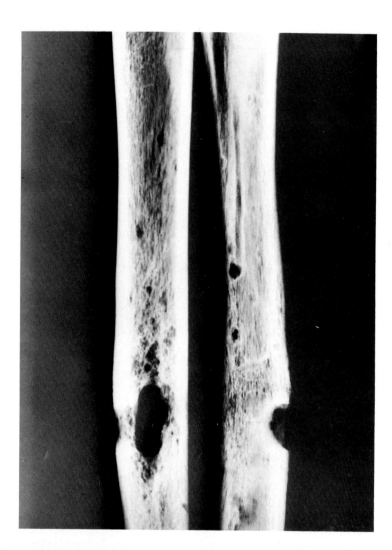

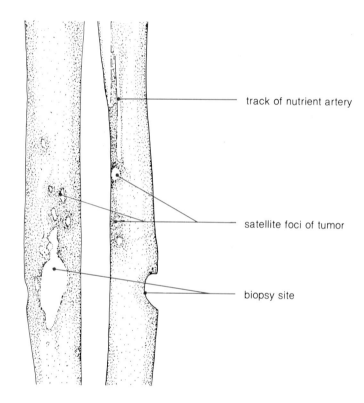

Fig. 13.34 Anteroposterior (left) and lateral (right) roentgenograms of a portion of the tibial diaphysis removed from a 9-year-old boy with adamantinoma of the tibia. Small punched-out lesions not connected with the main tumor mass are clearly evident; on histologic examination, each of these lesions contained tumor. When such satellite lesions are found, a radical resection is necessary if recurrence is to be avoided.

track of nutrient artery

satellite foci of tumor

biopsy site

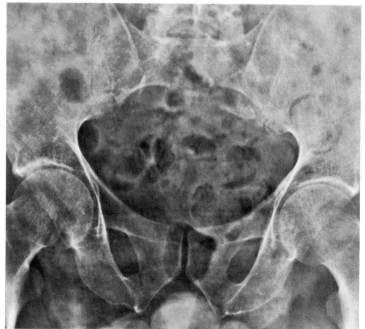

Fig. 13.35 Roentgenogram of a 60-year-old man who complained of pain in the coccygeal region reveals destruction of the sacrum and the coccyx by a large, lytic, expansile lesion, which on biopsy proved to be a chordoma.

whereas those with sacrococcygeal tumors may experience pain, paresthesia, or even paralysis. Roentgenograms show marked bone destruction. Lucent defects with irregular margins and calcification are typical radiologic findings (Fig. 13.35).

Chordomas appear grossly lobulated and well encapsulated, ranging in color from gray to blue. The bulk of the lesion has a gelatinous texture, but extensive evidence of hemorrhage and cystic degeneration is usually present. On microscopic examination, one may note both large vacuolated cells with a soap-bubble (or physaliphorous) appearance (Fig. 13.36), and polyhedral cells with eosinophilic cytoplasm, often arranged in lines or cords (Fig. 13.37). The intercellular matrix consists of mucinous material.

Although radiation may lead to significant tumor regression, the treatment of choice is complete surgical resection (where possible). Less than 50 per cent of all chordomas metastasize, and if they do, it is usually late in the course of the disease.

Reviews of large numbers of spheno-occipital chordomas have revealed a significant cartilaginous component in some of them. These tumors are referred to as "chondroid chordomas" and appear to carry a more favorable prognosis than those lesions with the classic microscopic presentation of chordoma (Fig. 13.38).

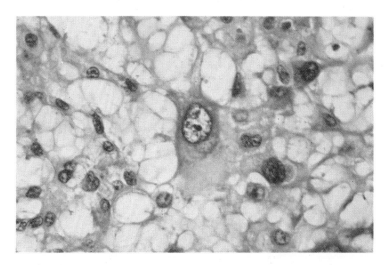

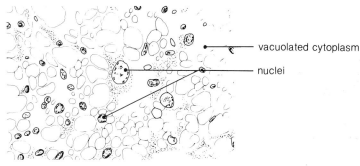

Fig. 13.36 Photomicrograph shows the large variegated and vacuolated cells characteristic of chordoma (physaliphorous cells).

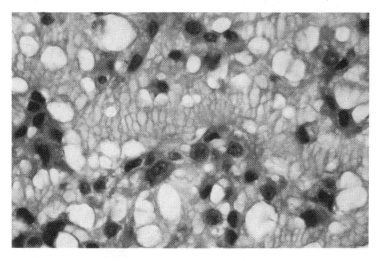

Fig. 13.37 In some areas of chordoma, large mucoid foci are present; in these mucoid areas, cords of eosinophilic cells may be seen (as in this photomicrograph).

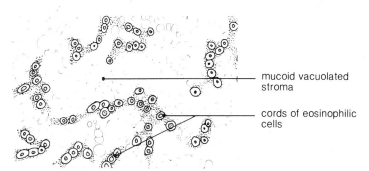

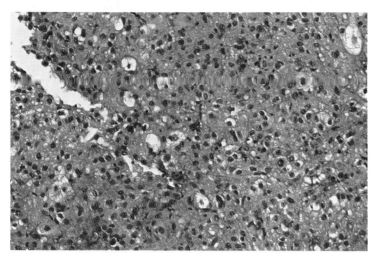

Fig. 13.38 In some patients with chordomas arising in the area of the clivus, the tumor shows a distinctly chondroid appearance (as seen in this photomicrograph). This chondroid pattern is important to recognize, since the prognosis for patients with chondroid chordomas in the base of the skull is much better than for patients with a conventional pattern of chordoma in that area.

Synovial Sarcoma

Synovial sarcomas are rare, malignant neoplasms of unknown histogenesis that involve soft tissue around the joints (Fig. 13.39). Although usually sharply circumscribed, these tumors may extend along fascial planes and invade bone. Only a very small percentage of the lesions directly involve the synovium.

Patients with a synovial sarcoma present with pain or with a slow-growing mass. Most tumors are located in the lower extremity; the major sites of involvement are around the knee joint, the foot, and the thigh. Affected individuals are generally in their third or fourth decade of life; this tumor is decidedly rare in children. A lobulated soft-tissue shadow may be seen on roentgenograms, and irregular spotty calcification is often evident (Fig. 13.40). Although the lesion may grossly appear to be encap-

sulated, on microscopic examination it usually reveals diffuse infiltration of the surrounding tissues. The tumor has a rubbery consistency, and may contain evidence of hemorrhage and cysts. Calcifications are usually visible on gross inspection.

On histologic examination, a synovial sarcoma reveals a biphasic pattern of both pleomorphic spindle cells and well-differentiated cuboidal to columnar cells forming glandlike spaces (Fig. 13.41). The glandular zone contains mucus-like material that stains positively with PAS. Microscopic calcifications are usually found.

Synovial sarcoma has a high rate of local recurrence, as well as metastasis.

Recently, attention has been given to malignant soft-tissue tumors with a monophasic pattern (Fig. 13.42).

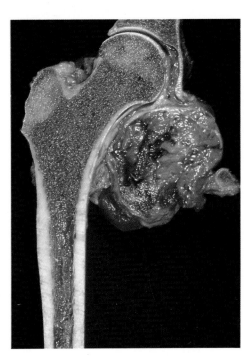

Fig. 13.39 Transected gross specimen of the upper end of the femur and acetabulum shows a soft-tissue solid tumor abutting against the neck of the femur. When examined histologically, this tumor proved to be a synovioma. (Typically, synoviomas do not involve the joint space.)

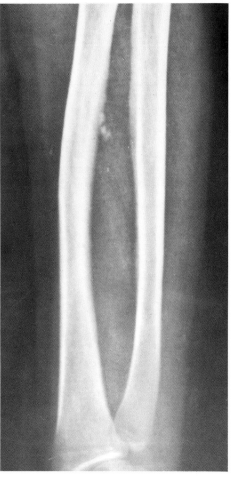

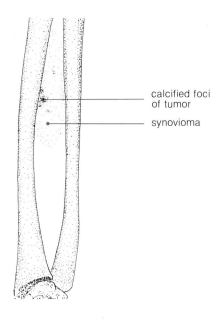

Fig. 13.40 Roentgenogram of a young adult patient who complained of pain and swelling in the right arm reveals a soft-tissue mass lying between the radius and the ulna; within this mass, focal areas of calcification are apparent. On biopsy, this lesion proved to be a synovioma.

calcified foci of tumor

synovioma

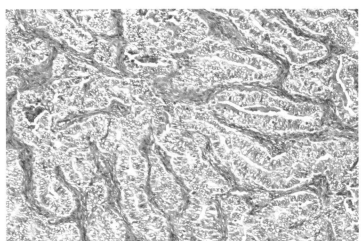

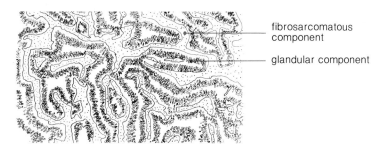

Fig. 13.41 Photomicrograph of a malignant synovioma demonstrates the biphasic appearance of such lesions. Glandlike spaces lined by tall columnar cells are seen, as are fibrosarcomatous stromata. The ratio of these two components may vary considerably; in this example, the glandular component is predominant.

fibrosarcomatous component

glandular component

These tumors are characterized by a malignant spindle cell population, but they lack the gland-forming components typically seen in the classic synovial sarcoma. Some clinicians report a poorer prognosis for patients with the so-called monophasic variant of synovial sarcoma.

The histogenesis of synovial sarcoma remains obscure, and, although the name implies origin from synovial lining cells, true intra-articular synovial sarcomas are distinctly rare.

EPITHELIOID SARCOMA

Epithelioid sarcomas are fully malignant, painless, soft-tissue sarcomas. These lesions occur in the superficial and deep fascia or tendon sheaths (Fig. 13.43) of the hand, wrist, or fingers, but the tumor may also extend to involve the skin. The histogenesis of this neoplasm remains obscure, but a synovial origin has been suggested.

On microscopic examination, an epithelioid sarcoma is found to be a nodular growth composed of a densely eosinophilic polyhedral cell population with prominent nucleoli and an epithelial appearance (Fig. 13.44). Pleomorphism is variable, and central necrosis may be evident. These tumors have a propensity to recur, and they may show lymphatic as well as vascular penetration, eventuating in lung metastases.

Because of the histologic appearance of an epithelioid sarcoma, the differential diagnosis includes a benign reactive granuloma. The treatment of choice is a wide excision.

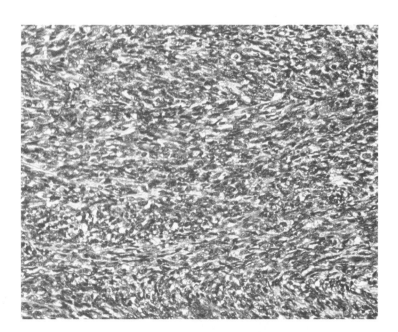

Fig. 13.42 Occasionally, soft-tissue lesions with the clinical presentation of a malignant synovioma have a histologic appearance similar to that demonstrated in this photomicrograph. A cellular spindle cell tumor is evident, without any of the biphasic glandular pattern seen in conventional synoviomas, leading some authors to designate these lesions as monophasic synoviomas. (They may also be considered poorly differentiated spindle cell tumors.)

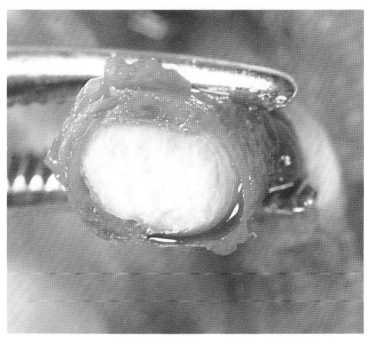

Fig. 13.43 In this patient with an epithelioid sarcoma, the tumor initially arose in the distal portion of the tendon sheath of the extensor policis longus. At amputation, as demonstrated in this photograph, the tumor was found to be in the subsynovial space of the tendon.

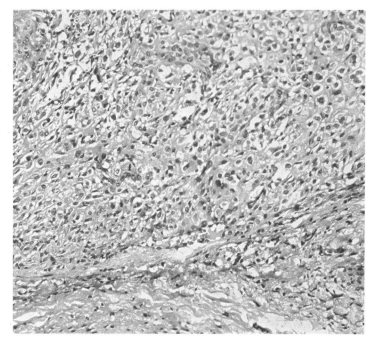

Fig. 13.44 Photomicrograph of an epithelioid sarcoma shows plump oval-to-polyhedral cells which have a dense eosinophilic cytoplasm. The predominant pattern seen here is epithelial, but in other areas a spindle fibrosarcomatous appearance is to be expected.

13.15

PIGMENTED VILLONODULAR SYNOVITIS
Giant-cell tumor of tendon sheath, benign synovioma
Pigmented villonodular synovitis (PVNS) is a locally aggressive synovial tumor of joints and tendon sheaths commonly seen in the knee and finger, but sometimes found in the hip, ankle, toe, and wrist. The lesion is either asymptomatic or only mildly painful; the pain appears to be more severe when the lesion is clinically diffuse in a major joint. In general, the condition is confined to one joint or tendon sheath. (These nodules may be discovered as an incidental finding at surgery, but this presentation is rare.)

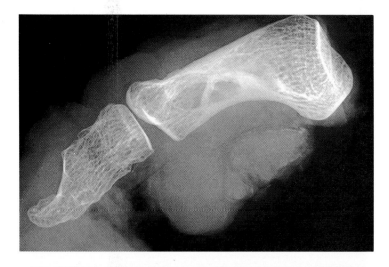

Fig. 13.45 Roentgenogram of a toe amputated because of a soft-tissue mass and intraosseous mass involving the proximal phalanx.

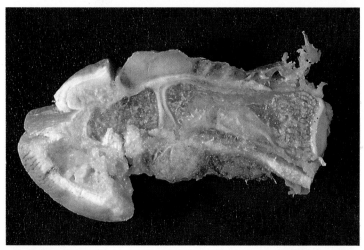

Fig. 13.46 Gross photograph of the specimen shown in Fig. 13.45. A soft-tissue tumor can be seen extending around, and involving, the distal interphalangeal joint. The lesion is also invading the medullary cavity of the phalanx. Focally, the tumor has a tan color. Histologically, this lesion proved to be PVNS.

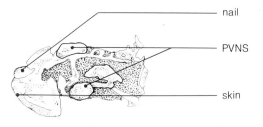

nail

PVNS

skin

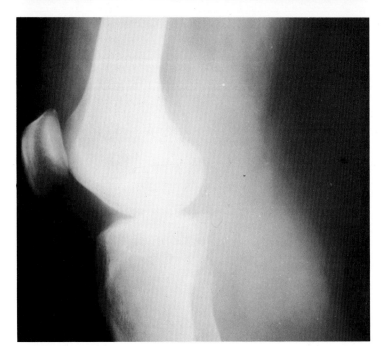

Fig. 13.47 Roentgenogram shows a large soft-tissue mass in the popliteal space in a young male patient with a history of recurrent pain and swelling of the knee. At surgery, the mass was found to result from the extensive infiltration of the synovium by PVNS.

The radiologic signs of PVNS depend on the site of occurrence. In the finger, only soft-tissue swelling may be evident, although cortical bone erosion may occur (Figs. 13.45 and 13.46). In the knee, the only consistently found roentgenographic change is soft-tissue swelling in and around the joint, which may be massive (Fig. 13.47). In the hip, one may note joint narrowing and lytic defects in the bone on both sides of the joint (Figs. 13.48 and 13.49). Local juxta-articular bone destruction may also be quite prominent in joints such as the wrist and ankle.

The lesion is usually solitary and well circumscribed when it occurs in the tendon sheath of a finger (Fig. 13.50). In the knee joint, it may consist of multiple

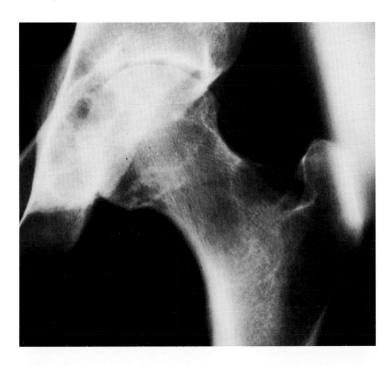

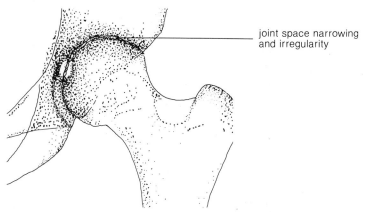

Fig. 13.48 Roentgenogram of a young woman with a history of rapid deterioration of function in the hip shows destructive changes on both sides of the joint, with marked narrowing of the joint space. Because of these roentgenographic findings, a diagnosis of tuberculosis was considered; however, at surgery, abundant hemosiderotic synovium with nodular fleshy areas within it was found.

joint space narrowing and irregularity

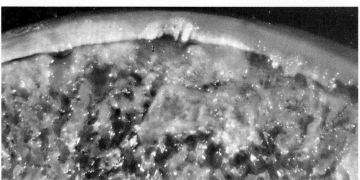

Fig. 13.49 Gross section of the femoral head *(left)* reveals the dissection of the articular cartilage, with a proliferation of soft tissue between the bone and cartilage. Histologic section of this tissue *(right)* reveals the presence of proliferating mononuclear cells and giant cells in the subchondral bone. A diagnosis of pigmented villonodular synovitis was confirmed in this patient.

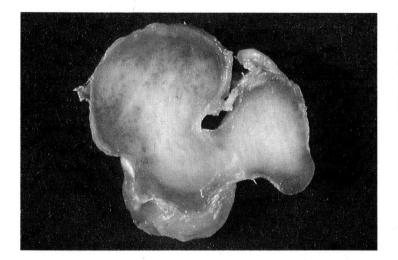

Fig. 13.50 Photograph of a transected nodule removed from a finger. The nodule is firm to palpation, the center of the nodule has a white-yellow appearance, and the pigment seems to be confined to the periphery of the lesion. This appearance is often found in the lesions of PVNS and, in fact, the pigment probably accumulates as a result of secondary hemorrhage into the lesion.

nodules, often with dramatic associated hyperplastic villous changes in the synovium and extensive hemosiderin deposition (Fig. 13.51). All lesions tend to have a tan color when viewed grossly.

On histologic examination, the lesion is found to be a nodule of proliferating, collagen-producing polyhedral cells, often with scattered, multinucleated giant cells (Figs. 13.52 and 13.53). Iron deposits and aggregates of foam cells may be present, but these are usually seen in the periphery of the lesion and are most consistent with secondary changes following hemorrhage into the lesion (Fig. 13.54). The abundant production of collagen may be evident in patients with long-standing disease.

The lesion appears to be localized below the synovial membrane lining cells, which suggests that it arises from a submembrane cell such as a fibrohistiocyte. In general, the lesion is noninflammatory, or only sparsely scattered with mononuclear cells, lymphocytes, and plasma cells. The differential diagnosis of pigmented villonodular synovitis includes hemosiderotic synovitis, which is seen in patients with chronic intra-articular bleeding (e.g., hemophilia). Although a hemosiderotic synovitis lesion contains a significant amount of pigment, it lacks the distinct submembranous mononuclear and giant-cell nodular cellular proliferation which characterizes pigmented villonodular synovitis.

The treatment of PVNS is excision; however, because complete surgical removal is very difficult, clinical recurrence is fairly frequent.

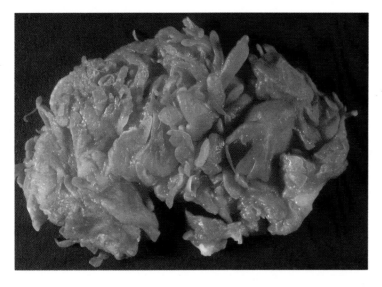

Fig. 13.51 Gross photograph of the synovium resected from the knee of a patient with PVNS. Note the reddish-brown staining due to hemosiderin deposition, as well as the plump papillary projections which result from cell proliferation. This appearance often causes diagnostic confusion with hemosiderotic synovitis (see Fig. 6.24).

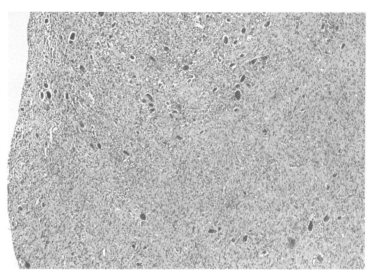

Fig. 13.52 Low power photomicrograph of an area of pigmented villonodular synovitis shows the subsynovial nodular accumulation of mononuclear cells with interspersed giant cells characteristic of PVNS.

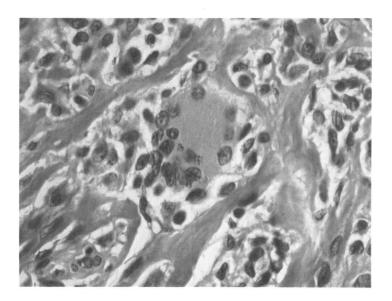

Fig. 13.53 High power photomicrograph of PVNS shows the mononuclear cells, together with the intercellular collagen production and occasional giant cells. Sometimes the collagen may be extremely dense.

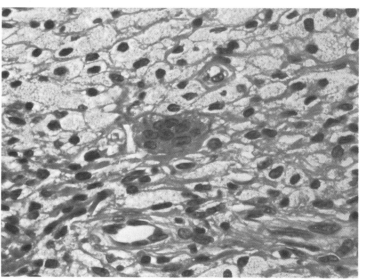

Fig. 13.54 Areas of lipid accumulation are sometimes seen in patients with PVNS. Associated with this condition, one sees the accumulation of foamy macrophages, which are readily apparent in this photomicrograph.

PRIMARY SYNOVIAL CHONDROMATOSIS

Primary synovial chondrometaplasia

Primary synovial chondromatosis is characterized by the proliferation of islands of irregularly cellular cartilage in the synovium of a joint (or tendon sheath) without any underlying arthritis. This finding distinguishes primary synovial chondromatosis from the much more commonly observed occurrence of articular cartilage fragment, often with associated reactive metaplastic cartilage, in the synovial tissues of patients with various types of arthritis. Patients have been observed with primary synovial chon-dromatosis in their second through seventh decades of life, and they usually report the gradual onset of pain, stiffness, or an enlarged mass around the affected joint. Pain and limitation of motion are characteristic findings on clinical examination.

The radiologic signs of this disorder include multiple loose bodies of variable sizes, which may or may not be radiopaque (Figs. 13.55 and 13.56). If the loose bodies are not radiopaque, contrast arthrography may be necessary to demonstrate the lesions (Figs. 13.57 and 13.58).

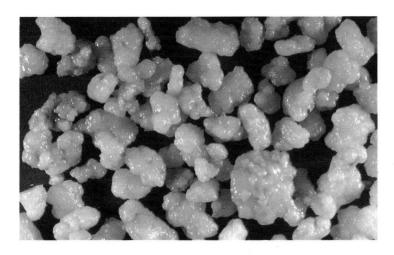

Fig. 13.55 Gross photograph of multiple loose bodies removed from a patient with synovial chondromatosis.

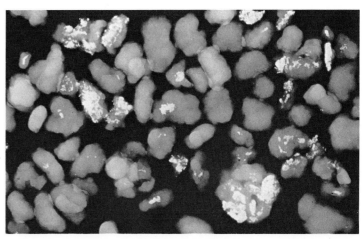

Fig. 13.56 Roentgenogram of the tissue shown in Fig. 13.55 demonstrates that only a few of the loose bodies contain calcium.

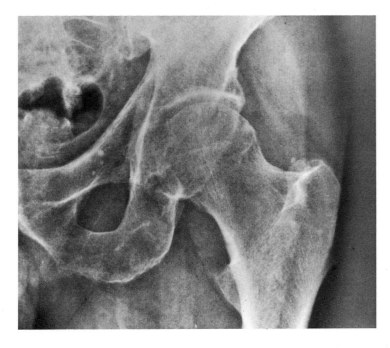

Fig. 13.57 Roentgenogram of a 65-year-old man who presented with an intermittent 20-year history of mild pain in the right hip shows no obvious lesion in the joint. (Courtesy of Dr. Alex Norman.)

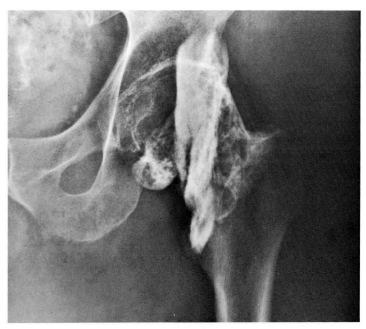

Fig. 13.58 Arthrogram of the patient shown in Fig. 13.57 demonstrates numerous, small, round filling defects in the synovium, symptomatic of synovial chondromatosis. The individual nodules of cartilage were neither calcified nor ossified, and therefore failed to show up on plain roentgenograms. (Courtesy of Dr. Alex Norman.)

Microscopic examination reveals foci of chondromatosis in the synovium, characterized by markedly disorganized cartilage cloning with cytologic atypia (Figs. 13.59 and 13.60). This disordered appearance helps to differentiate primary synovial chondromatosis from the much more common secondary chondromatosis, which occurs in association with traumatic loose bodies, osteochondritis dissecans, etc. (see Chapter 6). Although calcification and endochondral ossification of the cartilage nodules may occur, they are usually irregular and patchily distributed.

These lesions frequently recur after excision.

METASTATIC CANCER

Metastatic cancer is the most frequent malignant tumor found in bone. It is considerably more common than a primary bone tumor, and it usually causes pain. Reflecting the general prevalence of cancer in the population, most bone lesions are metastases from primary lesions in the breast, prostate, lung, or kidney. A diagnosis of neuroblastoma should be considered in patients under the age of five.

On roentgenograms, metastatic tumors may be seen to be sclerotic or lytic, solitary or multiple. In general, whereas purely blastic lesions are seen in the prostate and breast, kidney and thyroid metastases show lytic,

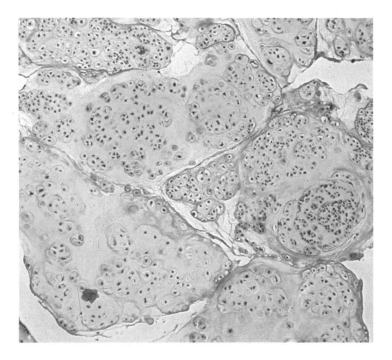

Fig. 13.59 Photomicrograph of the synovium removed from a patient with primary synovial chondromatosis shows nodules of irregular cellular cartilage within the synovium. Some of the cartilage nodules are undergoing endochondral ossification.

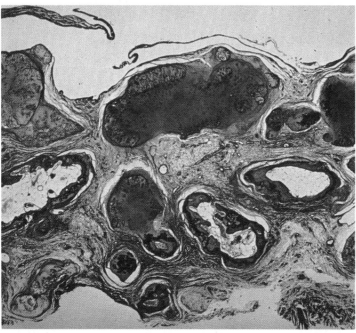

Fig. 13.60 Higher power view of a primary synovial chondromatosis lesion shows the atypical cells, which are crowded and clumped. This histologic picture helps to distinguish primary synovial chondromatosis from the secondary chondromatosis that is frequently seen in association with osteoarthritis and trauma.

often "expansile" qualities. It is not unusual for patients with an undiagnosed primary tumor (e.g., in the kidney) to present initially with a lytic lesion in the bone.

The diagnosis of metastatic disease is often aided by a fine-needle aspiration biopsy. In these circumstances, smears should be made to facilitate the interpretation of fine cytologic detail, and both core bone and blood (clot) should be processed and examined. The blood clot may produce evidence of cancer in many cases in which crushed tumor tissue precludes interpretation of the bone sample (Figs. 13.61 and 13.62).

The identification of the primary site from which the metastasis has originated may be difficult, especially in poorly differentiated neoplasms. Well-differentiated tumors may show squamous pearls if they are from a squamous carcinoma, and mucin-producing glands if they stem from an adenocarcinoma. (It should be noted that whereas gastrointestinal adenocarcinomas usually produce mucin, those from the lung may not, and those from the kidney rarely do.) The clear cells of renal cancer may create considerable diagnostic confusion, suggesting a clear-cell chondrosarcoma or chordoma.

The preferential deposition of tumor cells in bone marrow may be explained by the latter's rich vascularity and large sinusoidal channels.

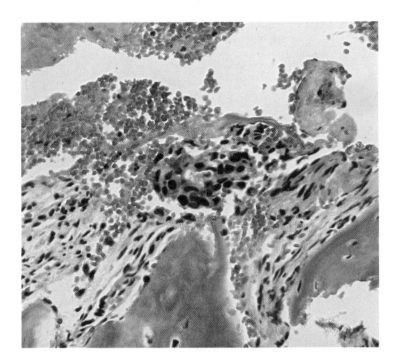

Fig. 13.61 Photomicrograph of a needle biopsy taken from a vertebral body with a sclerotic lesion suspected of arising from metastatic cancer. In the needle biopsy, there is obviously active new bone formation as well as fibrous scarring, and a clump of atypical cells is strongly suggestive of tumor. Definitive diagnosis may be difficult on this type of tissue; however, the aspirated clot seen in Fig. 13.62 is frequently diagnostic.

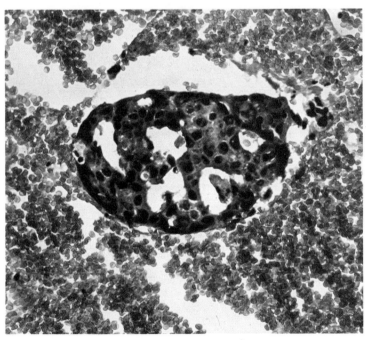

Fig. 13.62 Within the aspirated clot is seen evidence of adenocarcinoma. Often, in needle biopsies of bone, severe crushing artifacts preclude interpretation of the tissue sample. For this reason, aspirated blood should always be submitted for examination, and will frequently give positive results where the tissue is negative or equivocal.

14 Miscellaneous Orthopaedic Conditions

This chapter reviews a number of conditions frequently seen and treated by orthopaedic surgeons. In many of these conditions the etiology is unknown, but in others the causative factor is most likely trauma.

GANGLION

A ganglion is a fibrous, walled cyst filled with clear mucinous fluid, and usually lacking a recognizable lining of differentiated cells (Figs. 14.1 to 14.3). Ganglia occur in

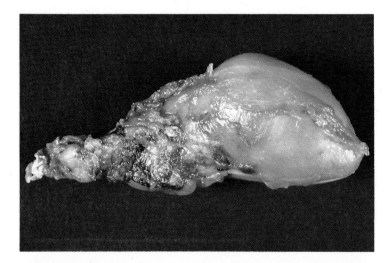

Fig. 14.1 Gross photograph of an intact, excised ganglion cyst. Note its smooth fibrous wall and translucent appearance.

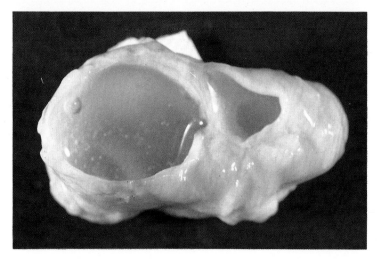

Fig. 14.2 Gross photograph of a bisected ganglion shows a multiloculated cyst filled with clear glairy fluid.

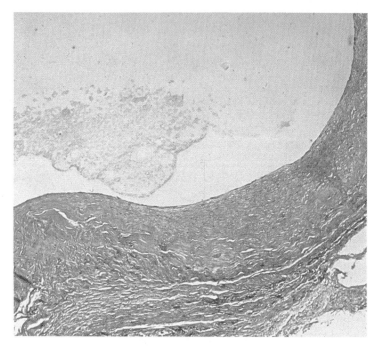

Fig. 14.3 Photomicrograph of a ganglion shows the dense fibrous connective tissue wall, with a thin layer of flattened cells lining the cyst.

the soft tissues, usually dissecting between tendon planes. They are often seen around the hands and feet, particularly on the extensor surfaces near joints. (The most common location is around the wrist joint.)

Ganglia may arise as herniations of the synovium or from mucinous degeneration within dense fibrous connective tissue, possibly secondary to trauma. Rarely, a communication with the joint cavity is demonstrable. On occasion, these lesions may erode the adjacent bone and become totally intraosseous. The most common site for such an intraosseous ganglion is the medial malleolus of the tibia (see Chapter 10).

On histologic examination, inflammation may be observed if the cyst has been previously ruptured. Similar cystic lesions are seen in the parameniscal tissue of the knee joint, usually in proximity to the lateral meniscus (Figs. 14.4 and 14.5).

If troublesome, surgical excision of the cyst is usually the treatment of choice.

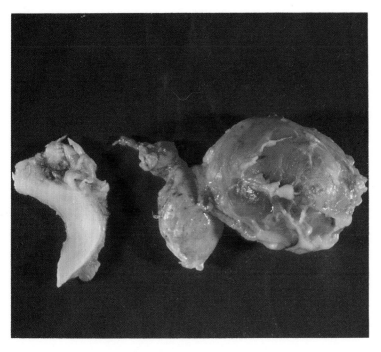

Fig. 14.4 Gross photograph of the lateral meniscus (*left*) and a parameniscal cyst (*right*). As is apparent here, cysts of the lateral meniscus may occasionally grow to a very large size.

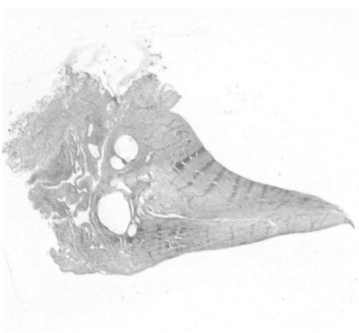

Fig. 14.5 Photomicrograph of a cross section of the lateral meniscus shows focal cystic degeneration in the outer third of the meniscus. Microscopic foci of myxoid degeneration and cystification are common findings in histologic sections of the meniscus.

BURSITIS

Bursitis is characterized by pain, redness, and swelling of one of the many bursae which lie between muscles, tendons, and bony prominences, especially around the joints. It commonly results from chronic trauma, and is frequently seen in the shoulders of professional athletes, and in the prepatellar and infrapatellar bursae of those who frequently kneel (e.g., housewives and the religiously inclined). Bursitis is sometimes seen as a complication of rheumatoid arthritis, particularly in the popliteal area in the form of a Baker's cyst. Occasionally this cyst may extend far into the calf (Fig. 14.6). Bursitis may also result from infection, an example of this being tuberculosis infection of the trochanteric bursae. Sometimes extensive calcification may complicate a chronically inflamed bursa.

On gross examination of an inflamed bursa, the wall of the bursal sac is usually markedly thickened, and the lining is often injected and shaggy in appearance due to fibrinous exudation into the cavity (Fig. 14.7).

Treatment depends on the etiology and extent of the lesion.

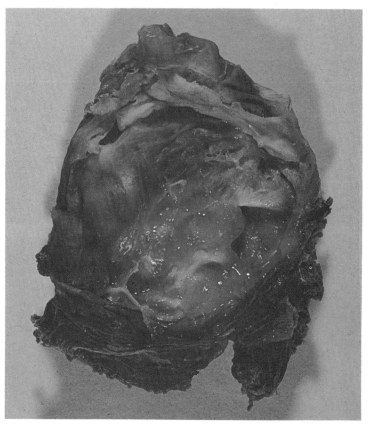

Fig. 14.7 Gross photograph of an excised popliteal cyst, which was opened to demonstrate a thick fibrous wall with a roughened lining, and a fibrinous exudate.

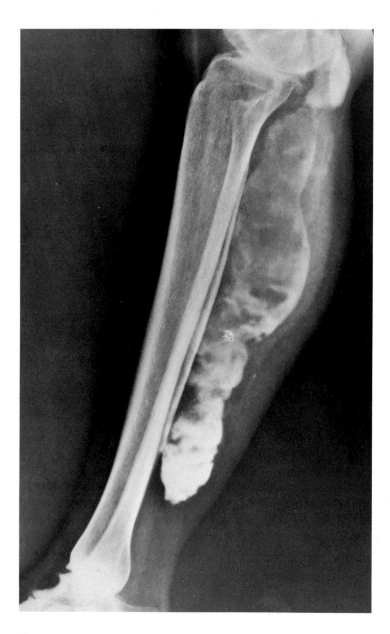

Fig. 14.6 Roentgenogram of a leg from a young woman with a history of juvenile rheumatoid arthritis who complained of fullness in the leg. The injection of a radiopaque dye clearly demonstrates the extent of a Baker's cyst in the popliteal region.

CARPAL TUNNEL SYNDROME

Carpal tunnel syndrome is an entrapment neuropathy caused by pressure on the median nerve as it passes under the transverse carpal ligament and over the hollow of the carpal bones (Fig. 14.8). The cause of the increased pressure varies, but most often it results from synovitis or posttraumatic fibrosis. Occasionally, carpal tunnel syndrome may herald rheumatoid arthritis, and, on rare occasions, it has been found to result from amyloid deposits.

Patients usually complain of night pain, often accompanied by paresthesia in the distribution of the median nerve. In advanced cases, wasting of the thenar muscles may occur.

This syndrome is treated by surgically dividing the transverse carpal ligament. Frequently, at operation, the nerve is seen to be congested above the ligament, and constricted and pale where it lies under the ligament (Fig. 14.9).

Two conditions related to carpal tunnel syndrome are trigger finger and de Quervain's disease (stenosing tenovaginitis of the common tendon sheath of the abductor pollicis longus and the extensor pollicis brevis). In both of these conditions, the free movement of the tendon is blocked due to a focal thickening of the tendon sheath resulting from fibrocartilaginous metaplasia (Fig. 14.10). The treatment is excision.

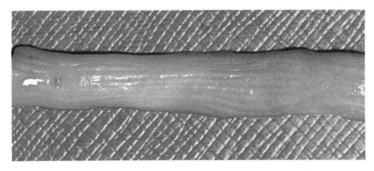

Fig. 14.9 Gross photograph of a segment of the median nerve, resected at autopsy from the part of the nerve that had entered the carpal tunnel. Note the slight constriction and pale appearance in the area of the nerve that had coursed under the transverse carpal ligament.

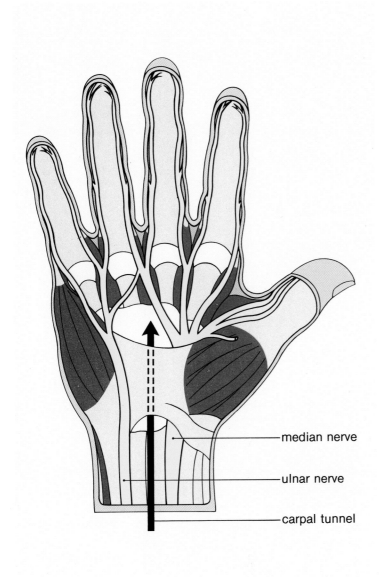

Fig. 14.8 This diagram of a dissected hand shows the median nerve passing through the carpal tunnel and under the transverse carpal ligament.

median nerve

ulnar nerve

carpal tunnel

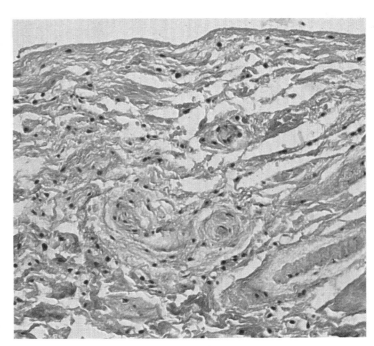

Fig. 14.10 Photomicrograph of a section of the tendon sheath from a patient with de Quervain's disease. Normally, the tenosynovium is a delicate structure consisting of a single layer of flattened synovial cells resting on a delicate fibroadipose tissue. Here, however, one sees extensive fibrocartilaginous metaplasia in the wall of the tendon sheath, characteristic of the foci of thickening normally seen in trigger finger and de Quervain's disease.

MORTON'S NEUROMA

Morton's neuroma is a distinct, clinicopathologic entity characterized by the thickening and degeneration of one of the interdigital nerves of the foot, most commonly that between the third and fourth metatarsal heads. The patient, usually a woman, experiences sharp shooting pains that are worse when standing. These pains characteristi-cally begin in the sole of the foot and radiate to the ex-terior surface. At surgery, a fusiform swelling proximal to the bifurcation of the plantar interdigital nerve is seen, and the resected specimen usually includes the neuro-vascular bundle (Fig. 14.11).

Histologic sections generally show three characteristic features: (1) endarterial thickening of the digital artery

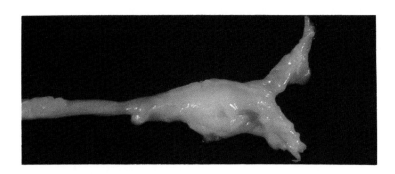

Fig. 14.11 Gross photograph of a segment of the plantar interdigital nerve resected from the space between the third and fourth metatarsal heads in a patient with Morton's neuroma shows fusiform swelling of the neurovascular bundle just proximal to the bifurcation.

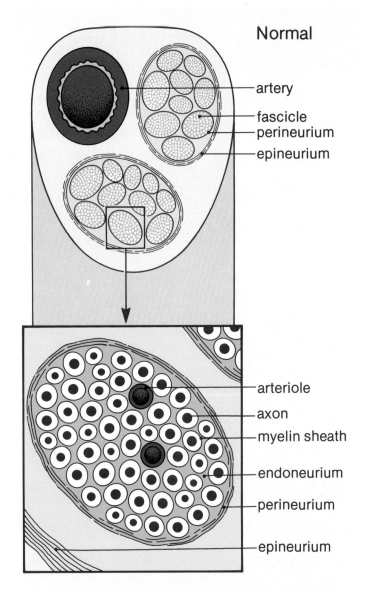

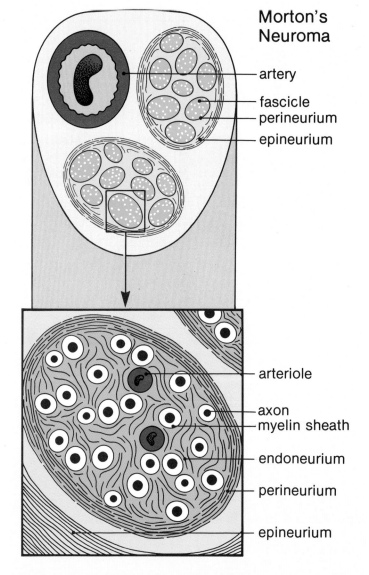

Fig. 14.12 (*Left*) Schematic diagram of a normal neurovascular bundle illustrating the relationship of the digital nerves and artery. (*Right*) Schematic diagram of the neurovascular bundle from a patient with a Morton's neuroma. Note the increased fibrosis in the epineurium, perineurium, and endoneurium. In addition, there is marked endothelial thickening of the artery, with narrowing of the lumen.

and, often, thrombosis and occlusion of its lumen; (2) extensive fibrosis both around and within the nerve, giving rise to demyelinization and a marked depletion of axons within the digital nerve; and (3) evidence of Schwann cell and fibroblast proliferation (Figs. 14.12 and 14.13). These findings are most consistent with recurrent nerve trauma, probably resulting from the wearing of poorly fitting shoes.

Morton's neuroma should be differentiated from an amputation or traumatic neuroma resulting from transection of a nerve bundle which is not immediately repaired. These lesions are frequently painful, and at operation a bulbous swelling is usually found at the severed nerve ending (Fig. 14.14). On microscopic examination, this nerve ending shows numerous proliferating nerve bundles within scar tissue (Fig. 14.15).

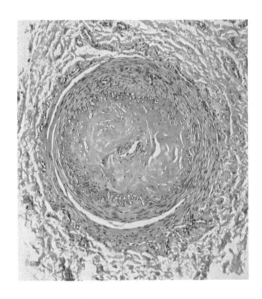
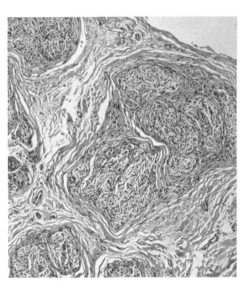
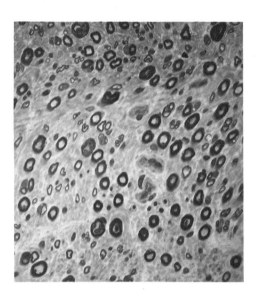

Fig. 14.13 (*Left*) Histologic section of a narrowed and occluded vessel from a patient with Morton's neuroma. (*Center*) The increased fibrosis of the nerve can be appreciated in this histologic section. (*Right*) High power photomicrograph of a single nerve fascicle shows the loss of myelinated nerve fibers together with increased endoneural fibrosis.

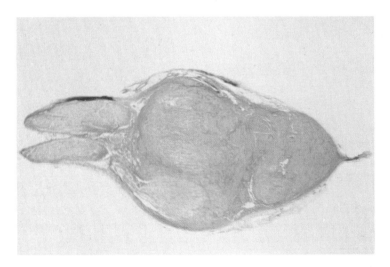

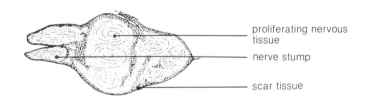

Fig. 14.14 Low power histologic section of an amputation neuroma stained with Masson trichrome shows the increased fibrous scar tissue. The proximal nerve stump is seen at left.

proliferating nervous tissue
nerve stump
scar tissue

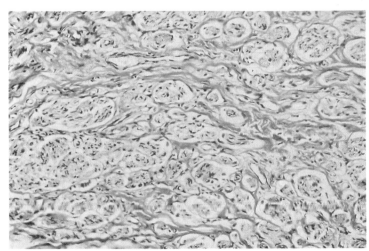

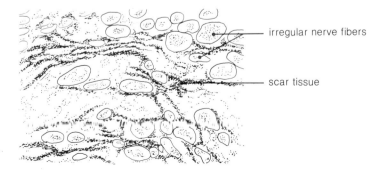

Fig. 14.15 High power photomicrograph of the section shown in Fig. 14.14 demonstrates the proliferating irregular nerve fibers coursing through the scar tissue, characteristic of an amputation neuroma.

irregular nerve fibers
scar tissue

14.7

COMPARTMENT SYNDROME
Volkmann's ischemic contracture

Compartment syndrome, i.e., swelling and ultimately loss of viability of a muscle group, results from compromised circulation within a confined anatomic space. Most commonly the condition is seen in the anterior tibial compartment and the deep posterior tibial compartment of the leg, in the volar compartment of the forearm, and in the interosseous compartments of the hand.

Generally, compartment syndrome results from trauma to an extremity (usually a fracture or crash injury), and recently the disorder has been noted in patients suffering from drug overdose. Vascular occlusion from either direct injury or increased pressure within the anatomic compartment results in diminished tissue function and viability. Muscle necrosis ensues and, eventually, the original tissue is replaced by dense, fibrous connective tissue, with subsequent deformity and loss of function (Figs. 14.16 to 14.18).

Treatment of the acute condition is aimed at relieving the pressure by fasciotomy, the removal of tight bandages, or whatever is appropriate to the circumstances.

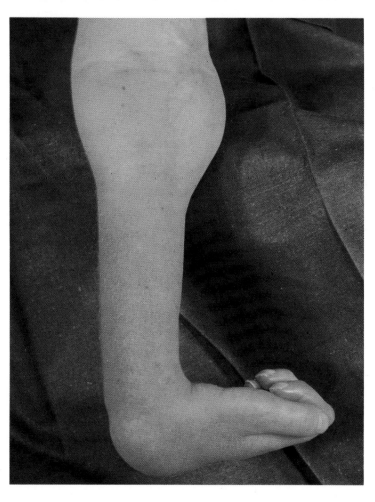

Fig. 14.16 Clinical photograph of the arm in a patient who developed compartment syndrome following multiple injuries to the elbow and forearm. Note the severe flexion contractures.

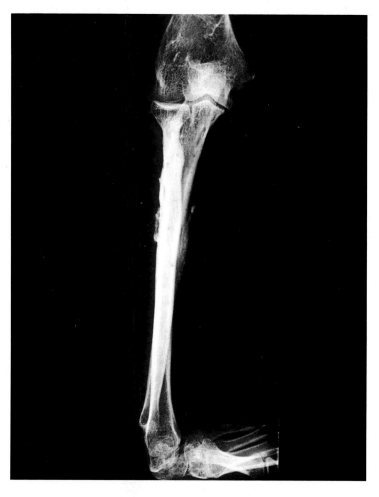

Fig. 14.17 Roentgenogram of the arm shown in Fig. 14.16. In addition to evidence of traumatic arthritis, there is also some shortening of the ulna, and mature bone formation around the ulna and radius in the upper third of the forearm.

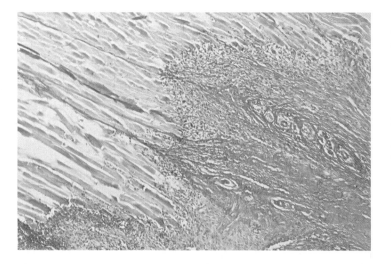

Fig. 14.18 Histologic section through a part of the muscle mass of the anterior tibial compartment involved in compartment syndrome reveals extensive muscle necrosis, with an inflammatory reaction and fibrous replacement.

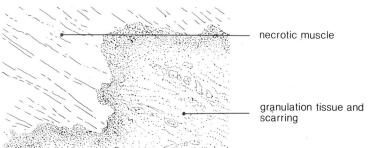

necrotic muscle

granulation tissue and scarring

CONGENITAL PSEUDARTHROSIS

A pseudarthrosis (false joint) developing in the shaft of the tibia (or of the ulna) may manifest at birth or during infancy. Usually the lesion is seen at the level of the junction of the middle and lower third of the bone shaft. This type of pseudarthrosis is considered congenital, and is a distinct orthopaedic entity.

Roentgenographic evaluation reveals a lucent defect in the diaphysis of the affected bone, which is associated with a characteristic tapering of the bone ends at the site of the pseudarthrosis (Fig. 14.19). Histologic examination reveals dense, fibrous connective tissue filling the defect (Fig. 14.20).

Neurofibromatosis is present in a high percentage of children with this condition, and as many as 10 per cent of patients with neurofibromatosis show the disorder. Nevertheless, neurofibromas are not usually seen in histologic specimens from the involved site.

These lesions usually prove to be very refractory to treatment.

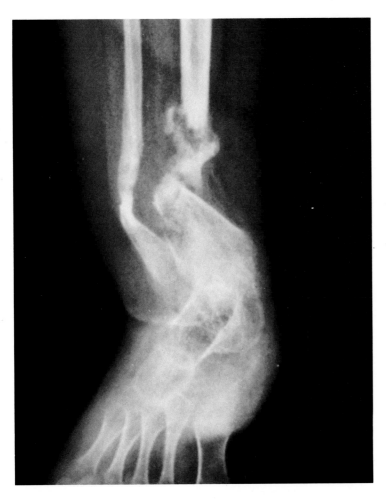 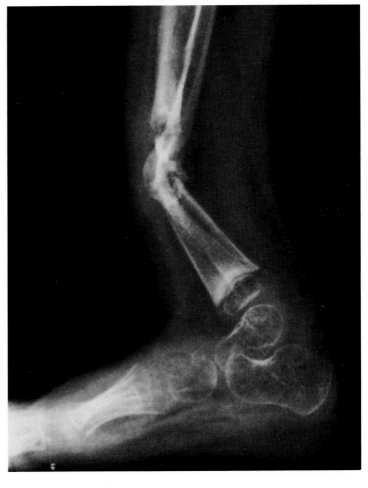

Fig. 14.19 Anteroposterior (*left*) and lateral (*right*) roentgenograms of a young boy with congenital pseudarthrosis of the tibia and fibula. The appearance of the lesion at the junction of the middle and lower third of the bones and the tapering of the bone ends are characteristically found in patients with congenital pseudarthrosis.

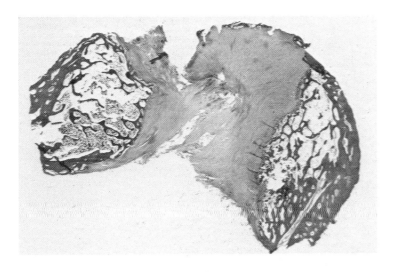

Fig. 14.20 Histologic section of a congenital pseudarthrosis of the clavicle shows that the gap in the bone is filled with dense. fibrous connective tissue, with no significant new bone formation.

14.9

SLIPPED CAPITAL FEMORAL EPIPHYSIS
Adolescent coxa vara

Slipped capital femoral epiphysis is the painful spontaneous disruption of the epiphyseal plate of the hip, usually in overweight adolescents, and occurring at the time of the growth spurt. The condition may be unilateral or bilateral. Early clinical complaints are pain or limping, with eventual limitation of mobility.

On roentgenograms, early displacement may be evident only as a backward (or dorsal) displacement on lateral films (Fig. 14.21). Eventually there is obvious separation of the femoral head and neck, with resultant coxa vara. Valgus presentation is rare.

The histologic appearance of the epiphyseal growth plate may be markedly irregular and thicker than normal. Orderly endochondral ossification is disturbed, and hemorrhage is often present between the growth plate and the primary spongiosa (Figs. 14.22 and 14.23).

The condition may result from the widening of the growth plate and increased vascularity at the time of accelerated skeletal growth. These circumstances would

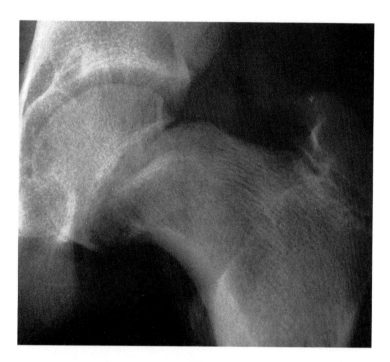

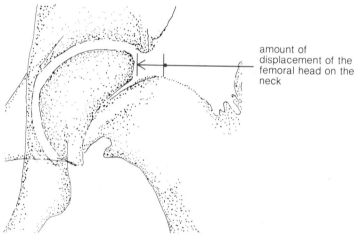

Fig. 14.21 Clinical roentgenogram of the hip joint in a patient with a significant slipped epiphysis. The displacement of the capital femoral epiphysis on the neck of the femur can be readily appreciated.

amount of displacement of the femoral head on the neck

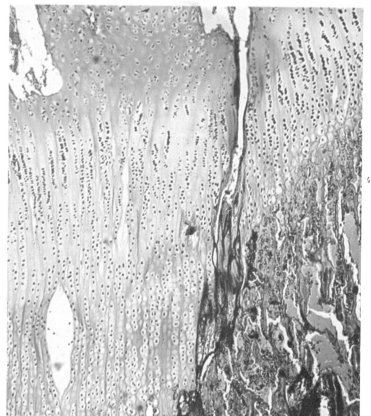

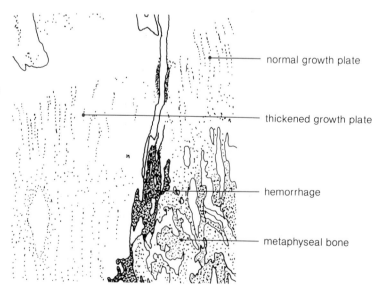

Fig. 14.22 In this low power photomicrograph taken during an early stage of slipped epiphysis, before extensive displacement has occurred, it is possible to see focal thickening of the growth plate, and separation of the growth plate from the underlying metaphysis by hemorrhagic tissue.

normal growth plate

thickened growth plate

hemorrhage

metaphyseal bone

lead to an increased propensity to shearing in the angulated growth plate of the femoral neck.

In blacks, an increased incidence of chondrolysis has been noted in association with a slipped epiphysis. Patients with the combined disorder have been shown to have elevated levels of immunoglobulins and the C3 component of complement. These findings suggest a localized antigen-antibody–mediated effect as part of a more systemic disorder.

Treatment of a slipped epiphysis is generally by internal fixation of the femoral head.

CONGENITAL DISLOCATION OF THE HIP

Congenital dislocation of the hip is a relatively uncommon abnormality in which the femoral head is not properly positioned in the acetabular fossa at the time of birth (Fig. 14.24). Not a true congenital malformation, it is a deformity subsequent to mechanical and/or physical factors that lead to instability of the hip in a newborn. These factors may include tight maternal abdominal and uterine musculature, breech presentation, maternal hormones such as estrogen and relaxin (which affect fetal as well as maternal ligamentous laxity), or forced hip extension

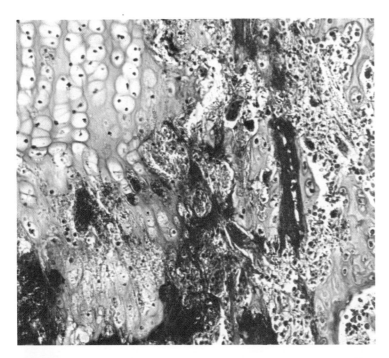

Fig. 14.23 High power photomicrograph of the tissue in Fig. 14.22 shows focal hemorrhage between the growth plate and the metaphysis. It is postulated that such hemorrhagic tissue serves to block continued endochondral ossification, and consequently the growth plate becomes thicker due to the lack of endochondral ossification and conversion to bone.

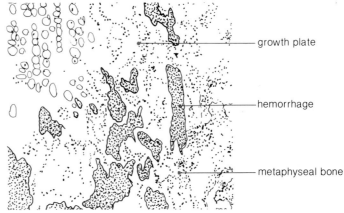

Fig. 14.24 Roentgenogram of a young child with untreated congenital dislocation of the hips reveals that both hips are dislocated, and the roof of the acetabulum appears poorly formed. Following reduction, this patient developed avascular necrosis of the right hip, a common complication.

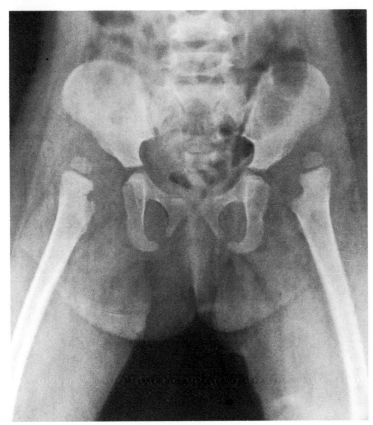

following birth. The left hip is more often involved, but bilateral occurrences may be observed in more than 25 per cent of patients.

Treatment consists of early detection and reduction, i.e., the return of the femoral head to its normal position as soon as possible after birth. However, in persistent dislocation resulting from delayed diagnosis, the bone and soft tissue adjacent to the joint undergo reactive changes that preclude easy reduction. Both the acetabulum and femoral head become irregularly contoured (Fig. 14.25). Forceful attempts at reduction may compromise the blood supply and lead to avascular necrosis.

In untreated patients, secondary osteoarthritis develops relatively early in life. Sometimes, hip dysplasia (malformation of the joint) occurs without an obvious cause like congenital dislocation of the hip (Fig. 14.26). This type of congenital malformation will also contribute to the early onset of secondary osteoarthritis.

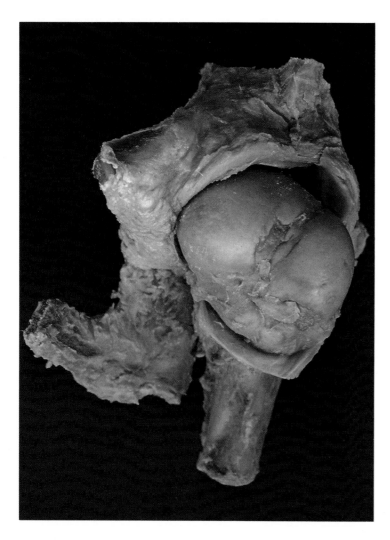

Fig. 14.25 An anatomic dissection from a young child with congenital dislocation of the hip that was not reduced. Note the deformity of the femoral head, which has developed a saddle-shaped groove across its superior portion. On clinical roentgenograms, this groove may give the appearance of a double head.

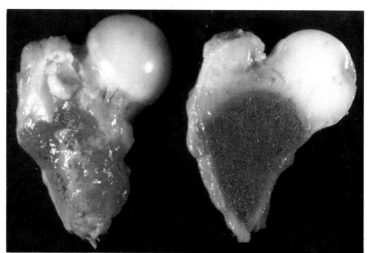

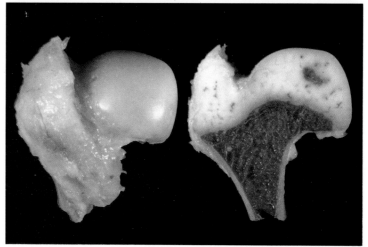

Fig. 14.26 (*Upper*) The upper end of the femur, whole and in coronal section, from a normally developed hip in a newborn. (*Lower*) The upper end of the femur, whole and in coronal section, from an infant with hip dysplasia shows the abnormal configuration of the femoral head and growth plate.

OSTEOCHONDRITIS DISSECANS

Osteochondritis dissecans is a benign noninflammatory condition of diarthrodial joints that affects young adults. The disorder is characterized by a demarcated fragment of bone and overlying articular cartilage that may be separated from the articular surface. The condition most commonly involves the lateral aspect of the medial femoral condyle and, less commonly, the posteromedial aspect of the talus and anterolateral aspect of the capitellum. Patients complain of joint pain, often with joint effusions and occasional locking of the joint.

Although osteochondritis dissecans is unilateral in most instances, it may be bilateral and symmetrical. Familial cases of osteochondritis dissecans have been reported, and the disorder is probably transmitted as an autosomal-dominant condition. Affected children are often short in stature and may have an endocrine dysfunction.

On roentgenograms one sees a well-demarcated defect in the articular surface of the affected joint (Fig. 14.27). The gross appearance is characterized by a flat, smooth nodule formed of avascular bone, with overlying viable articular cartilage (Fig. 14.28). A layer of dense, fibrous connective tissue or fibrocartilage usually forms on the bone surface (Fig. 14.29).

Treatment consists of either reattachment of the loose body (where feasible) or excision.

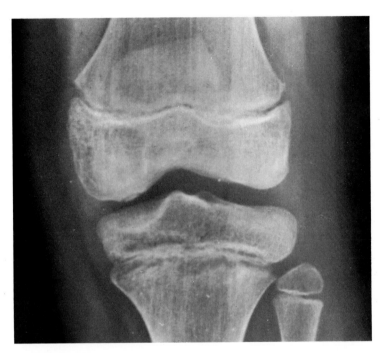

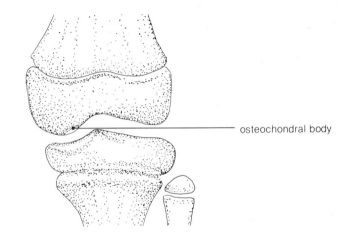

Fig. 14.27 Roentgenogram of the knee in a 12-year-old boy who complained of discomfort in the joint shows a well-demarcated defect on the articular surface of the medial femoral condyle. At this point the osteochondral body has not separated from the condyle and is still in situ.

osteochondral body

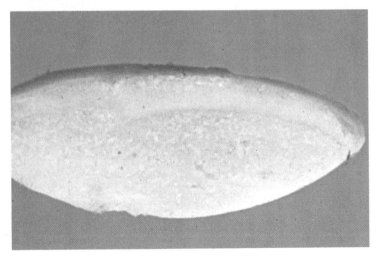

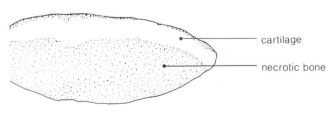

Fig. 14.28 Cross section of a loose body removed from a patient with osteochondritis dissecans shows a layer of apparently normal cartilage on one surface and, underlying the cartilage, a segment of necrotic bone having a smooth contour on its osseous surface.

cartilage

necrotic bone

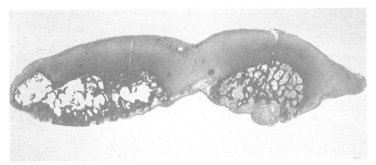

Fig. 14.29 Histologic section of an osteochondral loose body from a patient with osteochondritis dissecans shows a layer of intact fibrocartilage overlying a segment of necrotic bone.

PALMAR AND PLANTAR FIBROMATOSIS
Dupuytren's contracture

These conditions are characterized by fibroblastic tissue that, by their cellularity and capacity to infiltrate surrounding tissue, mimic a fibrosarcoma. However, these lesions do not metastasize. They occur in many parts of the body and are generally referred to as the fibroma-toses. Of particular interest to the orthopaedic surgeon are palmar fibromatosis (Dupuytren's contracture) and its plantar equivalent.

Palmar fibromatosis usually occurs in older adults; it is more common in men than women, and is frequently bilateral. In some instances it is associated with alcoholic cirrhosis of the liver. Patients present with nodular

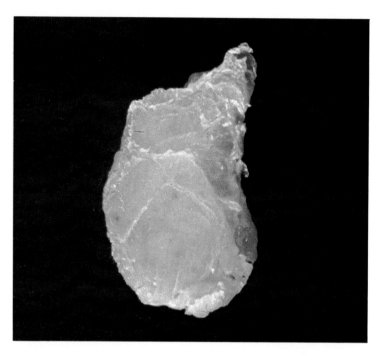

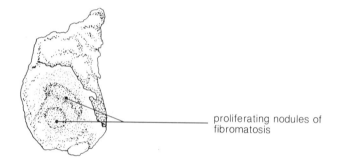

Fig. 14.30 Cross section of the thickened palmar fascia removed from a patient with Dupuytren's contracture. The aponeurotic tissue has a grayish-white, glistening appearance, and within this tissue can be seen thickened nodular areas having a more opaque, white-orange appearance. These areas represent the foci of proliferating fibromatosis. In long-standing Dupuytren's contracture, the entire aponeurosis may be scarred, and the proliferating nodules are no longer evident.

proliferating nodules of fibromatosis

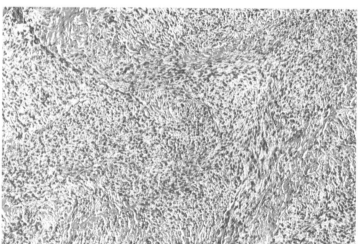

Fig. 14.31 Low power photomicrograph of one of the proliferative nodules found in Dupuytren's contracture shows strands of dense collagenized tissue passing through a cellular stroma.

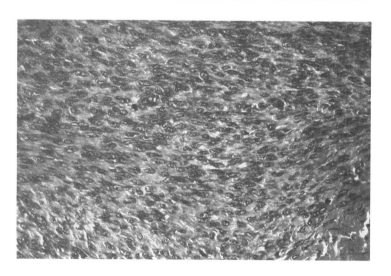

Fig. 14.32 High power photograph of Fig. 14.31 shows the packed but regular spindle cells characteristically found in Dupuytren's contracture. Mitoses are evident and may be quite numerous; however, atypical mitoses are not seen.

thickening of the palmar fascia (Fig. 14.30), and flexion contracture of the fingers (usually the third, fourth, and fifth). On histologic examination, the lesions are seen to vary in cellularity; some are very cellular and others are heavily collagenized (Figs. 14.31 and 14.32).

Plantar fibromatosis tends to occur in younger patients, is more aggressive, and presents with larger nodules than are usually found in patients with palmar fibromatosis (Figs. 14.33 to 14.36). However, plantar fibromatosis is not associated with the formation of contractures.

Surgical excision is the treatment of choice; however, due to the infiltrative nature of the lesion, local recurrence is common.

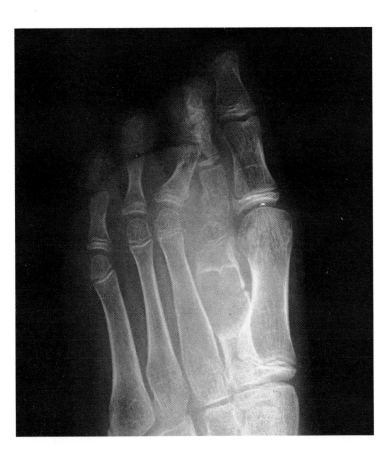

Fig. 14.33 Roentgenogram of a 13-year-old girl with a history of two excisions of plantar fibromatosis who was admitted to the hospital due to recurrence with bony involvement. Both soft-tissue swelling and invasion of the second metatarsal bone can be appreciated.

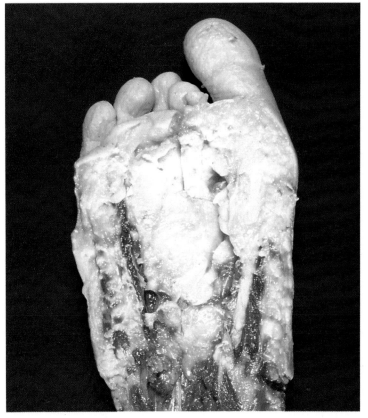

Fig. 14.34 This amputated specimen from the patient in Fig. 14.33, with plantar skin removed, clearly shows the extent of the tumor.

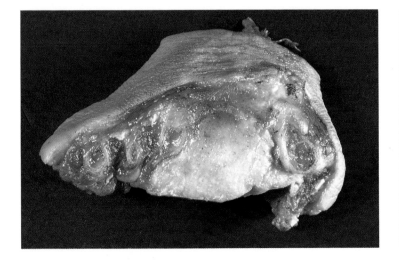

Fig. 14.35 Cross section of the foot shown in Fig. 14.34 demonstrates both the extent of tumor infiltration, and involvement of the second metatarsal bone.

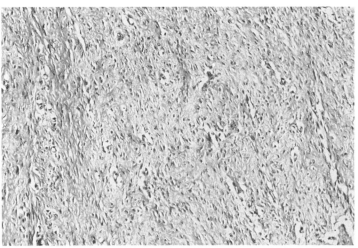

Fig. 14.36 Low power photomicrograph of the tumor illustrated in the previous three figures demonstrates the bland appearance of the plantar fibromatosis tissue.

MYOSITIS OSSIFICANS

Myositis Ossificans Progressiva. Two entirely separate conditions are described by the general diagnostic term "myositis ossificans." Myositis ossificans circumscripta will be discussed later. The other condition, myositis ossificans progressiva, is a rare progressive disease in which groups of muscles, tendons, and ligaments (usually the muscles of the back and those around major joints) become progressively ossified, thereby producing severe functional disability (Figs. 14.37 and 14.38). Symptoms of the disease usually begin in childhood or adolescence. In some cases the condition is inherited, and several members of a family may be affected.

Microscopic examination reveals poorly organized bone (both lamellar and woven), dense, fibrous scar

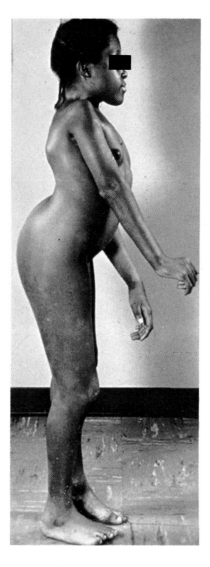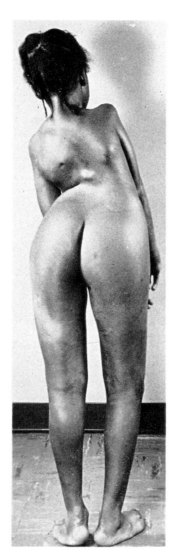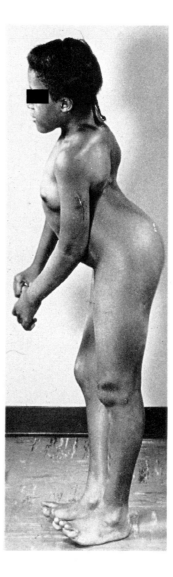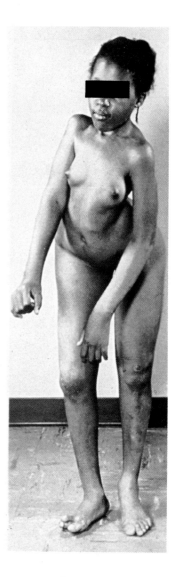

Fig. 14.37 These photographs demonstrate the severe deformities of the limbs, spine, and neck resulting from myositis ossificans progressiva.

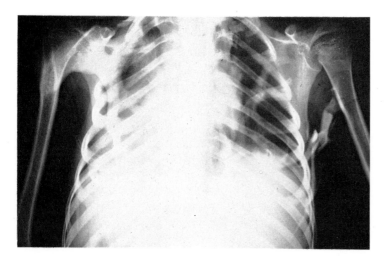

Fig. 14.38 Clinical roentgenogram of the patient in Fig. 14.37 shows ossification around both shoulder joints as well as in the paravertebral area.

tissue, and islands of poorly formed cartilage (Figs. 14.39 and 14.40). This disorder is generally fatal because of the progressive functional disability, including loss of pulmonary function.

Myositis Ossificans Circumscripta. Myositis ossificans circumscripta is a solitary, nonprogressive, benign ossifying lesion. The patient usually presents with a lump in a muscle that has been evident for some weeks and may have been somewhat painful. A history of trauma can usually be elicited, but the traumatic incidents are trivial in nature. A roentgenogram taken soon after the onset of symptoms may not reveal an opaque area, but within a week or two a poorly defined shadow will appear. Over succeeding weeks the periphery of this shadow becomes increasingly well delineated from the surrounding soft tissue (Fig. 14.41).

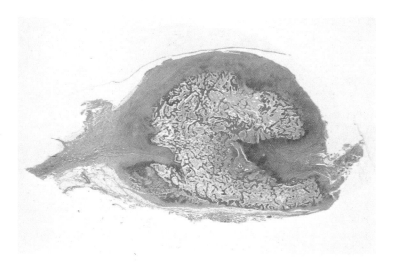

Fig. 14.39 Photomicrograph of a portion of ossified soft tissue taken from the hip joint of a patient with myositis ossificans progressiva demonstrates both immature bone and cartilage formation, with areas of dense fibrous connective tissue also in evidence.

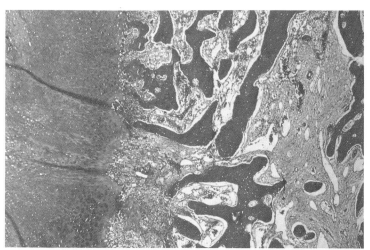

Fig. 14.40 Higher power photomicrograph of the tissue in Fig. 14.39 shows bone and cartilage formation within the soft tissue.

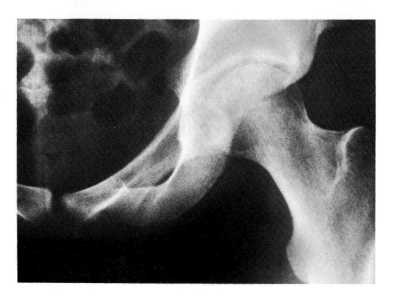
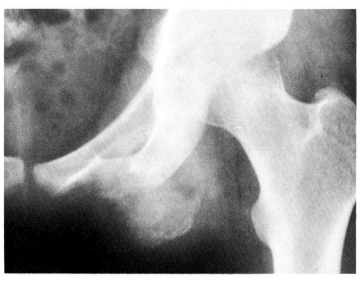

Fig. 14.41 (*Left*) Clinical roentgenogram of a young woman who developed pain in the region of the pubis following childbirth reveals no obvious abnormality. (*Right*) This roentgenogram, taken one month later, demonstrates a well-defined ossifying mass in the soft tissue adjacent to the pubis.

Gross examination of a focus of myositis ossificans circumscripta that has been present for a month or two reveals a shell of bony tissue with a soft reddish-brown central area. The lesion is usually 2 to 5 cm in diameter and is adherent to the surrounding muscle (Fig. 14.42).

Microscopic examination of myositis ossificans circumscripta reveals an irregular mass of active, immature fibroblastic cells in the center of the lesion, with foci of interstitial microhemorrhage that are rarely extensive (Fig. 14.43). At some distance from the center of the lesion, depending upon the age of the entity in question, one finds small foci of osteoid production. The resulting tissue may be disorganized and hypercellular (Fig. 14.44). Near the periphery more and more clearly defined trabeculae are evident (Fig. 14.45). The bone is usually the primitive

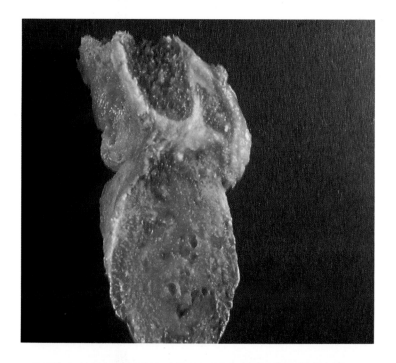

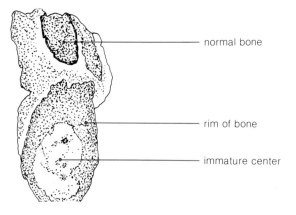

Fig. 14.42 Gross photograph of the specimen removed from the patient in Fig. 14.41. In the upper part can be seen a segment of normal bone, and immediately underlying this segment is a well-circumscribed ossified mass which had been attached to the periosteum, but did not arise from the bony tissue.

normal bone

rim of bone

immature center

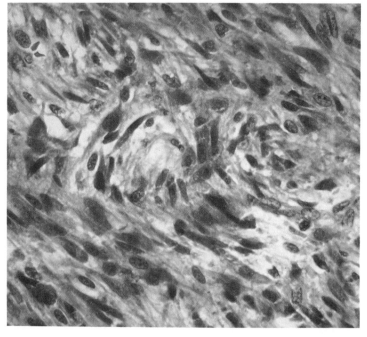

Fig. 14.43 High power photomicrograph of tissue taken from the center of the mass shown in Fig. 14.42 demonstrates a spindle cell lesion. The cells have a disorderly arrangement and are producing collagen.

woven type, with large, round, and crowded osteocytes; however, in long-standing lesions the bone is mature and has a lamellar pattern.

It may be difficult to differentiate a focus of myositis, especially in its acute stage, from a sarcoma by histologic evidence alone. A careful correlation of the clinical and radiologic findings is therefore essential. An important distinction to be emphasized is that, whereas myositis ossificans is most mature at its periphery and least mature at its center, the opposite is true of an osteosarcoma (see discussion of soft-tissue osteosarcoma in Chapter 12). Treatment of this condition is generally conservative, with excision of the mass an option.

ELASTOFIBROMA

An elastofibroma is an uncommon, unencapsulated but circumscribed lesion found in older adults which, with rare exceptions, occurs in the soft tissue between the rib fascia and the inferior portion of the scapula.

On microscopic examination, the lesion is found to be formed of dense collagen and fat interspersed with eosinophilic globules and fibers. These fibers consist histochemically and ultrastructurally of elastin (a fibrous protein) and elastin precursors (Fig. 14.46).

It is generally agreed that the lesion probably occurs posttraumatically. Treatment is usually by surgical excision.

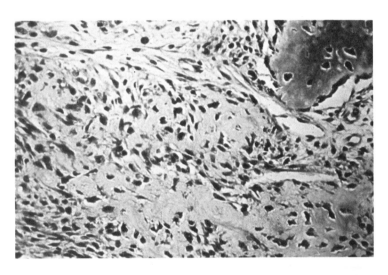

Fig. 14.44 Photomicrograph of an area adjacent to the tissue seen in Fig. 14.43 demonstrates bone formation. The cellularity of this tissue might cause concern and lead to an erroneous diagnosis of sarcoma.

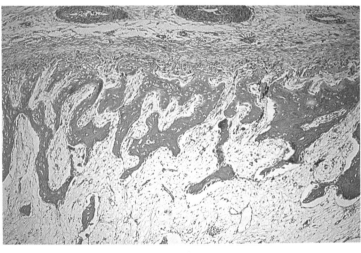

Fig. 14.45 Histologic section taken from the periphery of the lesion demonstrated in the previous three figures shows mature bone formation, characteristic of myositis ossificans circumscripta.

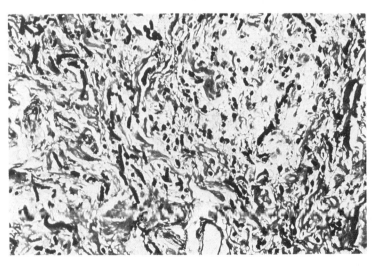

Fig. 14.46 Photomicrograph of an elastofibroma removed from the scapula region. The section, stained with an elastic tissue stain, shows the abundant elastic fibers mixed with fibroadipose tissue, characteristic of this lesion. (In a H & E section, the presence of the elastic fibers may be overlooked.)

INFANTILE CORTICAL HYPEROSTOSIS
Caffey's disease

Infantile cortical hyperostosis (ICH) is a disease of infants, who present with a classic triad of hyperirritability, soft-tissue swelling, and palpable hard masses over multiple and often symmetrical bones. Patients may be feverish and acutely ill, and the disease may often follow a recent upper respiratory infection. On roentgenograms one may note diffuse, usually symmetrical, cortical thickening. Many bones are affected, but especially the mandible, clavicle, and ribs (Fig. 14.47). Involvement of the long bones occurs less often, and the vertebral column and tubular bones of the hands and feet are usually spared altogether. Histologic examination of tissue from affected areas reveals a thickened periosteum, often with marked periosteal new bone formation and mild infiltration by acute chronic inflammatory cells (Fig. 14.48).

Laboratory data on patients with ICH may reveal an increased erythrocyte sedimentation rate, anemia, and leukocytosis with a shift to the left. These findings are highly suggestive of an infection; however, in the vast majority of cases no organism has been isolated.

Infantile cortical hyperostosis usually follows a protracted course with several exacerbations and remissions, but spontaneous recovery generally occurs in a few months.

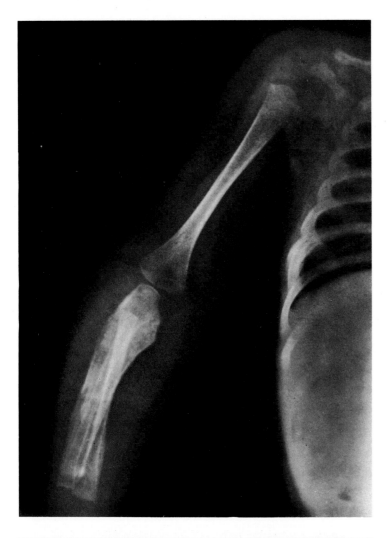

Fig. 14.47 Roentgenogram of an infant admitted to the hospital with fever and enlargement of the forearm shows extensive periosteal new bone formation causing enlargement of the ulna. In addition, there is thickening and widening of the seventh rib, as well as bilateral thickening of the mandible (not seen here).

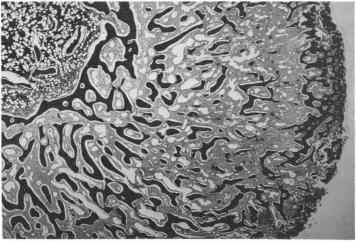

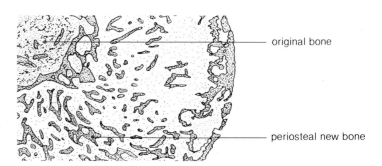

Fig. 14.48 Histologic section of tissue affected by ICH reveals extensive periosteal new bone formation, with vascularized fibrous tissue lying between the bone spicules. Although not seen here, a scattering of chronic inflammatory cells is commonly found.

original bone

periosteal new bone

14.20

Bibliography

GENERAL READINGS

Ackerman, L, Spjut H, Abell M (eds.): Bones and Joints. International Academy of Pathology Monograph. Williams & Wilkins, Baltimore, 1976.

Bourne G H (ed.): The Biochemistry and Physiology of Bone, 2nd ed. (4 volumes). Academic Press, New York, 1972–76.

Dahlin D: Bone Tumors: General Aspects and Data on 6,221 Cases, 3rd ed. Charles C Thomas, Springfield, Ill., 1978.

Hirohata K, Morimoto K, Kimura H: Ultrastructure of Bone and Joint Diseases, 2nd ed. Igaku-Shoin, New York, 1981.

Huvos A: Bone Tumors: Diagnosis, Treatment and Prognosis. Saunders, Philadelphia, 1979.

Jaffe, H L: Metabolic, Degenerative, and Inflammatory Diseases of Bones and Joints. Lea & Febiger, Philadelphia, 1972.

Jaffe, H L: Tumors and Tumorous Conditions of the Bones and Joints. Lea & Febiger, Philadelphia, 1958.

Management of Primary Bone and Soft Tissue Tumors. A collection of papers presented at the 21st Annual Clinical Conference on Cancer, 1976, at the University of Texas System Cancer Center, M. D. Anderson Hospital and Tumor Institute, Houston, Texas. Yearbook, Chicago, 1977.

Marcove R: The Surgery of Tumors of Bone and Cartilage. Grune and Stratton, New York, 1981.

Mirra J: Bone Tumors: Diagnosis and Treatment. Lippincott, Philadelphia, 1980.

Ortner D, Putschar W: Identification of Pathological Conditions in Human Skeletal Remains. Smithsonian Contributions to Anthropology, no. 28. Smithsonian Institution Press, Washington, D.C., 1981.

Owen R, Goodfellow J, Bullough P: Scientific Foundations of Orthopaedics and Traumatology. Saunders, Philadelphia, 1981.

Resnick D, Niwayama G: Diagnosis of Bone and Joint Disorders (3 volumes). Saunders, Philadelphia, 1981.

Schajowicz F: Tumors and Tumorlike Lesions of Bone and Joints. Springer-Verlag, New York, 1981.

Schmorl G, Junghanns H: The Human Spine in Health and Disease, 2nd Am. ed., Grune and Stratton, New York, 1971.

Sokoloff L (ed.): The Joints and Synovial Fluid (2 volumes). Academic Press, New York, 1978, 1980.

Spjut H J, Dorfman H D, Fechner R E, Ackerman L V: Tumors of Bone and Cartilage. Atlas of Tumor Pathology, 2nd series, fascicle 5. Armed Forces Institute of Pathology, Washington, D.C., 1971 (and Supplement, 1981).

Thompson, D'Arcy: On Growth and Form, abridged ed. by Bonner J T. Cambridge University Press, London, 1961.

Trueta J: Development and Decay of the Human Frame. Heinemann, London, 1968.

SUGGESTED READINGS

1 NORMAL BONE
The Matrix
Boskey A L: Current concepts of the physiology and biochemistry of calcification. Clin Orthopaed Rel Res 157:225, 1981.

Buckwalter J A: Proteoglycan structure in calcifying cartilage. Clin Orthopaed 172:207, 1983.

Weiss J B, Ayad S: An introduction to collagen. In Weiss J B, Jayson M V (eds.) Collagen in Health and Diseases. Churchill Livingstone, New York, 1982.

Cellular Control of the Matrix
High W B, Capen CC, Black H E: Effects of thyroxine on cortical bone remodeling in adult dogs. A histomorphometric study. Am J Pathol 102:438, 1981.

Vaughan J: The Physiology of Bone. Clarendon Press, Oxford, 1981.

The Bones
GROSS STRUCTURE AND FUNCTION

Burstein A H, Reilly D T, Martens M: Aging of bone tissue: Mechanical properties. J Bone Joint Surg 58-A:82, 1976.

Canoso J J: Bursae, tendons and ligaments. Clin Rheum Dis 7:189, 1981.

Murray P D F: Bones: A Study of the Development and Structure of the Vertebrate Skeleton. Cambridge University Press, London, 1936.

BLOOD SUPPLY

Brookes M: The Blood Supply of Bone. Butterworth, London, 1971.

Crock H V: The Blood Supply of the Lower Limb Bones in Man. Churchill Livingstone, Edinburgh, 1967.

Crock H V, Yoshizawa H: The Blood Supply of the Vertebral Column and Spinal Cord in Man. Springer-Verlag, New York, 1977.

Ogden J A: Changing patterns of proximal femoral vascularity. J Bone Joint Surg 56-A:941, 1974.

HISTOLOGY

Cooper R R, Misol, S: Tendon and ligament insertion. J Bone Joint Surg 52-A:1, 1970.

Fornasier V L: Osteoid: An ultrastructural study. Hum Pathol 8:243, 1977.

Ham A W, Cormack D H: Histology, 8th ed. Lippincott, Philadelphia, 1979.

The Joints
GROSS STRUCTURE

Goodfellow J W, O'Connor J J: The design of synovial joints. In Owen R, Goodfellow J, Bullough P (eds.) Scientific Foundations of Orthopaedics and Traumatology. Saunders, Philadelphia, 1980.

Cartilage
Freeman M A R: Adult Articular Cartilage, 2nd ed. Pitman Books, London, 1979.

Synovium
Soren A: Histodiagnosis and Clinical Correlation of Rheumatoid and Other Synovitis. Lippincott, Philadelphia, 1978.

Bone Growth and Development

Enlow D H: Principles of Bone Remodeling. Charles C Thomas, Springfield, Ill., 1963.

Ogden J A (ed.): Skeletal Injury in the Child. Lea & Febiger, Philadelphia, 1982, pp. 16–40.

Sillence D O, Horton W A, Rimoin D L: Morphologic studies in skeletal dysplasias. Am J Pathol 96:811, 1979.

Wuthier R E: Basic science and pathology—A review of the primary mechanism of endochondral calcification with special emphasis on the role of the cells, mitochondria and matrix vesicles. Clin Orthopaed Rel Res 169:219, 1982.

Method of Examination of Skeletal Tissue

Anderson C: Manual for the Examination of Bone. CRC Press, Boca Raton, Fl., 1982.

2 DISEASES RESULTING FROM DISTURBANCES IN THE FORMATION AND BREAKDOWN OF BONE I

Definition of Terms

Avioli L V, Krane S M: Metabolic Bone Disease, vols. I and II. Academic Press, New York, 1977, 1978.

Recker R R (ed.): Bone Histomorphometry: Techniques and Interpretation. CRC Press, Boca Raton, Fl., 1983.

Hyperparathyroidism

High W B, Casper C C, Black H E: The effects of 1,25 dihydroxychole calciferol, parathyroid hormone and thyroxine on cortical bone remodeling in adult dogs. A histomorphometric study. Am J Pathol 105:279, 1981.

Scholz D A, Purnell D C: Asymptomatic primary hyperparathyroidism: 10-year prospective study. Mayo Clin Proc 56:473, 1981.

Osteomalacia and Rickets

Frame B, Parfitt A M: Osteomalacia: Current concepts. Ann Intern Med 89:966, 1978.

Linovitz R J, Resnick D, Keissling P, et al.: Tumor-induced osteomalacia and rickets: A surgically curable syndrome. J Bone Joint Surg 58-A:419, 1976.

Mankin H J: Rickets, osteomalacia, and renal osteodystrophy, part I. J Bone Joint Surg 56-A:101, 1974.

Mankin H J: Rickets, osteomalacia, and renal osteodystrophy, part II. J Bone Joint Surg 56-A:352, 1974.

Hypophosphatemia

Moser C R, Fessel W J: Rheumatic manifestations of hypophosphatemia. Arch Intern Med 134:674, 1974.

Familial Hypophosphatemia

Scriver C R, Tenenhouse H S: On the heritability of rickets, a common disease (Mendel, mammals and phosphate). Johns Hopkins Med J 149:179, 1982.

Fanconi's Syndrome

Schneider J A, Schulman J D, Seelingmiller J E: Cystinosis and Fanconi's syndrome. In Stanbury J D, Wyngaarden J B, Fredrickson D S (eds.) The Metabolic Basis of Inherited Diseases, 4th ed. McGraw-Hill, New York, 1978.

Renal Osteodystrophy

Sherrard D J, Baylink D J, Wergedal J E, et al.: Quantitative histological studies on the pathogenesis of uremic bone disease. J Clin Endocrinol Metab 39:119, 1974.

Osteosclerosis

Genant H K, Baron J M, Straus F H, et al.: Osteosclerosis in primary hyperparathyroidism. Am J Med 59:104, 1975.

Soft Tissue Calcification

Anderson H C: Calcific diseases: A concept. Arch Pathol Lab Med (in press).

Tumoral Calcinosis

Boskey A L, Vigorita V J, Spencer O, et al.: Chemical, microscopic and ultrastructural characterization of the mineral deposits in tumoral calcinosis. Clin Orthopaed Rel Res (in press).

Hacihanefioglu U: Tumoral calcinosis. J Bone Joint Surg 60-A:1131, 1978.

Osteoporosis

Frost H M (ed.): Symposium on the Osteoporoses. Orthopaed Clin N Am, vol. 12, no. 3. Saunders, Philadelphia, July 1981.

Lane J M, Vigorita V J: Osteoporosis. J Bone Surg 65-A:274, 1983.

Massive Osteolysis

Bullough P G: Massive osteolysis. N Y S J Med 71:2267, 1971.

Heyden G, Kindblom L, Nielsen M: Disappearing bone disease. J Bone Joint Surg 59-A:57, 1977.

3 DISEASES RESULTING FROM DISTURBANCES IN THE FORMATION AND BREAKDOWN OF BONE II

Osteogenesis Imperfecta

Bullough P G, Davidson, D, Lorenzo J: The morbid anatomy of the skeleton in osteogenesis imperfecta. Clin Orthopaed Rel Res 159:42, 1981.

Scurvy

Minor R R: Collagen metabolism. A comparison of diseases of collagen and diseases affecting collagen. Am J Pathol 98:225, 1980.

Vitto J, Bauer E A: Diseases associated with collagen abnormalities. In Weiss J B, Jayson M V (eds.) Collagen in Health and Disease. Churchill Livingstone, New York, 1982, pp. 289–312.

Mucopolysaccharidosis

Lorincz A: The mucopolysaccharidoses: Advances in understanding and treatment. Pediatr Ann 7:104, 1978.

Hypophosphatasia

Anderton J M: Orthopaedic problems in adult hypophosphatasia. J Bone Joint Surg 61-B:82, 1979.

Whyte M P, Teitelbaum S L, Murphy W A, et al.: Adult hypophosphatasia: Clinical, laboratory, and genetic investigation of a large kindred with review of the literature. Medicine 58:329, 1979.

Hyperphosphatasia

Caffey J: Familial hyperphosphatasemia with ateliosis and hypermetabolism of growing membranous bone: Review of the clinical, radiographic and chemical features. Progr Pediatr Radiol 4:81, 1972.

Horwith M, Nunez E A, Krook L, et al.: Hereditary bone dysplasia with hyperphosphatasaemia: Response to synthetic human calcitonin. Clin Endocrinol 5 (suppl):341, 1976.

Fluorosis

Aggarwal N D: Structure of human fluorotic bone. J Bone Joint Surg 55-A:331, 1973.

Briancon D, Meunier P J: Treatment of osteoporosis with fluoride, calcium and vitamin D. In Frost H M (ed.) Symposium on the Osteoporoses. Orthopaed Clin N Am, vol. 12, no. 3. Saunders, Philadelphia, July 1981.

Riggs B L, Seeman E, Hodgson S F, et al.: Effect of the fluoride/calcium regimen on vertebral fracture occurrence in postmenopausal osteoporosis. N Engl J Med 306:446, 1982.

Vigorita V J, Suda M K: Histopathologic and histomorphometric analysis of transilial bone in sodium fluoride-calcium-vitamin D treated osteoporosis. Clin Orthopaed Rel Res 177:282, 1983.

Paget's Disease

Hamdy R C: Paget's Disease of Bone. Endocrinology and Metabolism Series, vol. 1. Praeger, New York, 1981.

Rebel A, Basle M, Pouplard A, et al.: Bone tissue in Paget's disease of bone. Arth Rheum 23:1104, 1980.

Osteopetrosis

Shapiro F, Glimcher M J, Holtrop M, et al.: Human osteopetrosis. J Bone Joint Surg 62-A:384, 1980.

Camurati-Engelmann Disease

Sparkes R S, Graham C B: Camurati-Engelmann disease. J Med Genet 9:73, 1972.

Van Buchem F S P, Hadders H N, Hansen J F, et al.: Hyperostosis corticalis generalisata. Am J Med 33:387, 1962.

Hypertrophic Pulmonary Osteoarthropathy

Epstein O, Ajdukiewicz A B, Dick R, et al.: Hypertrophic hepatic osteoarthropathy. Am J Med 67:88, July 1979.

4 INJURY AND REPAIR
Cell Injury and the Inflammatory Reaction

Hill R B Jr., La Via M F (eds.): Principles of Pathobiology, 3rd ed. Oxford University Press, New York, Oxford, 1980.

Surgical Wound Healing

Hunt T K (ed.): Wound Healing and Wound Infection. Appleton-Century-Crofts, New York, 1980.

Muscles

Allbrook D B: Muscle breakdown and repair. In Owen R, Goodfellow J, Bullough P (eds.) Scientific Foundations of Orthopaedics and Traumatology. Saunders, Philadelphia, 1980.

Tendons

Ver dan C: Tendon Surgery of the Hand. Churchill Livingstone, New York, 1979.

Peripheral Nerves

Sunderland S: The anatomic foundation of peripheral nerve repair techniques. Orthopaed Clin N Am 12:245, 1981.

Bone

Heppenstall R B (ed.): Fracture Treatment and Healing. Saunders, Philadelphia, 1980.

Cartilage

Bentley G: Repair of articular cartilage. In Owen R, Goodfellow J, Bullough P (eds.) Scientific Foundations of Orthopaedics and Traumatology. Saunders, Philadelphia, 1980.

The Menisci of the Knee

Bullough P G, Vosburgh F, Arnoczky S, et al.: Pathology of the meniscus. In Insall J N (ed.) Surgery of the Knee. Churchill Livingstone, New York, 1983.

Pavlov H, Ghelman B, Vigorita V J: Atlas of Knee Menisci. Appleton-Century-Crofts, New York, 1983.

5 DISEASE RESULTING FROM THE DEPOSITION OF METABOLIC PRODUCTS AND HEMATOLOGIC DISORDERS
Examination of Synovial Fluid for Crystals

Gatter R A: Use of the compensated polarizing microscope. Clin Rheum Dis 3:91, 1977.

Gout

Boss G R, Seegmiller J E: Hyperuricemia and gout. N Engl J Med 300:1459, 1979.

Chondrocalcinosis

McCarty D J: Calcium pyrophosphate dihydrate crystal deposition disease (pseudogout syndrome)—Clinical aspects. Clin Rheum Dis 3:61, 1977.

Markel S F, Hart W R: Arthropathy in calcium pyrophosphate dihydrate crystal deposition disease. Arch Pathol Lab Med 106:529, 1982.

Reginato A J, Schumacher H R, Martinez V: The articular cartilage in familial chondrocalcinosis: Light and electron microscopic study. Arth Rheum 17:977, 1974.

Resnick D, Niwayama G, Goergen T, et al.: Clinical, radiographic and pathologic abnormalities in calcium pyrophosphate dihydrate deposition disease (CPPD): Pseudogout. Radiology 122:1, 1977.

Oxalosis

Gherardi G, Poggi A, Sisca S, et al.: Bone oxalosis and renal osteodystrophy. Arch Pathol Lab Med 104:105, 1980.

Milgram J W, Salyer W R: Secondary oxalosis of bone in chronic renal failure. J Bone Joint Surg 56-A:387, 1974.

Ochronosis

Schumacher H R, Holdsworth D E: Ochronotic arthropathy. I. Clinicopathologic studies. Sem Arth Rheum 6:207, 1977.

Amyloidosis

Chapman R H, Cotter F: The carpal tunnel syndrome and amyloidosis. Clin Orthopaed Rel Res 169:159, 1982.

Glenner G G: Amyloid deposits and amyloidosis. N Engl J Med 302:1283, 1980.

Hemochromatosis

Schafer A I, Cheron R G, Dluhy R, et al.: Clinical consequences of acquired transfusional iron overload in adults. N Engl J Med 304:319, 1981.

Gaucher's Disease

Goldblatt J, Sacks S, Beighton P: The orthopedic aspects of Gaucher disease. Clin Orthopaed Rel Res 137:208, 1978.

Xanthomatosis

Fahey J J, Stark H H, Donovan W F, et al.: Xanthoma of the Achilles tendon. J Bone Joint Surg 55-A: 1197, 1973.

Seigelman S S, Schlossberg I, Becker N H, et al.: Hyperlipoproteinemia with skeletal lesions. Clin Orthopaed Rel Res 87:228, 1972.

Skeletal Manifestations of Hematologic Diseases

O'Hara A E: Roentgenographic osseous manifestations of the anemias and the leukemias. Clin Orthopaed Rel Res 52:63, 1967.

Thalassemia Major

Gratwick G M, Bullough P G, Bohne W H, et al.: Thalassemic osteoarthropathy. Ann Int Med 88:494, 1978.

Sickle Cell Disease

Bohrer S P: Radiology of Bone Ischaemia and Infarction in Sickle Cell Disease. Green, St. Louis, 1981.

Hemophilia

Arnold W D, Hilgartner M W: Hemophilic arthropathy. J Bone Joint Surg 59-A:287, 1977.

DePalma A F: Hemophilic arthropathy. Clin Orthopaed Rel Res 52:145, 1967.

Myelosclerosis and Myelofibrosis

Ellis J T, Peterson P: The bone marrow in polycythemia vera. Pathol Ann (Pt I) 14:383, 1979.

Killmann S A: Myelofibrosis. Clin Orthopaed Rel Res 52:95, 1967.

Laszlo J: Myeloproliferative disorders (MPD). Sem Hematol 12:409, 1975.

6 ARTHRITIS I

Commonly Observed Histologic Changes Seen in Association with Arthritis

Bullough P G: Pathologic changes associated with the common arthritides and their treatment. In Sommers S C, Rosen P P (eds.) Pathology Annual, vol. 14, part 2. Appleton-Century-Crofts, New York, 1979.

Cooper N S, Soren A, McEwen C, et al.: Diagnostic specificity of synovial lesions. Hum Pathol 12:314, 1981.

Macys J R, Bullough P G, Wilson P D Jr.: Coxarthrosis A study of the natural history based on a correlation

of the clinical, radiographic and pathologic findings. Sem Arth Rheum 10:66, 1980.

Mitchell N, Shepard N: The resurfacing of adult rabbit articular cartilage by multiple perforations through the subchondral bone. J Bone Joint Surg 58-A:230, 1976.

Rosenberger J L, Cooper N S, Soren A, et al.: A statistical approach to the histopathologic diagnosis of synovitis. Hum Pathol 12:329, 1981.

Rothwell A G, Bentley G: Chondrocyte multiplication in osteoarthritic articular cartilage. J Bone Joint Surg 55-A:588, 1973.

Watson M: Microfractures in the head of the femur. J Bone Joint Surg 57-A:696, 1975.

Wenger D R, Mickelson M R, Ponseti I V: Idiopathic chondrolysis of the hip. J Bone Joint Surg 57-A:268, 1975.

Rheumatoid Arthritis

American Rheumatism Association: Primer on the Rheumatic Diseases, 7th ed. Chicago, American Medical Association, 1973, pp. 661–812. Issued as a supplement to JAMA.

Williams H J, Biddulph E C, Coleman S S, et al.: Isolated subcutaneous nodules (pseudorheumatoid). J Bone Joint Surg 59-A:73, 1977.

7 ARTHRITIS II

Avascular Necrosis

Weil V H (ed.): Segmented Idiopathic Necrosis of the Femoral Head. Springer-Verlag, New York, 1981.

Legg-Calvé-Perthes Disease

Caterall A: Legg-Calvé-Perthes Disease. Churchill Livingstone, New York, 1982.

Osteoarthritis

Howell D S, Talbott J H (eds.): Osteoarthritis Symposium. Sem Arth Rheum 11 (suppl. 1), 1981.

Peyron J G (ed.): Epidemiology of Osteoarthritis. Symposium June 1980. Geigy.

Charcot's Joints

Eichenholtz S N: Charcot Joints. Charles C Thomas, Springfield, Ill., 1966.

8 ARTHRITIS III

Tissue Response to Artificial Joint Implants

Bullough P G: Pathologic changes associated with the common arthritides and their treatment. Pathol Ann 14 (pt 2):69, 1979.

Gordon M, Bullough P G: Synovial and osseous inflammation in failed silicone rubber prostheses. J Bone Joint Surg 64-A:574, 1982.

Kircher T: Silicone lymphadenopathy: A complication of silicon elastomer finger joint prostheses. Hum Pathol 11:240, 1980.

Diseases of the Spine

Schmorl G, Junghanns H: The Human Spine in Health and Disease, 2nd Am ed. Grune and Stratton, New York, 1971.

Diffuse Idiopathic Skeletal Hyperostosis (DISH)

Forestier J, Lagier R: Ankylosing hyperostosis of the spine. Clin Orthopaed Rel Res 74:65, 1971.

9 BONE AND JOINT INFECTIONS
Pyogenic Infections of Bones and Joints

Ashby M E: Serratia osteomyelitis in heroin users. J Bone Joint Surg 58-A:132, 1976.

Gifford D B, Patzakis M, Ivler D, et al.: Septic arthritis due to pseudomonas in heroin addicts. J Bone Joint Surg 57-A:631, 1975.

Greenspan A, Norman A, Steiner G: Case report 146: Squamous cell carcinoma arising in chronic, draining sinus tract secondary to osteomyelitis of right tibia. Skel Radiol 6:149, 1981.

Gustilo R B, Anderson J T: Prevention of infection in the treatment of one thousand and twenty-five open fractures of long bones. J Bone Joint Surg 58-A:453, 1976.

Miller J E (ed.): Symposium on Bone Infections. Clin Orthopaed Rel Res 96:2, 1973.

Waldvogel F A, Papageorgiou P S: Osteomyelitis: The past decade. N Engl J Med 303:360, 1980.

Granulomatous Inflammation of Bones and Joints

Bender B L, Yunis E J: Disseminated nongranulomatous *Mycobacterium avium* osteomyelitis. Hum Pathol 11:476, 1980.

Bjarnason D F, Forrester D M, Swezey R L: Destructive arthritis of the large joints. A rare manifestation of sarcoidosis. J Bone Joint Surg 55-A:618, 1973.

Chapman M, Murray R, Stoker D: Tuberculosis of the bones and joints. Sem Roentgenol 14:266, 1979.

Hooper J, McLean I: Hydatid disease of the femur. J Bone Joint Surg 59-A:974, 1977.

Tuli S M: Tuberculosis of the Spine. Published for the National Library of Medicine, U. S. Dept. of HEW, and the National Science Foundation, Washington, D.C., by Amerind Publishing Co. Put. Ltd., New Delhi, India, 1975.

Winter W G Jr., Larson R K, Honeggar M M, et al.: Coccidioidal arthritis and its treatment. J Bone Joint Surg 57-A:1152, 1975.

10 SKELETAL HAMARTOMAS AND OTHER BENIGN TUMOROUS CONDITIONS I
Epidermoid Inclusion Cyst

Roth S I: Squamous cysts involving the skull and distal phalanges. J Bone Joint Surg 46-A:1442, 1964.

Sugiura I: Intra-osseous glomus tumor. J Bone Joint Surg 58-B:245, 1976.

Ganglionic Cystic Defects of Bone

Kambolis C, Bullough P G, Jaffe H L: Ganglionic cystic defects of bone. J Bone Joint Surg 55-A:496, 1973.

Unicameral Bone Cyst

Boseker E H, Bickel W H, Dahlin D C: A clinicopath-ologic study of simple unicameral bone cysts. Surg Gynecol Obstet 127:550, 1968.

Aneurysmal Bone Cyst

Wise D W, Bullough P G: The natural history of aneurysmal bone cysts as shown in a review of twenty-six cases. J Hosp Spec Surg 1:1, 1975.

Giant-Cell Reparative Granuloma

Lorenzo J C, Dorfman H D: Giant-cell reparative granuloma of short tubular bones of the hands and feet. Am J Surg Pathol 4:551, 1980.

Hemangioma of Bone

Feldman F: Case 104. Skel Radiol 4:245, 1979.

Skeletal Hemangiomatosis/Lymphangiomatosis

Gutierrez R M, Spjut H J: Skeletal angiomatosis. Clin Orthopaed Rel Res 85:82, 1972.

Massive Osteolysis

Bullough P G: Massive osteolysis. N Y S J Med 71:2267, 1971.

Synovial Hemangioma

Moon N F: Synovial hemangioma of the knee joint. Clin Orthopaed Rel Res 90:183, 1973.

Fibrous Dysplasia

Harris W H, Dudley H Jr., Barry R J: The natural history of fibrous dysplasia. J Bone Joint Surg 44-A:207, 1962.

Henry A: Monostotic fibrous dysplasia. J Bone Joint Surg 51-B:300, 1969.

Ossifying Fibroma

Campanacci M, Laus M: Osteofibrous dysplasia of the tibia and fibula. J Bone Joint Surg 63-A:367, 1981.

Kempson R L: Ossifying fibroma of the long bones. Arch Pathol 82:218, 1966.

Nonossifying Fibroma

Spjut H J, Fechner R E, Ackerman L V: Benign fibrous histiocytoma. Supplement to Atlas of Tumor Pathology (2nd series). Tumors of Bone and Cartilage, fascicle 5. Armed Forces Institute of Pathology, Washington, D.C., 1981, p. 16.

11 SKELETAL HAMARTOMAS AND OTHER BENIGN TUMOROUS CONDITIONS II
Periosteal "Desmoid"

Kimmelstiel P, Rapp I: Cortical defect due to periosteal desmoids. Bull Hosp Joint Dis 12:286, 1951.

Enchondromatosis

Shapiro F: Ollier's disease. J Bone Joint Surg 64-A:95, 1982.

Osteochondroma

D'Ambrosia R, Ferguson A: The formation of osteochondroma by epiphyseal cartilage transplantation. Clin Orthopaed Rel Res 61:103, 1968.

Multiple Osteocartilaginous Exostoses

Voegeli E, Laissue J, Kaiser A, et al.: Case report 143. Skel Radiol 6:134, 1981.

Dysplasia Epiphysealis Hemimelica

Kettelkamp D B, Campbell C J, Bonfiglio M: Dysplasia epiphysealis hemimelica. J Bone Joint Surg 48-A:746, 1966.

Bone Island, Osteopoikilosis, Osteopathia Striata

Whyte M P, Murphy W A, Fallon M D, et al.: Mixed sclerosing-bone-dystrophy: Report of a case and review of the literature. Skel Radiol 6:95, 1981.

Melorheostosis

Campbell C J, Papademetriou T, Bonfiglio M: Melorheostosis. J Bone Joint Surg 50-A:1281, 1968.

Hove E, Sury B: Melorheostosis. Acta Orthopaed Scand 42:315, 1971.

Younge D, Drummond D, Herring J, et al.: Melorheostosis in children. J Bone Joint Surg 61-B:415, 1979.

Osteoid Osteoma

Sim F H, Dahlin D C, Beabout J W: Osteoid-osteoma: Diagnostic problems. J Bone Joint Surg 57-A:154, 1975.

Vigorita V J, Ghelman B: Localization of osteoid osteomas—Use of radionuclide scanning and auto-imaging in identifying the nidus. Am J Clin Pathol 79:223, 1983.

Osteomas of the Cranium and Facial Bones

Fallon M D, Ellerbrake D, Teitelbaum S L: Meningeal osteomas and chronic renal failure. Hum Pathol 13:449, 1982.

Hoffa's Disease

Weitzman G: Lipoma arborescens of the knee. J Bone Joint Surg 47-A:1030, 1965.

Eosinophilic Granuloma

Lieberman P H, Jones C R, Filippa D A: Langerhans cell (eosinophilic) granulomatosis. J Invest Dermatol 75:71, 1980.

12 NEOPLASMS I

Osteoblastoma

Marsh B W, Bonfiglio M, Brady L P, et al.: Benign osteoblastoma: Range of manifestations. J Bone Joint Surg 57-A:1, 1975.

Aggressive Osteoblastoma

Scully R E, Galdabini J J, McNeely B U: Case 40. N Engl J Med 303:866, 1980.

Osteosarcoma

Dahlin D C, Unni K K: Osteosarcoma of bone and its important recognizable varieties. Am J Surg Pathol 1:61, 1977.

Juxtacortical Osteosarcoma

Ahuja S C, Villacin A B, Smith J, et al.: Juxtacortical (parosteal) osteogenic sarcoma. Histological grading and prognosis. J Bone Joint Surg 59-A:632, 1977.

Bertoni F, Boriani S, Laus M, et al.: Periosteal chondrosarcoma and periosteal osteosarcoma. J Bone Joint Surg 64-B:370, 1982.

Paget's Sarcoma

Wick M R, McLeod R A, Siegal G P, et al.: Sarcoma of bone complicating osteitis deformans (Paget's disease). Am J Surg Pathol 5:47, 1981.

Enchondroma

Steiner G C: Ultrastructure of benign cartilaginous tumors of intraosseous origin. Hum Pathol 10:71, 1979.

Takigawa K: Chondroma of the bones of the hand. J Bone Joint Surg 53-A:1591, 1971.

Juxtacortical Chondroma

DeSantos L A, Spjut H J: Periosteal chondroma: A radiographic spectrum. Skel Radiol 6:15, 1981.

Chondroblastoma

Green P, Whittaker R P: Benign chondroblastoma. J Bone Joint Surg 57-A:418, 1975.

Schajowicz F, Gallardo H: Epiphysial chondroblastoma of bone. J Bone Joint Surg 52-B:205, 1970.

Chondromyxoid Fibroma

Schajowicz F, Gallardo H: Chondromyxoid fibroma (fibromyxoid chondroma) of bone. J Bone Joint Surg 53-B:198, 1970.

Fibromyxoma

Marcove R C, Kambolis C, Bullough P G, et al.: Fibromyxoma of bone. Cancer 17:1209, 1961.

Chondrosarcoma

Mankin H J, Cantley K P, Lippiello L, et al.: The biology of human chondrosarcoma I. J Bone Joint Surg 62-A:160, 1980.

Mankin H J, Cantley K P, Schiller A L, et al.: The biology of human chondrosarcoma II. J Bone Joint Surg 62-A:176, 1980.

Sanerkin N G, Gallagher P: A review of the behaviour of chondrosarcoma of bone. J Bone Joint Surg 61-B:395, 1979.

Dedifferentiated Chondrosarcoma

McCarthy E F, Dorfman H D: Chondrosarcoma of bone with dedifferentiation: A study of eighteen cases. Hum Pathol 13:36, 1982.

Mesenchymal Chondrosarcoma

Harwood A R, Krajbich J I, Fornasier V L: Mesenchymal chondrosarcoma: A report of 17 cases. Clin Orthopaed Rel Res 158:144, 1981.

Clear-Cell Chondrosarcoma

Unni K K, Dahlin D C, Beabout J W, et al.: Chondrosarcoma: Clear-cell variant. J Bone Joint Surg 58-A:676, 1976.

Desmoplastic Fibroma

Goldman A B, Bohne W H O, Bullough P G: Desmoplastic fibroma. Skel Radiol 4:102, 1979.

Sugiura I: Desmoplastic fibroma. J Bone Joint Surg 58-A:126, 1976.

Fibrosarcoma

Huvos A G, Higinbotham N L: Primary fibrosarcoma of bone. Cancer 35:837, 1975.

Giant-Cell Tumor

McCarthy E F: Giant cell tumor of bone: An historical perspective. Clin Orthopaed Rel Res 153:14, 1980.

13 NEOPLASMS II

Vascular Neoplasms

Enzinger F M, Smith B H: Hemangiopericytoma. Hum Pathol 7:61, 1976.

Larsson S E, Lorentzon R, Boquist L: Malignant hemangioendothelioma of bone. J Bone Joint Surg 57-A:84, 1975.

Unni K, Ivins J C, Beabout J W, et al.: Hemangioma, hemangiopericytoma and hemangioendothelioma and hemangioendothelioma (angiosarcoma) of bone. Cancer 27:1403, 1971.

Ewing's Sarcoma
Angervall L, Enzinger F M: Extracellular neoplasm resembling Ewing's sarcoma. Cancer 36:240, 1975.

Rosen G: Primary Ewing's sarcoma: The multidisciplinary lesion. Int J Rad Oncol Biol Phys 4:527, 1978.

Lymphoma
Sweet D, Mass D, Simon M, et al.: Histiocytic lymphoma (reticulum cell sarcoma) of bone. J Bone Joint Surg 63-A:79, 1981.

Multiple Myeloma
Kyle R A: Multiple myeloma: Review of 869 cases. Mayo Clin Proc 50:29, 1975.

Solitary (Localized) Myeloma
Valderrama J A F, Bullough P G: Solitary myeloma of the spine. J Bone Joint Surg 50-B:82, 1968.

Adamantinoma of Long Bones
Campanacci M, Laus M, Giunti A, et al.: Adamantinoma of the long bones. Am J Surg Pathol 5:533, 1981.

Chordomas
Mindell E R: Chordoma. J Bone Joint Surg 63-A:501, 1981.

Synovial Sarcoma
Krall R A, Kostianovsky M, Patchefsky A S: Synovial sarcoma. Am J Surg Pathol 5:137, 1981.

Wright P H, Sim F H, Soule E H, et al.: Synovial sarcoma. J Bone Joint Surg 64-A:112, 1982.

Epithelioid Sarcoma
Prat J, Woodruff J, Marcove R: Epithelioid sarcoma. Cancer 41:1472, 1978.

Pigmented Villonodular Synovitis
Docken W P: Pigmented villonodular synovitis. Sem Arth Rheum 9:1, 1979.

Primary Synovial Chondromatosis
Villacin A B, Brigham L N, Bullough P G: Primary and secondary synovial chondrometaplasia. Hum Pathol 10:439, 1979.

Metastatic Cancer
Levy R N: Metastatic disease of bone. Clin Orthopaed Rel Res 169:2, 1982.

Orr F W, Varani J, Gondek M D, et al.: Partial characterization of a bone-derived chemotactic factor for tumor cells. Am J Pathol 99:43, 1980.

14 MISCELLANEOUS ORTHOPAEDIC CONDITIONS

Ganglion
Kambolis C, Bullough P G, Jaffe H: Ganglionic cystic defects of bone. J Bone Joint Surg 55-A:496, 1973.

Carpal Tunnel Syndrome
Phalen G S: The birth of a syndrome, or carpal tunnel revisited. J Hand Surg 6:109, 1981.

Morton's Neuroma
Lassmann G: Morton's toe. Clinical, light and electron microscopic investigations in 133 cases. Clin Orthopaed Rel Res 142:73, 1979.

Compartment Syndrome
Hargens A R, Schmidt D A, Evans K L, et al.: Quantitation of skeletal muscle necrosis in a model compartment syndrome. J Bone Joint Surg 63-A:631, 1981.

Congenital Pseudarthrosis
Campanacci M, Nicoll E A, Pagella P: The differential diagnosis of congenital pseudarthrosis of the tibia. J Inter Orthopaed (SICOT) 4:283, 1981.

Slipped Capital Femoral Epiphysis
Boyer D W, Mickelson M R, Ponseti I V: Slipped capital femoral epiphysis. J Bone Joint Surg 63-A:85, 1981.

Congenital Dislocation of the Hip
Tachdjian M O (ed.): Congenital Dislocation of the Hip. Churchill Livingstone, New York, 1982.

Myositis Ossificans
Lagier R, Cox J N: Pseudomalignant myositis ossificans. Hum Pathol 6:653, 1975.

Noble T P: Myositis ossificans, a clinical and radiological study. Surg Gynecol Obstet 39:795, 1924.

Elastofibroma
Renshaw T S, Simon M A: Elastofibroma. J Bone Joint Surg 55-A:409, 1973.

Infantile Cortical Hyperostosis
Thornberg L P: Infantile cortical hyperostosis (Caffey-Silverman syndrome). Animal model: Craniomandibular osteopathy in the canine. Am J Pathol 95:575, 1979.

Index

deformities, F14.37
microscopic appearance, F14.39, F14.40

N

Necrosis, 4.4–4.5, F4.4, F4.5, F4.7
avascular, see Avascular necrosis
bone, and arthritis, F6.11
Nerves, peripheral, healing, 4.11, F4.18
Neurofibromatosis, 14.9
Neuroma, amputation, F14.14, F14.15
Nonossifying fibroma, 10.17–10.18
giant cells, F10.50, F10.51
gross appearance, F10.47
histiocytes, F10.48–F10.51
spindle cells, F10.50

O

Oblique fracture, 4.11, F4.20
Ochronosis, 5.10–5.11
gross appearance, F5.26
histologic appearance, F5.27
roentgenographic appearance, F5.23, F5.25
urine specimens, F5.22
Ollier's disease, see Enchondromatosis
Onion skin periostitis, 3.26, F3.67
Osgood-Schlatter disease, 4.13, F4.23
Ossification, endochondral, see Endochondral ossification
Ossifying fibroma, 10.16, F10.44–F10.46
Osteitis fibrosa cystica, see Hyperparathyroidism
Osteoarthritis, 7.10–7.15; see also Arthritis; Charcot's joints
and congenital hip dislocation, 14.12
cystic defects, F7.32–F7.35
fibrocartilage resurfacing, F7.41–F7.46
inflammatory osteoarthritis, 7.14
injury and repair balance, F7.47
joint space loss, F7.27
osteophytes, 7.12, F7.36, F7.37
secondary osteoarthritis, 7.10, F7.26
synovial membrane, F7.40
Osteoarthropathy, hypertrophic pulmonary, 3.26, F3.67, F3.68
Osteoarthrosis, see Osteoarthritis
Osteoblastic activity, and bone formation, F6.18
Osteoblastoma, 12.2–12.3
atypical, F12.4
Osteoblasts, 1.3
and bone matrix, 1.4, F1.5–F1.7
Osteocartilaginous exostoses, multiple, 11.6–11.7
deformities, F11.17, F11.18
Osteochondritis dissecans, 14.13, F14.27–F14.29
Osteochondroma, 11.4–11.5
cartilage cap, F11.10–F11.14
of the epiphysis, 11.8, F11.23
pedunculated, F11.13, F11.15
Osteoclastic resorption, 2.22, F2.59
Osteoclasts, 1.7, F1.13, F1.14
in osteopetrosis, 3.24, F3.63
in Paget's disease, 3.15, F3.37
Osteocytes, and bone matrix, 1.4–1.5, F1.8–F1.10
Osteocytic canaliculi, 1.5, F1.8–F1.10
Osteocytic osteolysis, 2.10
Osteodystrophy, renal, 2.14
Osteofibrous dysplasia, see Ossifying fibroma
Osteogenesis Imperfecta
bone hypercellularity, F3.18, F3.19
clinical evaluation, 3.2–3.3

congenita, type, F3.5
fracture cycle, F3.2
tarda type, F3.6
teeth appearance, F3.4
the epiphysis, 3.6–3.8
cartilaginous nodules, F3.14–F3.17
epiphyseal end irregularity, F3.13, F3.14
growth plate appearance, F3.14–F3.17
gross pathologic features, 3.5, F3.18, F3.19
lamellar pattern, F3.18, F3.19
Osteogenic sarcoma, see Osteosarcoma
Osteoid, 1.6, F1.11, F1.12
Osteoid osteoma, 11.13–11.15
bone density, F11.36–F11.41
immature bone formation, F11.45
nidus, F11.36–F11.41, F11.43, F11.46
stroma, F11.45
Osteolysis, massive, 2.22, F2.60, 10.11, F10.29, F10.30
Osteoma, osteoid, see Osteoid osteoma
Osteomalacia, 2.11
bilateral fractures and, F2.29
causes of, 2.10, 2.11
definition, 2.2
histologic examination, F2.30, F2.31
Osteomas of cranium and facial bones, 11.16–11.17
Osteomyelitis
amyloidosis in, 9.7
bacterial diagnosis, 9.9, F9.15
chronic, 9.7, F9.9–F9.11
hematogenous, 9.2–9.4
Batson's plexus, F9.3
and drug addiction, F9.2
metaphyseal veins in, F9.3
roentgenographic changes, F9.4
morbid anatomy, 9.9–9.11
Brodie's abscess, F9.17
inflammatory exudate extension, F9.19
involucrum, F9.20
necrotic bone, F9.18
polymorphonuclear leukocyte exudate, F9.16
sequestrum, F9.21
sickle cell anemia, F9.22
neonatal, 9.5, F9.6
roentgenographic changes, 9.8, F9.12–F9.14
and sickle cell disease, 5.20, F5.54
squamous cell carcinoma in, 9.7
Osteonecrosis, see Avascular necrosis; Legg-Calvé-Perthes disease
Osteopathia striata, 11.11, F11.31–F11.33
Osteopenia, F2.1
definition, 2.2
and rheumatoid arthritis, 6.20, F6.54
Osteopetrosis, 3.22–3.24
calcified cartilage, F3.62
Erlenmeyer flask deformity, 3.23, F3.59
gross appearance, 3.23, F3.59, F3.61
histologic appearance, 3.24, F3.62, F3.63
osteoclasts, F3.63
and osteomyelitis, 9.11
roentgenographic appearance, 3.22–3.23, F3.54–F3.58, F3.60, F3.61
Osteophytes, F6.19, F6.20
and osteoarthritis, 7.12, F7.36, F7.37
and rheumatoid arthritis, 6.15, F6.38, F6.39
Osteopoikilosis, 11.10, F11.29, F11.30
and osteopathia striata, 11.11
Osteoporosis, 2.18–2.20
alcohol, 2.21
biochemical makeup, 2.19
calcium supplementation in, 2.20

causes, 2.18
circumscripta, F3.38
compression fractures, F2.50, F2.51
definition, 2.2
and hemophilia, 5.21, F5.55
localized, 2.21–2.22, F2.57–F2.59
morphometric analysis, F2.54
and osteogenesis imperfecta, 3.4, F3.8
and sickle cell disease, 5.20, F5.51
and thalassemia major, 5.19, F5.49
treatment, 2.20–2.21
Osteoporotic bone, 3.14, F3.34
Osteosarcoma, 12.4–12.9
alkaline phosphatase, 12.5
bone matrix formation, F12.18–F12.20
Codman's triangle, F12.12, F12.13
in cortex of bone, F12.6–F12.8
gross appearance, F12.14
juxtacortical osteosarcoma, see Juxtacortical
    osteosarcoma
intramedullary, F12.5
and Paget's disease, 12.12, F12.33, F12.34
periosteal osteosarcoma, F12.24
in soft tissues, F12.9–F12.11
telangiectatic osteosarcoma, F2.1, F12.21–F12.23
Osteosclerosis, 2.15, F2.40–F2.42
Oxalosis, 5.9, F5.20, F5.21

P

Paget's disease, 3.15–3.21
arthritis and, 3.21, F3.50–F3.53
clinical assessment, 3.20–3.21
and immature bone, 1.14
juvenile, see Hyperphosphatasia
laboratory features, 3.19
microscopic features, 3.18–3.19, F3.45–F3.47
osteoblastic activity in, 3.18, F3.37, F3.46, F3.47
osteoclastic activity in, 3.18, F3.37, F3.45–F3.47
osteoporosis circumscripta, F3.38
radiologic features, 3.16–3.17, F3.36, F3.38,
    F3.39, F3.43, F3.44
sarcoma and, 3.20, F3.49
Paget's sarcoma, 12.12
Palmar fibromatosis, 14.14–14.15
nodules, F14.31, F14.32
palmar fascia, F14.30
spindle cells, F14.32
Parathyroid gland, see also Hyperparathyroidism
adenoma, F2.19
normal size and position, F2.16
Parosteal osteogenic sarcoma, see Juxtacortical osteosar-
    coma
Periosteal chondroma, 12.15, F12.41, F12.42
Periosteal desmoid, 11.2, F11.1, F11.2
Periosteal osteosarcoma, 12.9, F12.24
Periosteum, 1.10, F1.19, F1.20
and blood supply, 1.11, F1.21, F1.22
Periostitis, onion skin, 3.26, F3.67
Phagocytosis, 4.6
Phantom bone, see Osteolysis, massive
Pigmented villonodular synovitis, 13.16–13.17
finger manifestations, F13.50
foam cells, F13.54
hip manifestations, F13.48, F13.49
histologic appearance, F13.52–F13.54
knee manifestations, F13.47
Plantar fibromatosis, 14.14–14.15
Plasma cell myeloma, see Myeloma, multiple
Plasmacytoma, see Myeloma, solitary

Pott's disease, F9.28
Primary synovial chondromatosis, 13.19–13.20
atypical cells, F13.59, F13.60
cartilage cloning, F13.59, F13.60
loose bodies, F13.57, F13.58
roentgenographic appearance, F13.56
Primitive bone, 1.14, F1.28; see also Bone
Proteoglycan, 1.3, F1.3, F1.4
in cartilage, 1.17, F1.35
staining for, 1.28
Pseudarthrosis, congenital, 14.9, F14.19, F14.20
Pseudogout, 5.7; see also Chondrocalcinosis
Pseudotumor
and artificial joint implants, F8.9, F8.10
and hemophilia, F5.58
Psoriatic arthritis, 8.12
Pyogenic infections, bones and joints, 9.2–9.11
bacteriologic diagnosis, 9.9, F9.15
joint infection, 9.4–9.5
    following venereal disease, 9.6
osteomyelitis
    chronic, 9.7
    from inoculation of bacteria, 9.6–9.7
    hematogenous, 9.2–9.4
    morbid anatomy, 9.9–9.11
    neonatal, 9.5
roentgenographic changes, 9.8, F9.12–F9.14

R

Reed-Sternberg cell, see Sternberg-Reed cell
Reflex sympathetic dystrophy, 2.21–2.22; see also Atrophy,
    Sudeck's
Refractory rickets, see Hypophosphatemia
Reiter's syndrome, 8.12
Renal failure, chronic, see also Osteodystrophy, renal
causes, 2.14
and hyperparathyroidism, 2.8–2.9
Repair,
bones, 4.11–4.16
cartilage, 4.16–4.17
menisci of knee, 4.17–4.19
muscles, 4.9–4.10
peripheral nerves, 4.11
surgical would healing, 4.8–4.9
tendons, 4.10–4.11
Reticulum cell sarcoma of bone, 13.7
Rheumatoid arthritis, 6.14–6.22; see also Arthritis;
    Osteoarthritis
articular cartilage destruction, F6.53
bone sclerosis, F6.38
fibrinous tissue exudate, F6.46, F6.47
fibrous ankylosis, F6.51
hyperplastic inflamed synovium, F6.41
joint deformity, F6.35
joint destruction, F6.38, F6.39
lymphoid follicles, F6.45, F6.52
osteopenia of juxta-articular bone end, F6.54
osteophyte formation, F6.38
subcutaneous nodules, F6.55
synovial effusion, F6.36
synovial inflammation, F6.40, F6.41
synovial membrane infiltration, F6.42–F6.44
Rheumatoid factors, 6.22
Rheumatoid nodules, 6.20, F6.57, F6.58
Rickets, 2.12–2.13
causes, 2.12
costochondral junction beading, F2.32, F2.33
glycosuric, see Fanconi's syndrome
growth plate irregularity, F2.35–F2.38

proliferating cartilage, F2.38
wrist (and ankle) enlargement, F2.34
Rider's spur, 4.12–4.13
Russell's bodies, 6.16, F6.43, F6.44

S

Sarcoidosis, 9.16–9.17
  granulomas, F9.37
  lesions, F9.34
  synovial involvement, F9.35, F9.36
Sarcoma
  in Paget's disease, 3.20, F3.49
Schmorl's nodules, F8.22
Sclerosis
  in osteoarthritis, 7.12, F7.32–F7.35
  and rheumatoid arthritis, F6.38
  and sickle cell disease, F5.51
  and xanthomatosis, F5.43
Scoliosis, spine, 3.4, F3.8
Scurvy, 3.9
  fibroblastic proliferation, F3.23
  subperiosteal hemorrhage, F3.21–F3.23
Segmental infarction, see Avascular necrosis
Septic arthritis, see Joint infection
Shepherd's crook deformity, 10.14–10.15, F10.42; see
    also Fibrous dysplasia
Sickle cell anemia, 9.11, F9.22
Sickle cell disease, 5.20, F5.51–F5.54
Silicone elastomer, and joint implants, 8.7–8.8, F8.19
Simple bone cyst, see Unicameral bone cyst
Simple fracture, 4.14
Skeletal hemangiomatosis/lymphangiomatosis, 10.10–10.11,
    F10.24–F10.27
Slipped capital femoral epiphysis, 14.10–14.11
  displacement, F14.21
  growth plate, F14.22, F14.23
  hemorrhage, F14.22, F14.23
Slipped disc, F8.23, F8.24
Sodium fluoride, and osteoporosis, 2.20
Sodium urate crystal, 5.3, F5.2
Soft-tissue calcification
  in injured tissue, 2.16
  metastatic, 2.16–2.17
Solitary cyst, see Unicameral bone cyst
Solitary myeloma, see Myeloma, solitary
Spinal diseases, 8.8–8.12
  ankylosing spondylitis, 8.11–8.12
  degenerative disease, 8.10
  diffuse idiopathic skeletal hyperostosis, 8.10–8.11
  intervertebral disc disease, 8.9
Sporotrichosis, 9.16
Squamous cell carcinoma in chronic osteomyelitis, 9.7,
    F9.9–F9.11
Staining techniques, in skeletal tissue examination, 1.28
Staphylococcus aureus
  and hematogenous osteomyelitis, 9.2
  and neonatal osteomyelitis, 9.5
Sternberg-Reed cell, 13.8, F13.22
Steroid therapy, and avascular necrosis, 7.7–7.8
Streptococcus, and neonatal osteomyelitis, 9.5
Stress fracture, 4.12, 4.16, F4.21, F4.22
Subperiosteal hemorrhage, and scurvy, F3.21–F3.23
Subperiosteal resorption, and hyperparathyroidism,
    F2.20
Sudeck's atrophy, see Atrophy, Sudeck's
Surgical wound healing, 4.8–4.9
Synarthroses, 1.15
Synovial cells, 1.20, F1.44, F1.45

Synovial fluid
  and arthritis, 6.10
  examination, 5.2–5.3, F5.1–F5.4
Synovial hemangioma 10.12, F10.31–F10.33
Synovial membrane, 1.20, F1.43–F1.45
  and hemophilia, F5.56, F5.57
  and joint implants, F8.2, F8.7
  and osteoarthritis, 7.13, F7.40
Synovial sarcoma, 13.14–13.15
  fibrosarcomatous component, F13.41
  glandular component, F13.41
  gross specimen, F13.39
  roentgenographic appearance, F13.40
Synovioma, benign, see Pigmented villonodular synovitis
Synovitis
  and carpal tunnel syndrome, 14.5
  crystal diagnosis, 5.2–5.3, F5.1–F5.3
  pigmented villonodular, see Pigmented villonodular
    synovitis
Synovium
  and arthritis, 6.8–6.10
    cartilage and bone fragments, F6.25
    giant cells, F6.23, F6.25
    hemosiderin staining, F6.24
    villous pattern, F6.21
  and rheumatoid arthritis, 6.15–6.17
Syringomyelia, 7.16

T

Telangiectatic osteosarcoma, 12.9, F12.21–F12.23
Tendon repair, 4.10–4.11
Tetracycline-labeling analysis, bone, 2.7, F2.15
Thalassemia major, 5.18–5.19
  gross appearance, F5.45, F5.48
  hair-on-end appearance, F5.46
  honeycomb appearance, F5.47
  iron deposits, F5.50
  and osteoporosis, F5.49
  vertebral column, F5.48
Tidemark, cartilage, 1.17, F1.36–F1.38
Total hip replacement, see Artificial joint implants
Transverse fracture, 4.11, F4.20
Traumatic arthritis, 6.13, F6.33; see also Arthritis
Trevor's disease, 11.8, F11.23
Trigger finger, 14.5
  and rheumatoid arthritis, 6.19
Tuberculosis, 9.12–9.15
  atypical mycobacteria, F9.30
  hip manifestations, F9.25, F9.26
  knee manifestations, F9.27
  Langerhans giant cells, F9.29
  Pott's disease, F9.28
  spinal manifestations, F9.23, F9.24
Tubular dysfunction
  and hypophosphatemia, 2.14
  and rickets, 2.12
Tumoral calcinosis, 2.17, F2.46
Tunneling resorption, 2.10, F2.25, F2.26

U

Unicameral bone cyst, 10.4–10.5
  calcific matrix, F10.13
  fibrous membrane, F10.10, F10.11
  in proximal humerus, F10.8, F10.9
  secondary changes, F10.12
Urinary phosphate, and hypophosphatemia, 2.14
Uveitis, 8.12

V

Vascular insufficiency, and hematogenous osteomyelitis, 9.3

Vascular invasion, and bone development, 1.24–1.25, F1.56–F1.58

Vascular neoplasms, 13.2–13.3
  hemangiopericytoma, 13.3
  poorly differentiated endothelial tumors, 13.2–13.3
  well-differentiated endothelial tumors, 13.2

Vasculitis, 6.21

Venereal disease, joint infection following, 9.6

Vertebral bodies, and hyperparathyroidism, F2.23

Vertebral crush fracture, 2.18–2.19, F2.50

Vitamin C, and scurvy, 3.9

Vitamin D
  and hypophosphatemia, 2.14
  and osteomalacia, 2.10, 2.11
  and osteoporosis, 2.21
  and rickets, 2.2

Volkmann's ischemic contracture, *see* Compartment syndrome

Von Recklinghausen's disease of bone, *see* Hyperparathyroidism

Voorhoeve's disease, *see* Osteopathia striata

W

Whipple's disease, 8.12

Wolff's law, 1.9, F1.18

Wormian bones, 3.4, F3.9

Woven bone, 1.14, F1.28, 2.10; *see* also Bone

Wrist enlargement, and rickets, 2.12, F2.34

X

Xanthomatosis, 5.16–5.17
  Achilles tendon thickening, F5.39
  cholesterol clefts, F5.42
  histiocytes, F5.42, F5.44
  sclerotic bone, 5.17

X-ray, skeletal tissue, 1.28

Z

Zeiss MOP-AM03 computer, 2.4–2.5, F2.6